ENVIRONMENTAL AND OCCUPATIONAL EXPOSURES

REPRODUCTIVE IMPAIRMENT

ENVIRONMENTAL AND OCCUPATIONAL EXPOSURES

REPRODUCTIVE IMPAIRMENT

– Editor –

Dr. Sunil Kumar

Dr. R.R. Tiwari

2018

Daya Publishing House®

A Division of

Astral International Pvt. Ltd.

New Delhi - 110 002

First Published, 2010
Reprinted, 2018

ISBN: 978-81-7035-646-2 (Hardbound)

Publisher's note:

Every possible effort has been made to ensure that the information contained in this book is accurate at the time of going to press, and the publisher and author cannot accept responsibility for any errors or omissions, however caused. No responsibility for loss or damage occasioned to any person acting, or refraining from action, as a result of the material in this publication can be accepted by the editor, the publisher or the author. The Publisher is not associated with any product or vendor mentioned in the book. The contents of this work are intended to further general scientific research, understanding and discussion only. Readers should consult with a specialist where appropriate.

Every effort has been made to trace the owners of copyright material used in this book, if any. The author and the publisher will be grateful for any omission brought to their notice for acknowledgement in the future editions of the book.

Published by : **Daya Publishing House®**
A Division of
Astral International Pvt. Ltd.
– ISO 9001:2008 Certified Company –
4736/23, Ansari Road, Darya Ganj
New Delhi-110 002
Ph. 011-43549197, 23278134
E-mail: info@astralint.com
Website: www.astralint.com

From Editors

This is an introductory book in the area of occupational and environmental toxicology. It addresses the role of occupational and environmental exposure in reproductive impairments in both male and female. It is useful to the researchers working in the area of occupational, environment health and reproductive toxicology as well as to the postgraduate students of toxicology, environmental, reproductive and allied sciences.

This book includes a total of seventeen chapters. The first two chapters deal with the general structure and function of both male and female reproduction and third chapter on "Reproductive toxicity testing of chemicals under REACH Legislation". These chapters will provide the insight to the subject. The later part of the book mainly deals with the environmental and occupational exposure such as exposure to air pollutants, extreme heat, heavy metals, radiations, persistent chemicals, solvents etc., and reproductive impairments in both male and female.

In addition a chapter deal with the long working hours or shift work and reproduction. A few examples are also there about the role of oxidative stress on reproductive system and its mechanism in causing reproductive toxicity. Role of changing lifestyle such as dietary pattern changes in reproductive impairment is also extensively dealt with in another chapter. Further miscellaneous exposures such as detergents and visual display terminal use and their effect on reproductive function and pregancy outcomes are also informative.

Owing to the recent concern about the role of environmental and occupational exposure to persistent chemicals, the proposed book is very timely.

Dr. Sunil Kumar, ***PhD***

Dr. R.R. Tiwari, ***MD***

Contents

Environmental & Occupational Exposures (2010) ***Pages 1–43***
Editors: **Sunil Kumar & R.R. Tiwari**
Published by: **DAYA PUBLISHING HOUSE, NEW DELHI**

Chapter 1

Structure and Physiology of Mammalian Testis

M. Rajalakshmi[1], R.S. Sharma[2] and P.C. Pal[3]*

[1]*Formerly Professor and Head, Department of Reproductive Biology, All India Institute of Medical Sciences, New Delhi and Currently, Director (Academic Cell), Medical Council of India, New Delhi*
[2]*Scientist F, Indian Council of Medical Research, New Delhi*
[3]*Department of Biochemistry, All India Institute of Medical Sciences, New Delhi*

ABSTRACT

Research done nearly sixty years back has shown that male specific development of the bipotential gonad occurs under the influence of hormones like anti-Mullerian hormone, testosterone and insulin-like 3. A number of transcription factors are involved in sex determination; these include general transcription factors involved in early genital ridge development (*e.g.*, Lim 1, SF1, WT1 and Emx2), promoters of testis development (*e.g.*, SRY and SOX9) and factors that act against development of male gonad (DAX1). The available information on the role of these factors in sex determination is reviewed. This review also describes the structure of human testis, pattern

* E-mail: profraj@hotmail.com

of testicular blood supply and details of the process of spermatogenesis including spermatogonial renewal and differentiation, maintenance and differentiation of spermatogenic stem cells, and formation of spermatids and their differentiation into spermatozoa. The kinetics of spermatogenesis in rodent and primate models has been described. The epigenetic changes in gene expression during spermatogenesis involve DNA methylation, histone methylation, histone acetylation and phosphorylation and chromatin modeling. These have an impact on chromatin structure. Epigenetic regulation is an essential aspect of male germ cell development. The structure of Sertoli and Leydig cells and their role in maintaining blood-testis barrier and androgen production, respectively, have been described.

Gonadal and Sexual Determination and Differentiation

In eutherian mammals, sex determination begins with the initiation of testis development from the bipotential gonad (genital ridge). Gonads originate from the genital ridge, which develops as a thickening on the ventro-lateral surface of the primitive mesonephros. In mice, uro-genital ridges are visible at the embryonic age of day 10. The genital ridges are composed of somatic cells derived from the mesonephros and primodial germ cells that have migrated, via the hidgut and mesonephros, from the extraembryonic mesoderm at the base of the allantois[1].

Germ cells have no role in sex determination. Following the gonadal determination, sex differentiation occurs which is defined as the phenotypic development of structures due to the action of hormones and is gonad-dependent only in males[2,3]. The mammalian gonad has three bipotential cell lineages, in addition to germ cells: (1) supporting cell lineage giving rise to Sertoli cells in testis or follicle cells in the ovary which surround the germ cells and provide a suitable environment for growth, (2) steroidogenic cell lineage producing sex hormones responsible for development of secondary sex characters, and (3) connective cell lineage responsible for the formation of gonads as an entity. The first sign of testis determination occurs when aggregation of pre-Sertoli cells (probably derived from the adjacent mesonephros) occurs around the germ cells at about 6-7 weeks of gestation. This aggregation results in the formation of primary sex cords. By the end of week 9, interstitial cells are formed from the mesenchyme that separates the seminiferous cords. The primordia for male genital ducts are derived from the mesonephric ducts.

Nearly 60 years ago, Jost has shown that male specific development of the bipotential gonad occurs when fetal testis secretes two hormones, anti-Mullerian hormone (AMH) and testosterone at a critical period in early gestation[4,5]; another hormone, the insulin-like 3 (Insl 3) is also implicated in this process[6]. Regression of Mullerian ducts begins at 8 weeks of gestation by the action of AMH, secreted by the Sertoli cells, which bind to type II AMH receptors present in the mesenchyme of the Mullerian ducts[7,8]. Testosterone secreted by the interstitial cells induces the development and differentiation of Wolffian duct derivatives such as epididymis, vas deferens and seminal vesicles. The development of male external genitalia is under the control of dihydrotestosterone. The final inguino-scrotal descent of testis completes sex development in male and is mediated by insulin-like 3 (Insl 3)[9].

The transfer of testis from the site of its origin at the urogenital ridge into the scrotum is a critical event in male sexual differentiation. Failure of testis to decend into the scrotum resulting in cryptorchidism is one of the most frequent congenital abnormalities in male children at birth. During the transabdominal phase of testicular descent in male mice embryos (15.5-17.5 days post coitum; dpc), testosterone induces regression of the Cranial Suspensory Ligaments (CSL). Insl 3 promotes contraction of the gubernacular cord and outgrowth of the gubernacular bulb occurs along with elongation of the embryonic rostro-caudal axis, which results in the location of the testes at the base of the abdomen at birth[6]. Inguino-scrotal descent of testes is regulated by hormonal and mechanical factors. It has been suggested that the regression of gubernaculum, its altered visco-elastic properties combined with increased abdominal pressure caused by the growth of the viscera push the testes down through the inguinal canal[10]. Inguino-scrotal descent starts around week 26 of gestation in human and testes reach the scrotum at ~ 35 weeks.

Genes Controlling Sex Determination and Differentiation

Even though several genes have been identified as essential for early gonadal development, the role of these in sex determination is not completely clarified. The transcription factors involved in mammalian sex determination have been classified into three groups[2].

The first group consists of general transcription factors which are likely to be involved from early genital ridge development until differentiation of specific cell types in the gonads and include a) Lim I (a member of the LIM class of homeobox genes), b) SFI (Steroidogenic factor I–member of the subfamily of nuclear orphan receptors), c) WTI (Wilms tumour-associated gene), and d) Emx 2. The steroidogenic transcription factor SF1 has a role as a regulator of endocrine differentiation at multiple levels; gonads lacking in SF1 stop development between 11 and 11.5 dpc and undergo apoptosis[2]. Adrenals also do not develop but the exact role of SF1 in the development of gonads and adrenals has not been delineated. It is stated that SF1 is needed for the differentiation and/or maintenance of and growth of somatic cells already present in the early indifferent gonad[2]. The role of *Lim1* in gonad development has not been investigated in detail but it has been reported that mice homozygous for deletions in *Lim1* do not have kidneys or gonads[11]. The Wilm's tumor-associated gene (WT1) encodes a variety of protein products with different functions, has many functional domains and can regulate transcription in different ways (S and L). This gene is involved in male urogenital development. Mice deficient for encoding transcription factor EMX2 also show impaired gonadal and kidney development. Thus, SF1, WT1, Lim1 and Emx2 are the genes involved in formation of genital ridge and primordial of adrenal and kidneys but their precise role has not been established.

The second group consists of promoters of testis development eg., SRY and SOX9. After the formation of gonads, testis differentiation is controlled by the presence of a gene in the sex-determinig region of the Y-chromosome–Sry (mouse) or SRY (human)[12–14]. SRY encodes a high-mobility group (HMG) box-type DNA binding domain and exerts its effects by genetically switching the development of the indifferent gonad from the female to male pathway. Sry is expressed first around 10.5 dpc, shortly after the genital ridges emerge and peak levels of expression occurs by 11.5 dpc and disappears shortly after 12.5 dpc in the mouse[15–16]. The primary function of Sry is to induce Sertoli cells differentiation. It triggers Sertoli cell lineage in the testis which in turn initiates the differentiation of rest of testicular cell types. SRY switches on a male specific cascade of molecular events but its continued expression is not necessary for future events. One of the earliest effects of Sry expression is the induction of somatic cell migration from the mesonephros into the male gonad, mediated by Platelet Derived Growth Factors (PDGF) which act as signalling molecules[17]. PDGF signalling is considered an indirect effect of Sry expression. The migrating cells are mostly endothelial cells but also include some interstitial cells and peritubular myoid cells, which cooperate with pre-Sertoli cells to form testis cords[18–19]. Cool *et al.*[20] have reported recently that peritubular myoid cells are induced within the gonad and endothelial cells are the migrating cell types. Sry gene expression regulates mechanisms of morphogenesis including extra-cellular matrix remodelling, cell associations, cell movements and vascularisation of the developing testes. As a result, germ cells get surrounded successively by epithelial Sertoli cells and peritubular myoid cells with Leydig cells between the cords. The vasculature becomes branching[21]. The down regulation of Sry expression at 12.5 dpc is by Sox9 but the mechanism by which Sox9 shuts down Sry expression has not been clarified. Polanco and Koopman[22] have concluded that threshold levels of Sry must be achieved in individual cells during a critical time window to appropriately activate Sox9 and trigger testis determination before the ovarian determining pathway engages.

As a result of these changes, the testis cord structure becomes visible by ~ 12.5 dpc. Sox9 is present in low levels in both male and female gonadal ridges in mice but by 11.5 dpc, it is upregulated in the male gonad (absent in female gonad) and by 12.5 dpc, Sox9 is expressed in Sertoli cells and remains throughout life[23,24]. It has been concluded that Sox9 is essential for early testis development and its upregulation is due to direct effect of SRY action[2]. Polanco and Koopman[22] have presented strong evidence that SOX9 is the agent of Sry down regulation. But, the overlapping expression pattern of Sry and Sox9 makes it difficult to discriminate between the cellular roles of each gene[22].

The third group consists of factors that act against the development of the male gonad and includes DAXI, an X-linked member of the Nuclear Hormone Receptor Superfamily. DAX1 is expressed in both sexes in the genital ridge, is down regulated in the male as differentiation proceeds but remains in the ovary[2]. Thus, DAXI is not required for testis formation.

Histoacrhitecture of Adult Testis

The adult human testis is oval in shape lying within the scrotal sac and is covered on all sides, except at its posterior border, by a thick fibrous testicular capsule, generally mentioned as the tunica albuginea. The testicular capsule is composed of three layers, *viz.*, an outer tunica vaginalis visceral, a middle tunica albuginea and an inner thin delicate layer called *tunica vasculosa* (Figure 1.1). The tunica albuginea is the most predominant layer and is composed of interlocking collagen fibres, fibroblasts and smooth muscles. The tunica albuginea is covered everywhere by the tunica vaginalis visceral except where it is reflected over the epididymis and along the posterior border of the testis where the blood vessels enter. The tunica vasculosa is very thin, loose and forms the innermost layer of the testicular capsule. It consists of a network of minute blood vessels held together by delicate areolar tissue. It forms an internal coat for all spaces of the testicular parenchyma. The functional role of the testicular capsule is not known.

The human testis is approximately 4.5-5.1 cm long with an average volume of 20cc in healthy young men. The testicular parenchyma is divided into lobules by very thin septa called trabeculae arising from the tunica albuginea (Figure 1.1). These septa form a connective tissue support for the passage of blood vessels. The septa are absent in the rat testes. On the posterior aspect of the testis, the tunica albuginea is widened to form an incomplete septum called the mediastinum testis. The trabeculae radiate from the mediastinum testis to the tunica albuginea to form testicular lobules. Each lobule contains 1-4 highly convoluted seminiferous tubules, which are 150-250 ìm in diameter, 30-70 cm long and highly tortuous. At the apex of each lobule, the seminiferous tubules are straight and have only Sertoli cells, narrow abruptly and pass into the first part of the system of excurrent ducts called tubuli recti or vasa recta, which are lined by simple cuboidal epithelium. These converge on the rete testis, which is an anastamosing network of tubules in the connective tissue of the mediastinum. From the upper part of the rete testis, about 6-12 efferent ductules join to form a single canal, which

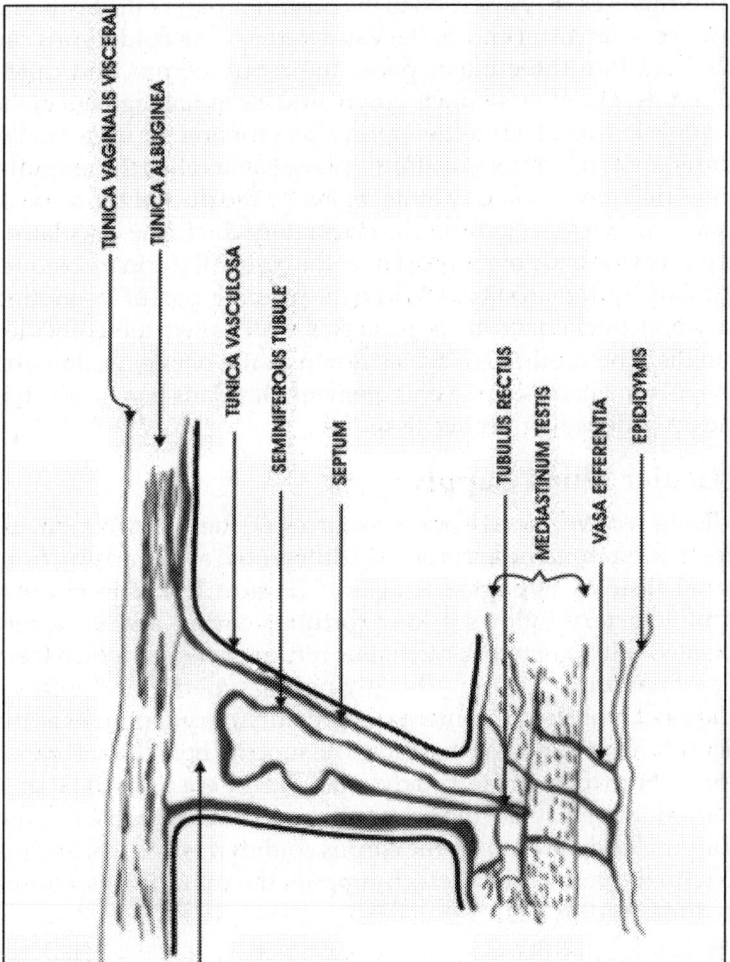

Figure 1.1: Diagrammatic Representation of Testicular Capsule

by its convolutions make up the epididymis (Figure 1.2). The epididymis is embedded in the adipose tissue of the fat pad. The epididymis is closely apposed to the posterior part of the testis and continues at its distal end as the vas deferens. The epididymis can be divided into three major parts, the caput, corpus and cauda epididymis. The efferent ducts empty into the initial segment of the caput epididymis. The vas deferens, after crossing the ureter in the abdominal cavity forms a fusiform enlargement called the ampulla. The vas deferens is joined at this region by the duct of the seminal vesicle, on each side, to form the ejaculatory duct. The ejaculatory duct pierces the body of the prostate at the base of the urinary bladder and finally by a small slit opens into the prostatic part of the urethra on a small thickening of its posterior wall called the colliculus seminalis. The urethra continues down as the penile urethra and ends with an acorn-shaped enlargement, the glans penis, which is made up of dense connective tissue.

Testicular Blood Supply

Testis receives blood from two sources: (1) the internal spermatic artery arising from the aorta and (2) differential artery arising from internal ileac or hypogastric artery[25] (Figure 1.3). The internal spermatic artery follows a long tortuous course and is closely associated with a network of venous return channels, which form the pampiniform plexus. After giving off superior and inferior epididymal branches, the internal spermatic artery continues as the testicular artery supplying the testis. The superior epididymal branch supplies the proximal caput epididymis and the epididymal fat pad. The inferior epididymal branch sends branches to the distal caput epididymis and descends to the corpus epididymis where it forms a loop with the vasal artery, which supplies the vas deferens, corpus and cauda epididymis.

The blood in the testicular artery cools as it approaches the testis loosing heat to the adjacent venous system of pampiniform plexus by counter-current heat exchange. This vascular counter-flowing arrangement facilitates not only exchange of heat but also small molecules including testosterone. Due to the counter-current exchange of heat in the spermatic cord, the temperature of the blood in the testis of a normal individual is 2-4°C lower than the rectal temperature. In men with cryptorchidism (undescended testis), this temperature differential is lost resulting in testicular dysfunction.

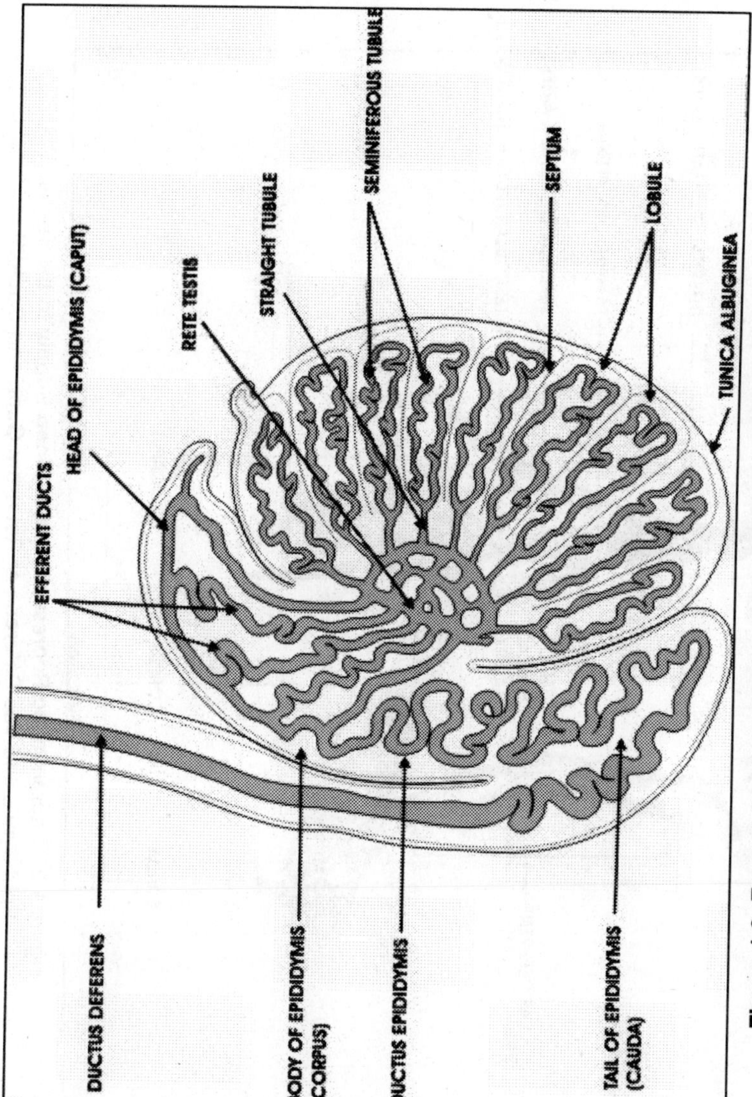

Figure 1.2: Frontal Section of Mammalian Testis and Epididymis (from internet)

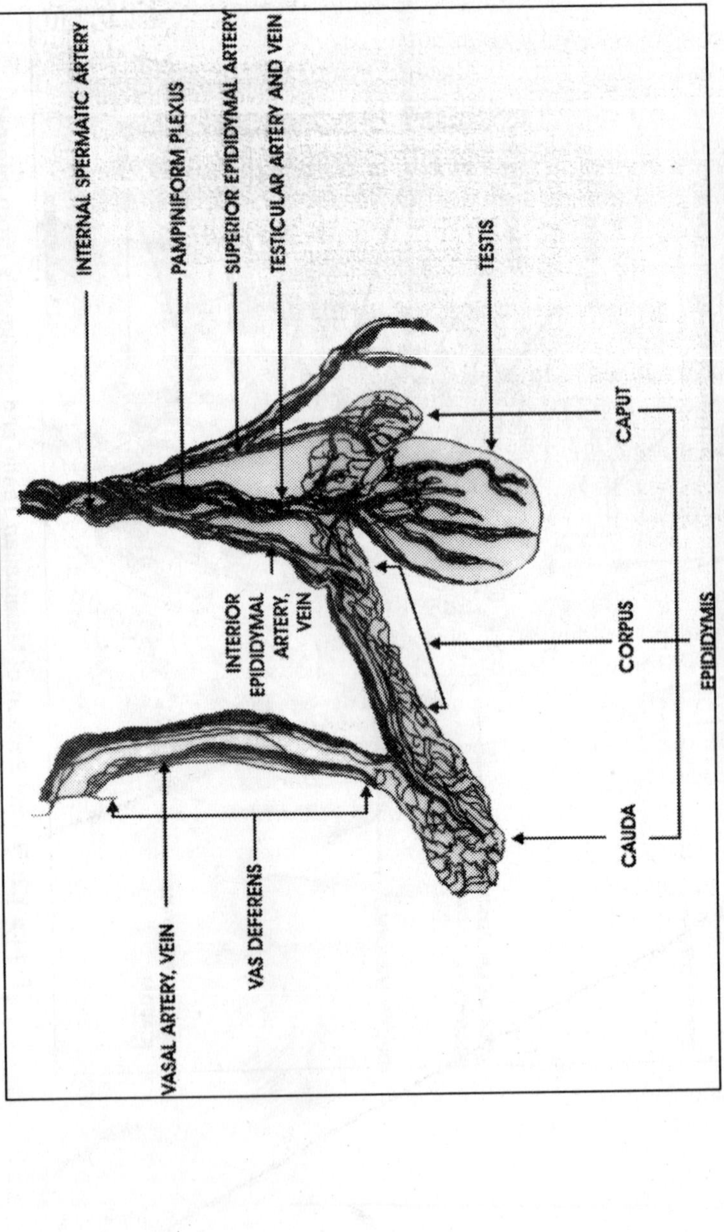

Figure 1.3: Diagrammatic Representation of Blood Supply to the Testis, Epididymis and Vas Deferens of Rat (from Gunn and Gould[25])

The spermatic veins are thin-walled with poorly developed musculature and effective valves are present only at the inflow points into the inferior vena cava or the renal vein. The right spermatic vein drains into the vena cava. The renal vein on the left side is compressed as it passes between the superior mesenteric artery and the aorta and may impair flow through the left renal and spermatic veins, which is considered to be a possible reason for the higher prevalence of varicocele on the left side.

Spermatogenesis

The seminiferous tubules provide the milieu for the production of spermatozoa by a complex series of divisions of the precursor cells termed as spermatogonia. The seminiferous epithelium has two main types of cells, *viz.*, the germ cells and the supporting cells. The supporting cells include the peritubular cells of the basement membrane which form the myoid layer and the Sertoli cells. The germinal elements are composed of (1) a slowly dividing population of primitive stem cells, (2) the rapidly dividing spermatogonia, (3) spermatocytes which undergo meiosis, and (4) spermatids which undergo differentiation to form the spermatozoa.

The gonocytes or primitive germ cells are located in a central position at the time of differentiation of gonad into testes and are called as spermatogonia when they migrate to the periphery of the seminiferous tubules. Mitotic activity in gonocytes is visible from 7-9 years of life of the child. Spermatogonia populate the base of the seminiferous tubule in numbers equal to that of Sertoli cells.

Spermatogenesis is a cytological process in which spermatogonia by a series of divisions form spermatozoa. Spermatogenesis takes place in the seminiferous epithelium which has two major types of cells, the germ cells and Sertoli cells. Sertoli cells extend from the basement membrane to the lumen of the seminiferous tubules and have a close morphological and physiological relationship with the germ cells. The process of spermatogenesis can be divided into four major phases: (1) proliferation and division of spermatogonia to form spermatocytes, (2) formation of spermatids by reduction division (meiosis) of spermatocytes, (3) differentiation of the round spermatid arising from the final division of meiosis into the complex structure called the spermatozoon–a process termed spermiogenesis, and (4) spermiation, the process of release of spermatozoon from the Sertoli cell. These four processes are inter-dependent but each process is also dependent on regulatory molecules from other components of the testis like Sertoli cells, Leydig cells and peritubular cells.

Proliferation and Division of Spermatogonia

Spermatogonial Divisions: Renewal and Differentiation

During the normal adult life of a male, a continuous proliferation of germinal epithelial cells occurs. This requires a continuous supply of the precursors of these cells and the mechanism of this renewal is called stem cell renewal[26]. According to this theory, at the beginning of each spermatogenic cycle, stem cell divisions result in the formation of additional stem cells, which remain "dormant" until the subsequent cycle and in the formation of spermatogonia which ultimately form the spermatozoa. The dormant gonia divide to form a new generation of type A gonia.

Mitotic divisions of spermatogonia give rise to a population of spermatogonia that are destined to enter the process of meiosis. Well characterized markers are not available to identify the different types of spermatogonia. The cytological characteristics of the nuclei, particularly their chromatin pattern have been used for identification of different types of spermatogonia. Spermatogonial renewal has been studied using ^{3}H-thymidine labeling followed by autoradiography at different times after labeling. In the monkey, two main types of spermatogonia have been identified on the basis of their chromatin pattern. Type A_1 spermatogonia, considered as reserve stem cells, have fine pale dust-like chromatin whereas type A_2 spermatogonia, considered as renewing stem cells, have coarse crust-like chromatin and are found close to the basement membrane[27]. Five morphologically distinct types of A spermatogonia, designated A_0, A_1, A_2, A_3 and A_4, have been reported at specific stages of spermatogenesis in the rat[28] (Figure 1.4). Of these, A_0 spermatogonia were considered as reserve stem cells and A_1-A_4 as renewing stem cells. In the monkey, Clermont proposed two classes of A spermatogonia, the A_{dark} spermatogonia (considered as reserve stem cells) with low proliferative activity during normal spermatogenesis and A_{pale} spermatogonia which proliferate continuously (renewing stem cells) during each spermatogenic cycle[27]. Based on histological characteristics, the existence of a population of $A_{transition}$

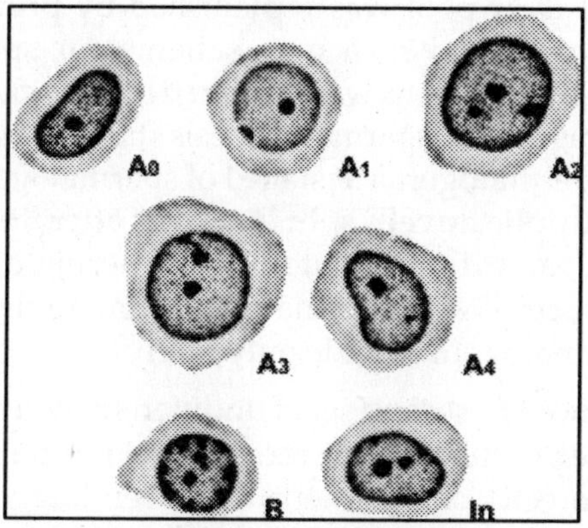

Figure 1.4: Various Types of Spermatogonia (from Clermont and Bustos-Obregon[28])

spermatogonia also has been proposed. The pattern of spermatogonial expansion is identical in various macaques. A_{dark} spermatogonia now are considered the reserve stem cells which proliferate only when significant loss of A_{pale} spermatogonia occurs due to X-ray irradiation or cytotoxic exposure, in which case the A_{pale} spermatogonia population is restored from A_{dark} pool of spermatogonia[29–30]. It is now confirmed that A_{pale} spermatogonia are the cells that cycle in a regular manner and replenish their own number as well as give rise to B spermatogonia. Using *in vivo* and *in vitro* models, a new clonal model of spermatogonial expansion has been proposed[31]. According to this model, spermatogenesis in rhesus monkey is initiated by a first meiotic division of A_{pale} spermatogonia at stage VII of the seminiferous cycle. The A_{pale} spermatogonia produce both A_{pale} and B_1 spermatogonia after two mitotic divisions at stage VII and IX of the cycle of the seminiferous epithelium. Single proliferating spermatogonia are very rare and proliferate independently of the seminiferous epithelial cycle. But, Ehmcke *et al.*[31] have concluded that the identity of the cell which acts as the primate male germline stem cells has not been unequivocally demonstrated.

The model of kinetics of spermatogonial proliferation in man suggested by Clermont[32–33] included that A_{pale} spermatogonia do not self-renew and their pool was replenished by proliferating A_{dark} spermatogonia. However, a new scheme for spermatogonial proliferation in human testis was prepared by Ehmcke and Schlatt[34]. According to this model, spermatogenesis starts with the division of a pair of A_{pale} spermatogonia at stage I of spermatogenesis to give 4 cells. The quadruplicate cells split into pairs after first division and three of these pairs differentiate into B spermatogonia and the remaining one acts as A_{pale} spermatogonia and replenishes its own pool. A_{dark} spermatogonia divide only rarely.

The existence of a second set of undifferentiated spermatogonia that possess the potential to self-renewal but normally do not do so (potential stem cell compartment) has been suggested by pulse labeling experiments of a subset of "undifferentiated spermatogonia" using transgenic approaches[35]. The results suggest that these potential stem cells turn over rapidly and act as transit amplifying cells in normal conditions. But, the potential stem cells change their mode from transient amplification to self-renewal upon transplantation, regeneration or loss of actual stem cells during the long reproductive period[35].

Maintenance and Differentiation of Spermatogenic Stem Cells

The spermatogenic stem cells can renew their own number and produce a large number of differentiated germ cells[36]. For normal spermatogenesis and fertility, a balance between spermatogonial stem cell renewal and differentiation is necessary, which are in turn regulated by intrinsic gene expression in stem cells and extrinsic signals including soluble factors and adhesion molecules from the surrounding environment, known as niche[37]. The techniques of spermatogonial stem cell transplantation, their long-term culture and study of mutant and knockout mice[36,38,39] have generated data on spermatogonial stem cell biology.

Plzf (Promyelocytic Leukaemia Zinc Finger), a transcriptional repressor protein is considered essential for spermatogonial stem cell renewal. The loss of Plzf function shifts the balance between spermatogonial stem cell self-renewal and differentiation[40]. TAF-4b, a germ cell specific component of the RNA polymerase complex is shown to be essential for maintenance of spermatogenesis[41]. The transcription factors Sohlh 1 and 2 are reported to be essential for spermatogonial differentiation[42,43].

The presence of germ line niches in mammalian testis has been shown[37]. A niche is a subset of tissue cells and extracellular substrates which can house one or more stem cells indefinitely and control their self-renewal and progeny production[37]. Sertoli cells play a major role in stem cell niche regulation by providing Glial Cell line-Derived Neurotrophic Factor (GDNF) and Stem Cell Factor (SCF) for spermatogonial stem cell and by segregating the spermatogonia to the basal compartment[44-46]. ERM, a transcription factor of mature Sertoli cell origin, is required for spermatogonial stem cell renewal and maintenance of spermatogenesis in adult mice[47].

While these transcription factors are considered essential for spermatogonial stem cell renewal and differentiation, the Sertoli cell-germ cell interaction in the niche is of great importance in the maintenance and differentiation of spermatogonial stem cell.

Formation of Spermatids by Meiosis

Type B spermatogonia form preleptotene primary spermatocytes, when they lose contact with the basement membrane. The preleptotene primary spermatocytes begin DNA synthesis, their chromosomes condense and appear as two thin filaments or chromatids of the leptotene stage. The chromatids undergo thickening and the pairing of the homologous chromosomes occur. During the pachytene stage, exchange of genetic material between homologous chromosomes derived from maternal and paternal sources occur. The chiasmata formed at the site of exchange of genetic material involving DNA strand breakage and repair become clear when the homologous chromosomes begin to separate at the diplotene stage of meiosis. The nuclear membrane is dissolved and the homologous chromosomes align on the spindle and move to opposite poles of the spindle during anaphase, leading to the formation of secondary spermatocytes containing haploid number of chromosome[48]. Since each chromosome has a pair of chromatids, secondary spermatocytes have a diploid DNA content. After a short interphase of approximately six hours in the human, a second meiotic division takes place in the secondary spermatocytes. During the second meiosis, the chromatids in each chromosome move to opposite poles of the spindle. The resulting cells are called spermatids.

In the human, the duration for meiosis from preleptotene spermatocytes to round spermatids is approximately 24 days.

Spermiogenesis: Differentiation of Round Spermatid into Spermatozoon

Spermiogenesis is the process by which the round spermatid, formed at the end of meiosis, undergoes a series of transformations to form the spermatozoon. Le Blond and Clermont[49], using Periodic Acid Schiff staining technique, observed characteristic morphological changes in the acrosome of the spermatid in rat during spermiogenesis leading to a description of 19 well-defined steps. These 19 steps were classified under four phases, (1) Golgi phase (steps 1-3), (2) cap phase (steps 4-7), (3) acrosome phase (steps 8-14), and (4) maturation phase (steps 15-19). The changes taking place in rat spermatids during these different steps of spermiogenesis are well characterized and are described below.

Golgi Phase

This phase is characterized by the formation of PAS-positive granules within the Golgi apparatus, coalescence of granules into a single acrosomal granule, adherence of the acrosomal granule to the nuclear envelope and early stages of tail development at the pole opposite that of the adherence of acrosomal granule.

Cap Phase

The acrosome granule spreads over the surface of spermatid nucleus until two-thirds of the anterior portion of each spermatid nucleus is covered by a thin double layered membranous sac that closely adheres to the nuclear membrane. Development of the tail filament continues. The migration of centrioles from the periphery of the cell to a position at the pole of nucleus opposite from the developing acrosome takes place. The proximal centriole migrates closest to the nucleus where it perhaps forms the basis for attachment of tail to head. The tail formed from the distal centriole elongates.

Acrosome Phase

The rotation of the spermatid so that acrosome faces the basement membrane of the seminiferous tubule takes place. Nucleus migrates from centre to near the periphery of the cell. Chromatin condenses into dense granules. Nucleus changes from spheroidal to an elongate flattened structure. Acrosome also condenses and elongates to correspond to the shape of the nucleus. The cytoplasm is developed caudally and surrounds the proximal portion of the developing tail. Within this cytoplasm, microtubules associate to form a temporary cylindrical sheath called the manchette which projects from the caudal border of acrosome posteriorly where it loosely surrounds the acrosome. Within this, a specialized structure called chromatoid body condenses around the axoneme to form ring-like annulus. Mitochondria begin to concentrate close to the axoneme.

Maturation Phase

The chromatin undergoes condensation to form a homogeneous material that uniformly fills the entire nucleus. Fibrous sheath with nine coarse fibres form around the axoneme from annulus to the beginning of the tailpiece. Mitochondria get arranged around midpiece to form a sheath. Manchette disappears.

de Kretser and Kerr[48], using light and electron microscopic observations, classified the major events during spermiogenesis, into five major categories, which is essentially common to all species. These changes are: (a) acrosome formation, (b) nuclear modifications, (c) development of the flagellum, (d) reorganization of the cytoplasm and cell organelles, and (e) final release of the spermatozoon from the Sertoli cell, called spermiation.

Acrosome Formation

As early as 1922, Bowen[50] reported the origin of the acrosome from the Golgi complex. The proacrosome granules are elaborated in the Golgi apparatus of the newly formed spermatids and coalesce to form a single granule which gets deposited at one pole of the nucleus and spreads to form the acrosomal cap. The acrosomal cap occupies approximately 25-60 per cent of the nuclear surface, depending on the species. During this phase, additional material appears to be transferred from the Golgi complex to the acrosome by vesicles[51–52]. Glycoproteins are transferred from the Golgi complex to the acrosome[53]. In many species, a conspicuous thickening of the acrosomal cap extending beyond the nucleus is formed and is called the apical segment. In many species including the human, the caudal region of the acrosome becomes partially attenuated and is called the equatorial segment[54–55]. The equatorial segment persists even after the acrosome reaction is completed and is involved in binding with the oocyte during fertilization[56]. The acrosome becomes closely apposed to the spermatid membrane. A thin layer of moderately electron-dense material is present between the inner and outer acrosomal membranes, which is stated to represent the perfaratorium.

Changes in Spermatid Nucleus

The changes in the spermatid nucleus during spermiogenesis include: (a) shift in the position of the nucleus from the central to an eccentric position where it gets covered with the acrosomal cap, (b) condensation of chromatin to form large electron-dense granules and eventually into an electron-dense mass, (c) changes in chemical characterization of DNA and its stabilization, (d) reduction in nuclear volume, and (e) changes in shape of sperm head. During spermiogenesis, lysine-rich histones are replaced with transitional proteins and later by arginine-rich protamines[57–58]. The single protamine is rich in arginine and cystine and is species-specific. Further, a number of non-protamine proteins, several transiently appearing basic nuclear proteins and loss of virtually all non-histone nuclear proteins occur during spermiogenesis[59]. The diversity in shape of sperm head is considered to be due to genetically determined patterns of molecular aggression taking place during chromatin condensation[60].

Formation of the Tail

The axial filament which forms the central core of the tail originates from the distal centriole. The axial filament consists of 9 peripheral doublet microtubules arranged equidistant from each other around a circle (Figures 1.5 and 1.6). Two single microtubules are present at the centre. Each doublet has two subfibres, subfiber A and B. Subfiber A is complete and circular in cross section. Subfiber B is C-shaped; the concavity of the C is attached to subfiber A. The subfibers are composed of tubulin. Each subfiber A has a hook-like arm, called dynein arm, which protrudes towards subfiber B of the adjacent doublet. The doublets are connected by nexin links and to the central sheath surrounding the two central microtubules by radial spokes. In infertile men with sperm immotility, the dynein arms are absent.

During early spermiogenesis, the axial filament projects from the surface of the round spermatid. Subsequently, centrioles and axial filament form the neck or connecting piece. The connecting piece is in the form of a truncated cone and contains both the proximal and distal centrioles (Figure 1.7). The arched base is called the

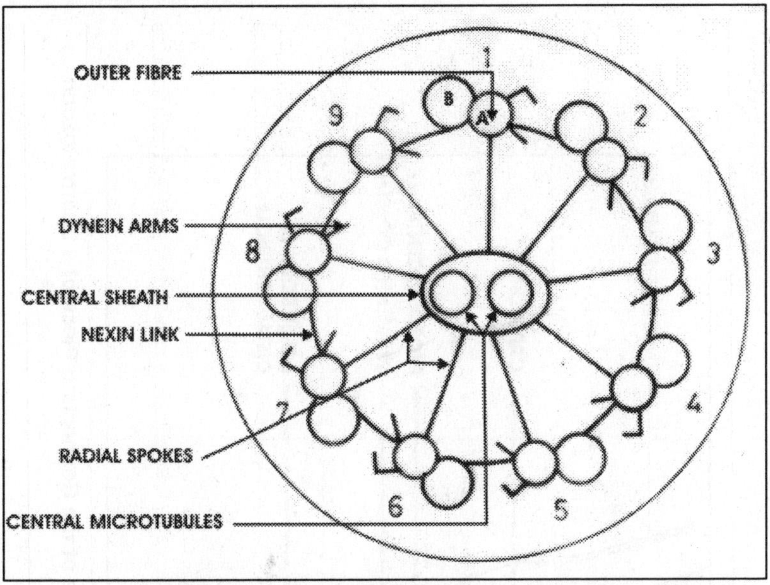

Figure 1.5: Diagrammatic Representation of the Structure of the Axial Filament of the Tail of Spermatozoon

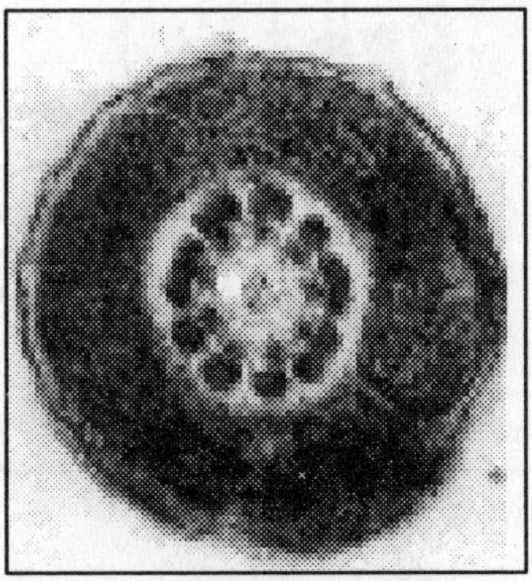

Figure 1.6: Transmission Electron Microscopic Structure of the Tail of an Ejaculated Spermatozoon of Rhesus Monkey

capitulum lodged in a shallow depression called the implantation fossa. The truncated apex has nine longitudinal cross-striated columns, which arise from electron-dense material near the distal centriole. The connecting piece is connected to the nucleus at the

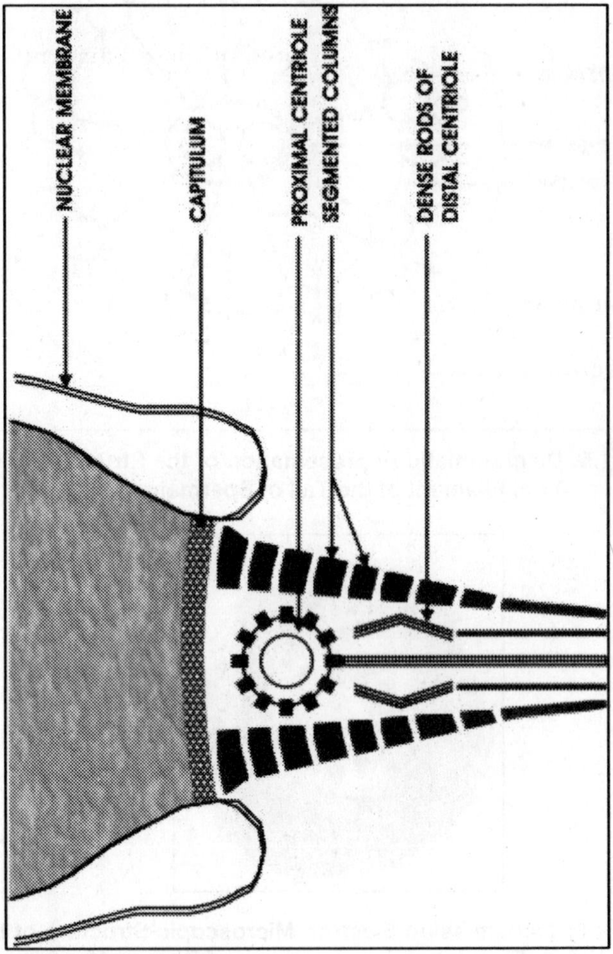

Figure 1.7: Diagrammatic Representation of the Structure of the Connecting Piece of a Spermatozoon

implantation fossa, where the nuclear membranes are closely apposed.

During spermiogenesis, the outer dense fibres and fibrous sheath of the midpiece and principal piece develop. These provide structural stability to the tail. Proteins involved in sperm motility like A-kinase Anchoring Protein, and the calcium ion regulating proteins, CatSper 1, and CRISP 2, are located in this region[61-63]. The principal piece of the tail consists of a series of rib-like structures joined to two longitudinal columns. In the human, the ribs have a microtubular origin[64].

The formation of the midpiece occurs late in spermiogenesis. The mitochondria, located at the periphery of the spermatid, aggregate aound the proximal part of the flagellum to form a helical structure[65]. In the coming years, it is likely that investigators may be able to report subtle changes in nucleus and acrosome using glutaraldehyde-fixed plastic sections stained with toluidine blue, which could not be discerned using PAS or haematoxylin-eosin stained sections.

Spermiation

The Sertoli cell is believed to play an active role in spermiation. The cytoplasm migrates to the caudal portion around the tail and is shed. These cytoplasmic remnants are called the residual bodies and contain Golgi complex, mitochondria, lipids and ribosomes. These are phagocytosed by lysosomal activity at the base of the Sertoli cells. The microtubules are incorporated in the residual body. During spermiation, the spermatozoon leaves the seminiferous epithelium. The small amount of cytoplasm that remains as a droplet surrounding the midpiece of the spermatozoon is called the cytolasmic droplet. It has been suggested that finger-like projections of the Sertoli cell cytoplasm invaginate the cell membrane of the spermatid cytoplasm and "pull" the residual cytoplasm off the spermatid[48]. Simultaneously, a progressive movement of the spermatid towards the seminiferous tubule lumen takes place. A gradual attenuation of the cytoplasm attached to the spermatid is followed by loss of the connection and the residual body is retained within the Sertoli cell. Loss of final contact with the Sertoli cell completes the process of spermiogenesis and the released cell with the cytoplasmic droplet attached is called the spermatozoon[66]. The cytoplasmic droplet is lost during migration of the spermatozoon through the epididymal tubule. This process is under androgenic control and is considered as an index of attainment of maturational capabilities by the sperm[67].

Kinetics of Spermatogenesis

Cycle of the Seminiferous Epithelium

Le Blond and Clermont[49] reported that in each cross section of the seminiferous tubule containing spermatids in one of the 14 steps of spermatid development, the remaining cells of the seminiferous epithelium form a precisely defined association of specific germ cell types. A set of spermatids in a certain phase of spermiogenesis are always associated with the same type of spermatocytes and spermatogonia. Such cellular associations are called "stages" of the seminiferous epithelium and are shown by Roman numerals. A number of stages recur in the seminiferous epithelium sequentially in a cyclic manner and forms the "cycle of the seminiferous epithelium" (Figure 1.8). Le Blond and Clermont[49] defined the *cycle* of the seminiferous epithelium as "the series of changes in a given area of the seminiferous epithelium between two appearances of the same developmental stage". It is a dynamic time-dependent change occurring in one area of the seminiferous epithelium. Le Blond and Clermont[49] also demonstrated that the duration of any one stage was proportional to the frequency with which it was observed in the testis. As type A spermatogonia in any one area of the seminiferous epithelium progress through meiosis and spermiogenesis to form spermatozoa, the specific area of the tubule would pass through the 14 *stages* four times. During each cycle, the spermatogonial progeny progressively move toward the lumen of the seminiferous epithelium. But, the duration of cycle varied for each species[68–69]. In the rat, it is possible to dissect lengths of the seminiferous tubules at the same *stage* of spermatogenesis under transillumination[70]. The stages of spermatogenesis were sequentially arranged along the seminiferous tubule to form a "wave"[68] (Figure 1.9). The *wave* of the seminiferous epithelium has no kinetic significance and refers to the more or less orderly distribution of cellular associations along the seminiferous tubules at any time. In rat, each seminiferous tubule has 12 complete waves, each approximately 2.6 cm in length. The cycle of the seminiferous epithelium is a process whose kinetics is time-

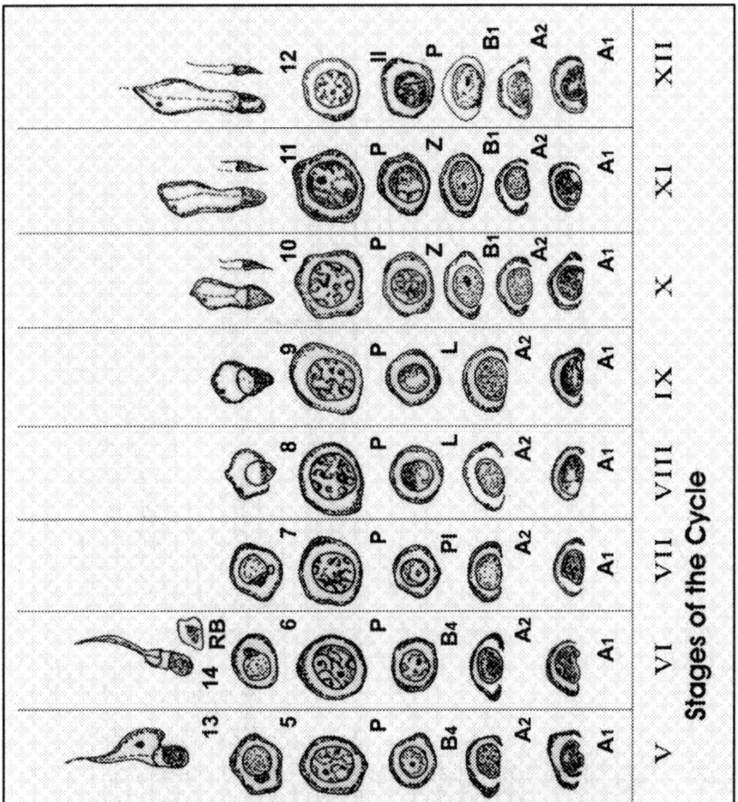

Figure 1.8: Diagrammatic Representation of the 12 Stages of the Seminiferous Epithelium in the Monkey (from Clermont[27])

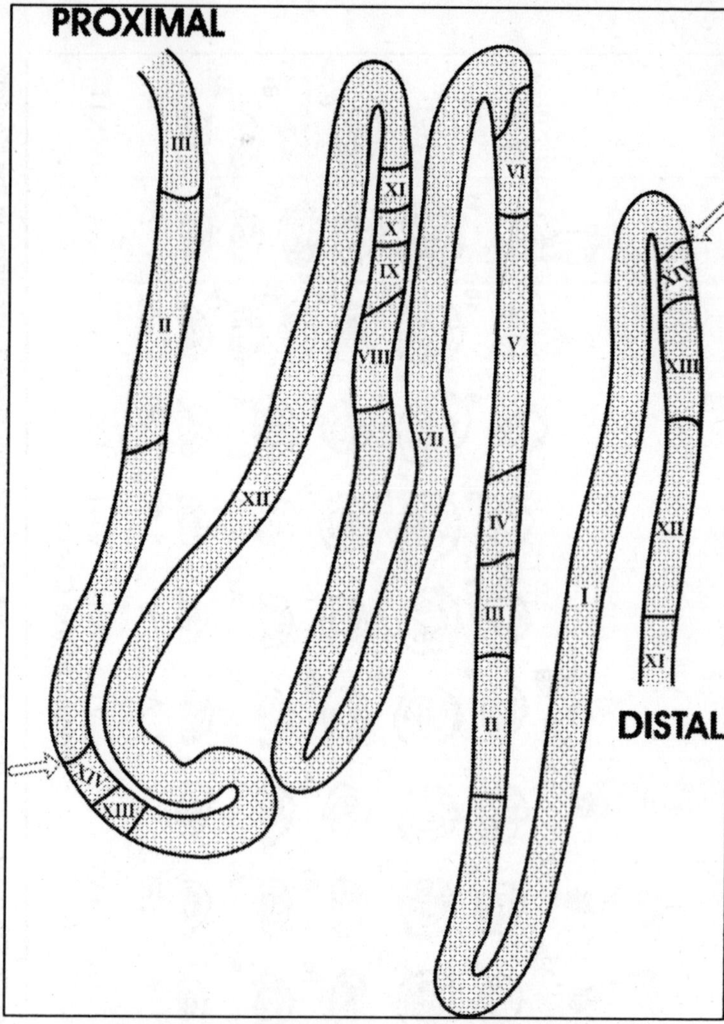

Figure 1.9: Wave of the Seminiferous Epithelium showing Continuity in Order. Limits of a wave are shown by arrows (from Perey *et al.*[68]).

dependent while the wave refers to spatial arrangement of stages. It has been stated by Regaud as early as in 1901 that "a wave is in space what the *cycle* is in time". In the human, spermatogenesis could be divided into 6 cellular associations or stages and took ~70 days for completion from the time A_{pale} spermatogonium is committed to proliferate until release of spermatozoon (spermiation) occurs. The formation of specific cellular associations and the sequence of their appearance in a given area of the seminiferous tubule are synchronized. The numerical relationships between the various cell types within a cellular association and their absolute numbers within a cross section of the seminiferous tubule are highly consistent.

Gene Expression during Spermatogenesis

Epigenetic changes *i.e.*, mitotically and or meiotically heritable changes in gene expression without changes in underlying DNA sequence taking place, have an impact on chromatin structure. These epigenetic alterations involve DNA methylation, histone methylation, histone acetylation and histone phosphorylation, and chromatin remodeling. These epigenetic modifications are essential for several aspects of meiotic chromosome packing, pairing and recombination[71]. DNMT3L, a DNA methyl transferase, is involved in facilitating the methylation pattern required during male meiosis. In the absence of DNMT3L, meiotic chromosomes fail to form heterochromatin appropriately and fail to pair at the zygotene stage[72–73]. Studies have clarified that DNMT3L-mediated methylation is needed for meiotic cells to progress through spermatogenesis. In addition to dynamic changes in histone modifications, successful meiosis during spermatogenesis also requires the use of specialized histone variants like H2AX[74]. In the pachytene stage of meiosis, the X and Y chromosomes form an XY (or sex) body and become transcriptionally silent in a process known as meiotic sex chromosome inactivation (MSCI)[75,76]. After meiosis, post-meiotic sex chromosome repression (PMSR) occurs[77]. It was found that 87 per cent of genes on the X-chromosome remain suppressed post-meiotically compared to 92 per cent genes repressed in pachytene spermatocytes[77]. Spermiogenesis involves re-shaping and condensation of the nucleus to transcriptionally inactivate and protect the DNA. This is assisted by double strand breaks (DSBs) and the histone-to-protamine transition; this has been reviewed[78,79]. The histone-to-protamine transition involves the replacement of the histones with transition nuclear proteins (TP1, TP2 and TP4) which appear only during steps 12-15 of spermiogenesis and the subsequent replacement of the TPs with protamines (PRM1 and PRM2) during steps 16-19. But, 10 per cent of sperm chromatin still retains nucleosomal histones in rodents and human. The histone-to-protamine transition is associated with hyperacetylation of histone H4[80]. Protamines are small basic proteins rich in arginine and cysteine and are found only in spermatids[81]. Most mammals produce two forms of protamine, PRM1 and PRM2, which are responsible for the DNA being packaged into a very compact arrangement. In fact, the molecular compaction of mammalian sperm DNA is so designed that sperm chromatin has become the most condensed eukaryotic nucleus. In addition to the histone to protamine transition, spermiogenesis is critically dependent on changes in H1 linker histones. H1T2 is a H1 variant specifically expressed in round through to elongated spermatids[82,83]. During male germ cell development, epigenetic regulation is crucial in silencing of transportable elements (TE), imprinting of paternal genes, chromatin remodeling, meiotic sex chromosome inactivation (MSCI), histone-protamine transition and postmeiotic sex chromosome repression (PMSR). Several genes show transgenerational epigenetic inheritance through the male germline[84].

Sertoli Cell

Sertoli cells, the only non-germinal part of the seminiferous epithelium, was first described by the Italian physiologist, Enrico Sertoli, in 1865 as extending from the basement membrane to the lumen of the seminiferous tubule and enveloping the germ cells. The existence of a physiological symbiotic relationship between Sertoli cells and germ cells was first proposed by von Ebner[85,86] and he named this unit, the "spermatoblast". Fawcett and Burgos[87] showed that each Sertoli cell has distinct cellular boundaries. Sertoli cells alter their morphology (nuclear morphology, quantity of cytoplasmic liquid, variation in enzyme number) in relation to the stages of the spermatogenic cycle to accommodate the changes in structure and movement of germ cells from the base to the surface of the seminiferous epithelium[70]. The margins of the Sertoli cell undergo transformation to remain associated with the different types of germ cells and the changes taking place in them during different stages of spermatogenesis including spermiation. In the monkey, ultrastructural studies showed that the volume occupied by the Sertoli cells in the seminiferous epithelium ranged from 24 per cent in stage I to 32 per cent in stage VII of the cycle[88]. In the rat, the proportion occupied by Sertoli cells during spermatogenic cycle ranges from 19-28 per cent with lowest volume during stage VII[48]. This changing shape and volume of Sertoli cells are believed to be due to their motor activity to accommodate the changing volume of germ cells.

The Sertoli cell is characterized by a large and irregular nucleus located at the basal region of the cell (Figure 1.10). The nuclei of the Sertoli cells are seen more or less in a single row towards the basement membrane of the seminiferous tubule. The nucleus is highly infolded. But in the rat, its shape and position are variable according to the spermatogenic cycle. The nucleoplasm is of fine fibrogranular texture, and has a homogeneous distribution of euchromatin. The nucleus is very prominent. The heterochromatin is confined usually to either side of the nucleolus as densely stained compact masses to form the nucleolus-associated heterochromatin, called the Satellite karyosomes. The nucear envelope has a number of pores, which are very uniformly distributed. In the human, the large nucleolus which stains intensely with basophilic dyes can be used to distinguish the Sertoli cell in the seminiferous epithelium.

The cytoplasmic components are usually found at the basal region of the Sertoli cell whereas the apical region is relatively devoid of inclusions. But, the apical portion of the Sertoli cell in the human testis has mitochondria, endoplasmic reticulum and glycogen. The mitochondria are usually slender and often long with the cristae usually arranged transversely. The mitochondria in the basal cytoplasm are randomly oriented while those in the supranuclear portion are parallel to the cell axis.

The Golgi complex in rat testis consists of a network of perforated membrane sheets interconnected with narrow bridges, located in the basal cytoplasm and occasionally in the supranuclear region. Numerous membrane-limited dense bodies of various sizes are seen in the cytoplasm and include homogeneous dense bodies presumed to be primary lysosomes, larger heterogeneous autophagic vacuoles and dense lipochrome pigment.

Granular endoplasmic reticulum is found mostly in the basal cytoplasm. The smooth endoplasmic reticulum which is in great abundance does not have specific morphology and is often associated with lipid droplet. The functional significance of this is

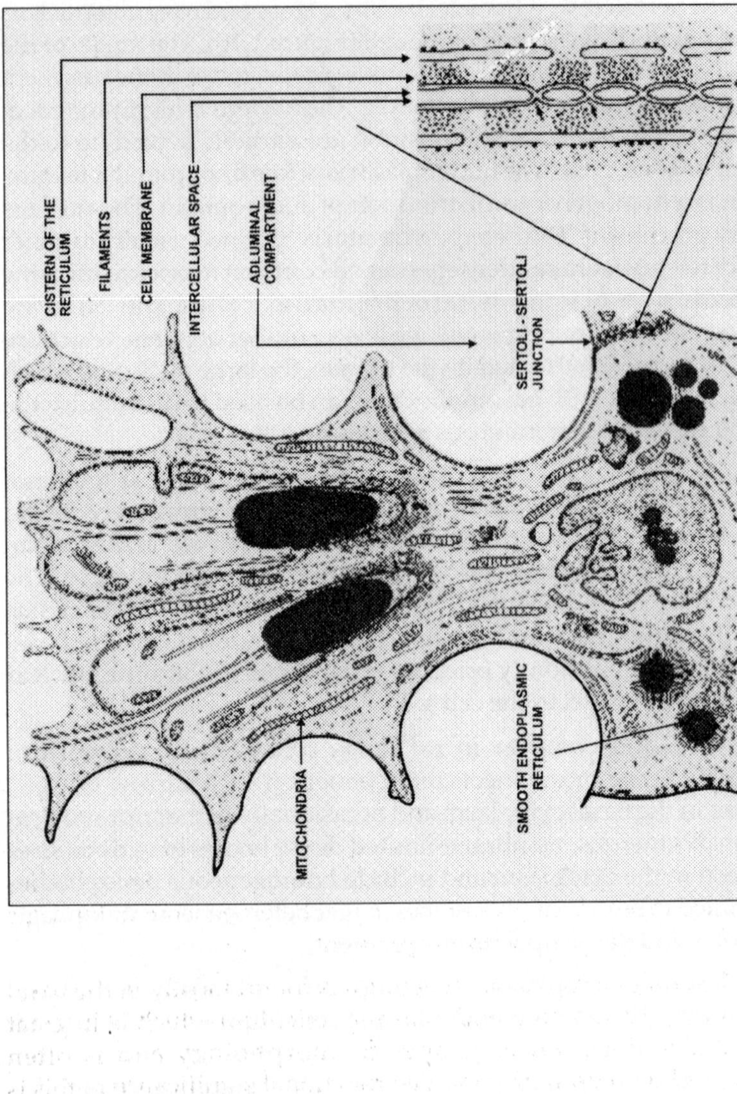

Figure 1.10: Diagrammatic Representation of a Sertoli Cell and the Composition of Sertoli-Sertoli Cell Functional Complex (from Fawcett[91])

not known. The lipid inclusions in Sertoli cells of rat show cyclic accumulation and decline, during the spermatogenic cycle[89] and is considered to represent a balance between lipolysis and synthesis. In human testis, two types of crystals, based on their length and thickness, are found in the perinuclear region of the Sertoli cell cytoplasm and are called Charcot-Böttcher crystals[87,90]. Sertoli cells also contain variable amounts of dense bodies which are considered as collection of lysosomes, multivesicular bodies and vacuoles[48]. Sertoli cells play an important role in phagocytosis and destruction of foreign particulate matter, degenerating germ cells and excess residual cytoplasm. Sertoli cells have an elaborate cytoskeleton and contractile elements in the cytoplasm[91].

Role of Sertoli Cell in Maintaining Blood Testis Barrier

One of the earliest observations on the existence of a blood-testis barrier was the observations of Ribbert[92], Bouffard[93] and Pari[94] that intravenously injected dyes did not gain entry into the testis. These and subsequent studies by a number of investigators established the existence of a blood-testis barrier. Waites and Setchell[95] and Setchell[96] studied the blood-testis barrier in conscious rams by measuring rate of passage of substances from blood plasma into testicular lymph and into rete testis fluid. All substances tested passed rapidly into lymph while only a few passed into testicular fluid. Therefore, these investigators concluded that the barrier is not the capillary wall but in or around the seminiferous tubules.

Tracer substances that reach seminiferous epithelium remain in the basal region of the epithelium and rarely penetrate beyond the zone occupied by spermatogonia. The extent to which tracer penetrates is limited by the zone of specialized junctional complexes[97] where the lateral cytoplasmic processes of adjacent Sertoli cells arch over the spermatogonia but below the spermatocytes. These Sertoli cell-Sertoli cell junctions consist of symmetrical specializations of neighbouring Sertoli cells each having subsurface cisternae of endoplasmic reticulum separated from opposing cell membranes by parallel bundles of filaments (Figure 1.10). The distance between membranes is usually ~200A^0 resembling gap junctions or at regular intervals along the junctional complex, the membranes are fused to form tight junctions. Electron opaque tracers stop at these sites. In laboratory rodents, there are two compartments to the blood-testis barrier: (1) the adventitial compartment–an incomplete barrier constituted by the myoid cells, and (2) the Sertoli cell-Sertoli cell junction forming a more effective intraepithelial compartment. In primates, the adventitial compartment is absent. The Sertoli cell-Sertoli cell junctional complexes divide the seminiferous epithelium into two compartments: a basal compartment containing spermatogonia and preleptotene and leptotene spermatocytes and an adluminal compartment beyond the level of the tight junctions that sequesters the more differentiated germ cells like more advanced spermatocytes and spermatids. Substances from blood reach directly the basal compartment but due to the occluding junctions, substances have to pass through the Sertoli cell cytoplasm to reach the germ cells in the adluminal compartment.

The actual physiological function of the blood-testis barrier is not known. In rodents, germ cell surface-specific antigens appear on pachytene spermatocytes and subsequent stages of germ cell differentiation[98] and on surface of Sertoli cells[99]. The process of meiosis and spermiogenesis occur in an immunologically privileged adluminal compartment, ensured by the presence of Sertoli cell-Sertoli cell junctions[100]. But, the barrier is flexible accommodating the needs of the germ cells as they migrate from basal to adluminal compartment.

The Sertoli cell also plays a major role in conferring stability to the seminiferous epithelium. The germ cells are prevented from detachment and extrusion into the lumen of seminiferous tubules by regions of ectoplasmic stabilizations of the Sertoli cell that face the surface of the germ cells. These consist of a dense band of filaments that are rich in actin and are present between the Sertoli cell plasma membrane and the cisternae of endoplasmic reticulum and constitute the inter-Sertoli cell tight junctions at the base of the Sertoli cells[91,101]. These ectoplasmic specializations are seen facing mid-pachytene spermatocytes and round spermatids but during elongation of spermatids, a covering of the ectoplasmic specialization is seen around the spermatid head[102]. The ectoplasmic specializations have been implicated in (a) adhesion between Sertoli and germ cells, (b) as structural support, (c) in spermiation, and (d) as contractile elements[48,102]. During spermiation, the cytoplasm of the elongated spermatid gets gradually attenuated along the long axis of the sperm and forms a slender lobe, the future residual cytoplasm.

Other types of junctional specializations in the seminiferous epithelium include desmosomes, hemi-desmosomes and gap junction. Desmosomes, seen between Sertoli cells and round germ cells form adhesion sites between cells and help in the orderly upward movement of germ cells during maturation. Hemidesmosomes seen at the site where Sertoli cell rests on the basal lamina is believed to help in anchoring Sertoli cells. Gap junction are absent in human Sertoli cells[103] but are present in laboratory animals and may have a role in intercellular communication.

Sertoli cells secrete a number of products including Androgen Binding Protein (ABP), transport proteins like transferrin and ceruloplasmin, acidic glycoprotein, inhibin, activin, growth factors (fibroblast growth factor, somatomedin), H-Y protein, CMB-21, Eppin, anti-Mullerian hormone etc[104–106]. In rat, 80 per cent of the ABP is secreted into the lumen of the seminiferous tubule and remaining 20 per cent into blood[107]. Readers may refer to various articles published for further information.

Peritubular Cells

Myoid cells, which lie external to the basement membrane of the seminiferous tubules, by their contractions, help to propel the secretions of the Sertoli cells and spermatids into the seminiferous lumen and further to the rete testis. The myoid cells have been reported to produce growth factors like activin A and platelet derived growth factors[108–109].

Leydig Cell

The Leydig cell was first described by Leydig in 1850 in which he described that the space between seminiferous tubules was occupied by cells containing vacuoles and pigments. The intertubular space has blood vessels surrounded by Leydig cells, loose connective tissue, fibroblasts, macrophages, lymphocytes and lymphatic sinusoids or vessels[110]. The arrangement of these components shows species variations.

The human Leydig cell is polygonal in shape and 15-20 ìm in diameter. It is surrounded by a plasma membrane, which is thrown frequently into folds or microvilli. The nucleus is large, round or irregularly oval with a thin peripheral rim of heterochromatin broken at the sites of the pores in the nuclear membrane. One or two prominent nucleoli are seen.

The most distinctive character of the cytoplasm of the Leydig cells is the presence of large amounts of smooth endoplasmic reticulum which shows diversity in its architecture. Smooth endoplamic reticulum is most abundant in guinea pig and mouse whereas it is moderate in the rat and human[111–112]. The surface area of the smooth endoplasmic reticulum is vast and usually consists of a random network of interconnected tubules or form more regular arrays of fenestrated cisternae. Studies have shown a strong correlation between testosterone secretion and amount of smooth endoplasmic reticulum and Golgi membranes indicating the role of Leydig cell in testosterone production[113]. These investigators have also suggested that conversion of pregnenolone to progesterone may be located in specialized regions of the Leydig cell.

The rough endoplamic reticulum is scattered and in patches. Mitochondria vary in size and number and are usually lamellar. Golgi is well developed and consists of 4-6 flattened sacs closely pressed together with small vesicles at their periphery. Cytoplasm contains lipid droplets, microtubules and filaments and lysosomes. Species differences occur in the amount of lipid inclusions in the Leydig cell. While it is abundant in rhesus monkey, very few inclusions are seen in the Leydig cells of African green monkey, squirrel monkey or human[48]. The changes in lipid content reflect changes in Leydig cell function. In the human Leydig cells, rod-shaped structures of 20 μm length termed crystals of Reinke are seen but their functional role is not clear.

Leydig cells are continuously but slowly lost from the testis with increasing age. It has been reported that after 20 years of age, 8 million Sertoli cells are lost per paired testes per annum[114] but the mechanism of attrition is still to be described.

Testicular Production of Androgens

Leydig cells are the source of almost all of androgen produced by the tesis. Cholesterol for steroid biosynthesis is sourced from plasma and also by local production. The plasma cholesterol required for steroid hormone biosynthesis is obtained from lipoproteins. Cholesterol enters the mitochondria for side chain cleavage and is converted to pregnenolone (C_{27} side chain cleavage) which is converted to progesterone by enzymes in the microsomes. Testosterone biosynthesis involves multi-functional cytochrome

P450 complexes involving C20 and C22 hydroxylases, C20,22 lyases and 17-hydroxylase/17,20 lyase. Hall[115] has shown that trophic hormones like LH act on cholesterol transport to the mitochondrial side chain cleavage cytochrome P-450 cholesterol side-chain cleavage enzyme complex located on the inner mitochondrial membrane complex. The supply of cholesterol is governed by sterol carrier protein 2[116], StAR[117] and peripheral benzodiazepine receptor[118]. Once side chain cleavage has occurred, the resulting pregnenolone must pass through the mitochondrial membrane into the cytoplasm for further biosynthesis into testosterone. The necessary enzymes are bound to the smooth endoplasmic reticulum mostly.

References

1. Ginsburg M, Snow MH and McLaren A (1990). Primordial germ cells in the mouse embryo during gastrulation. Development, 110: 521-528.

2. Swain A and Lovell-Badge R (1999). Mammalian sex determination. A molecular drama. Genes and Dev, 13: 755-767.

3. Hughes IA (2001). Minireview: Sex differentiation. Endocrinology, 142: 3281-3287.

4. Jost A (1947). Recherches sur le différentiation sexuelle de l'embryon de lapin III. Rôle des gonads foetales dans la différentiation sexuelle somatique. Arch Anat Microsc Morphol Exp, 36: 271-315.

5. Jost A (1953). Problems of fetal endocrinology: the gonadal and hypophyseal hormones. Recent Prog Horm Res, 8: 379-418.

6. Nef S and Parada LF (2000). Hormones in male sexual development. Genes and Dev, 14: 3075-3086.

7. Baarends WM, van Helmond MJL, Post M, van der Schoot PJ, Hoogerbrugge JW, de Winter JP, Uilenbroek JT, Karels B, Wilming LG, Meijers JH, *et al.* (1994). A novel member of the transmembrane serine/threonine kinase receptor family is specifically expressed in the gonads and in mesenchymal cells adjacent to the Müllerian duct. Develoment, 120: 189-197.

8. Allard S, Adin P, Gonedard L, di Clemente N, Josso N, Orgebin-Crist MC, Picard JY, Xavier F (2000). Molecular mechanisms of

hormone mediated Mullerian duct regression: involvement of β-catenin. Development, 127: 3349-3360.

9. Nef S and Parada LF (1999). Cryptorchidism in mice mutant for Insl3. Nat Genet, 22: 295-299.

10. Frey HL, Peng S and Rajfer J (1983). Synergy of abdominal pressure and androgens in testicular descent. Biol Reprod, 29: 1233-1239.

11. Shawlot W and Behringer RR (1995). Requirement for *Lim 1* in head-organizer function. Nature, 374: 425-430.

12. Gubbay J, Collignon J, Koopman P, Capel B, Economou A, Munsterberg A, Vivian N, Goodfellow P and Lovell-Badge R (1990). A gene mapping to the sex-determining region of the mouse Y chromosome is a member of a novel family of embryonically expressed genes. Nature, 346: 245-250.

13. Sinclair AH, Berta P, Palmer MS, Hawkins JR, Griffiths BL and Smith MJ, Foster JW, Frischauf AM, Lovell-Badge R, Goodfellow PN. (1990). A gene from the human sex-determining region encodes a protein with homology to a conserved DNA-binding motif. Nature, 346: 240-244.

14. Capel B and Lovell-Badge R (1993). The Sry gene and sex determination in mammals. In: Wasserman PM (ed): Advances in Developmental Biology, vol 2, pp. 1-35, JAI Press, Greenwich.

15. Koopman P, Munsterberg A, Capel B, Vivian N and Lovell-Badge R (1990). Expression of a candidate sex-determining gene during mouse testis differentiation. Nature, 348: 50-52.

16. Hacker A, Capel B, Goodfellow P and Lovell-Badge R (1995). Expression of Sry, the mouse sex determining gene. Development, 121: 1603-1614.

17. Smith CA, McClive PJ, Hudson Q and Sinclair AH. (2005). Male-specific cell migration into the developing gonad is a conserved process involving PDGF signaling. Dev Biol, 284: 337-350.

18. Martineau J, Nordqvist K, Tilmann C, Lovell-Badge R and Capel B (1997). Male-specific cell migration into the developing gonad. Curr Biol, 7: 958-968.

19. Capel B, Albrecht KH, Washburn LL and Eicher EM (1999). Migration of mesonephric cells into the mammalian gonad depends on Sry. Mech Dev, 84: 127-131.

20. Cool J, Carmona FD, Szucsik JC and Capel B (2008). Peritubular myoid cells are not the migrating population required for testis cord formation in the XY gonad. Sex Dev, 2: 128-133.

21. Pelliniemi LJ and Dyn M (1993). The fetal gonad and sexual differentiation. In: Tulchinsky D and Little B (eds): Maternal-fetal Endocrinology, pp. 297-320, Saunders, Philadelphia.

22. Polanco JC and Koopman P (2007). Sry and the hesitant beginnings of male development. Dev Biol, 302: 13-24.

23. Kent J, Wheatley SC, Andrews JE, Sinclair AH and Koopman P (1996). A male-specific role for SOX9 in vertebrate sex determination. Development, 122: 2813-2822.

24. Morais de Silva S, Hacker A, Harley V, Goodfellow P, Swain A and Lovell-Badge R (1996). Sox9 expression during gonadal development implies a conserved role for the gene in testis differentiation in mammals and birds. Nat Genet, 14: 62-68.

25. Gunn SA and Gould TC (1975). Vasculature of the testes and adnexia. In: Hamilton DW and Greep RO (eds): Handbook of Physiology, Section 7, Endocrinology, Vol 5, Male Reproductive System, pp. 117-142, Williams and Wilkens, Baltimore.

26. Clermont Y and Le Blond CP (1953). Renewal of spermatogonia in the rat. Am J Anat, 93: 475-502.

27. Clermont Y (1969). Two classes of spermatogonial stem cells in the monkey (Cercopithecus aethiops). Am J Anat, 126: 57–71.

28. Dym M and Clermont Y (1970). Role of spermatogonia in the repair of the seminiferous epithelium following X-irradiation of the rat testis. Am J Anat, 128: 265–282.

29. van Alphen MM, van de Kant HJ and de Rooij DG (1988a). Depletion of the spermatogonia from the seminiferous epithelium of the rhesus monkey after X irradiation. Radiat Res, 113: 473–486.

30. van Alphen MM, van de Kant HJ and de Rooij DG (1988b). Repopulation of the seminiferous epithelium of the rhesus monkey after X irradiation. Radiat Res, 113: 487–500.

31. Ehmcke J, Simorangkir DR and Schlatt S (2005). Identification of the starting point for spermatogenesis and characterization of the testicular stem cell in adult male rhesus monkeys. Human Reproduction, 20: 1185-1193.

32. Clermont Y (1966a). Renewal of spermatogonia in man. Am J Anat, 118: 509-524.

33. Clermont Y (1966b). Spermatogenesis in man: a study of the spermatogonial population. Fertil Steril, 17: 705-721.

34. Ehmcke J and Schlatt S (2006). A revised model for spermatogonial expansion in man: lessons from non-human primates. Reproduction, 132: 673-680.

35. Yoshida S, Nabeshima Y and Nakagawa T (2007). Stem cell heterogeneity: actual and potential stem cell compartments in mouse spermatogenesis. Ann N Y Acad Sci, 1120: 47-58.

36. Oatley JM and Brinster RL (2006). Spermatogonial stem cells. Methods in Enzymology, 419: 259-282.

37. Dadoune JP (2007). New insights into male gametogenesis: what about the spermatogonial stem cell niche? Folia Histochem et Cytobiol, 45: 141-147.

38. McLean DJ (2005). Spermatogonial stem cell transplantation and testicular function. Cell Tissue Res, 322: 21-31.

39. Ogawa T, Ohmura M and Ohbo K (2005). The niche for spermatogonial stem cells in the mammalian testis. Int J Hematol, 82: 381-388.

40. Costoya JA, Hobbs RM, Barna M, Cattoretti G, Manova K, Sukhwani M, Orwig KE, Wolgemuth DJ and Pandolfi PP (2004). Essential role of Plzf in maintenance of spermatogonial stem cells. Nat Genet, 36: 653-659.

41. Falender AE, Freiman RN, Geles KG, Lo KC, Hwang K, Lamb DJ, Morris PL, Tjian R and Richards JS (2005). Maintenance of spermatogenesis requires TAF4b, a gonad-specific subunit of TFIID. Genes Dev, 19: 794-803.

42. Ballow D, Meistrich ML, Matzuk M and Rajkovic A (2006a). Sohlh 1 is essential for spermatogonial differentiation. Dev Biol, 294: 161-167.

43. Ballow DJ, Xin Y, Choi Y, Pangas SA and Rajkovic A (2006b). Sohlh2 is a germ cell-specific bHLH transcription factor. Gene Expr Patterns, 6: 1014-1018.

44. Meng X, Lindahl M, Hyvonen ME, Parvinen M, de Rooij DG, Hess MW, Raatikainen-Ahokas A, Sainio K, Rauvala H, Lakso

M *et al.* (2000). Regulation of cell fate decision of undifferentiated spermatogonia by GDNF. Science, 287: 1489-1493.

45. Rossi P, Sette C Dolci S and Geremia R (2000). Role of c-kit in mammalian spermatogenesis. J Endocrinol Invest, 23: 609-615.

46. Tadakoro Y, Yomogida K, Ohta H, Tohda A and Nishimune Y (2002). Homeostatic regulation of germinal stem cell proliferation by the GDNF/FSH pathway. Mech Dev, 113: 29-39.

47. Chen WS, Xu PZ, Gottlob K, Chen ML, Sokol K, Shiyanova T, Roninson I, Weng W, Suzuki R, Suzuki R, Tobe K *et al.* (2005). Growth retardation and increased apoptosis in mice with homozygous disruption of the Akt1 gene. Genes Dev, 15: 2203-2208.

48. de Kretser DM and Kerr JB (1994). The cytology of the testis. In Knobil E, Neill JD (eds). The Physiology of Reproduction, 2nd ed. pp. 1177-1290, New York, Raven Press.

49. Le Blond and Clermont Y (1952). Definition of the stages of the cycle of the seminiferous epithelium in the rat. Ann N Y Acad Sci, 55: 548-573.

50. Bowen RH (1922). On the idiosome, Golgi apparatus and acrosome in the male germ cells. Anat Record, 24: 158-180.

51. Holstein AF (1976). Ultrastructural observations on the differentiation of spermatids in men. Andrologia, 8: 157-165.

52. Hermo L, Rambourg A and Clermont Y (1980). Three-dimensional architecture of the cortical region of the Golgi apparatus in the rat spermatids. Am J Anat, 157: 357-373.

53. Clermont Y and Tang XM (1985). Glycoprotein synthesis in the Gogi apparatus of spermatids during spermiogenesis of the rat. Anat Record, 213: 33-43.

54. Pederson H (1972a). The postacrosomal region of ram and Macaca artoides. J Ultrastr Res, 40: 366-377.

55. Pederson H (1972b). Further observations on the fine structure of the human spermatozoon. Z Zellforsch, 123: 305-315.

56. Stefanini M, Oura C and Zamboni L (1969). Ultrastructure of fertilization in the mouse. 2. Penetration of sperm into ovum. J Submicr Cytol, 1: 1-23.

57. Oko RJ, Jando V, Wagner CL, Kistler WS and Hermo LS (1996). Chromatin reorganization in rat spermatids during the disappearance of testis-specific histone, Hlt, and the appearance of transition proteins TP1 and TP2. Biol Reprod, 54: 1141-1157.

58. Steger K, Klonisch T, Gavenisk K, Drabent B, Doenecke D and Bergmann M (1998). Expression of mRNA and protein of nucleoproteins during human spermiogenesis. Mol Hum Reprod, 10: 939-945.

59. Bellve AR (1979). The molecular biology of mammalian spermatogenesis. In: Finn CA (ed). Oxford Reviews in Reproductive Biology. Vol I, pp. 159-261, Clarendon Press, Oxford.

60. Beatty RA (1970). The genetics of the mammalian gamete. Biol Rev, 45: 73-119.

61. Mei X, Singh IS, Erlichman J and Orr GA (1997). Cloning and characterization of a testis-specific developmentally regulated A-kinase-anchoring protein (TAKAP-80) present on the fibrous sheath of rat sperm. Eur J Biochem, 246: 425-432.

62. Vijayaraghavan S, Liberty GA, Mohan J, Winfrey VP, Olson GE and Carr DW (1999). Isolation and molecular characterization of AKAP110, a novel sperm-specific protein kinase A-anchoring protein. Mol Endocrinol, 13: 705-717.

63. Kirichok Y, Navarro B and Clapham DE (2006). Whole-cell patch-clamp measurements of spermatozoa reveal an alkaline-activated calcium channel. Nature, 439: 737-740.

64. Wartenberg H and Holstein AF (1975). Morphology of the "spindle-shaped body" in the developing tail of human spermatids. Cell Tissue Res, 159: 435-443.

65. de Kretser DM (1969). Ultrastructural features of human spermiogenesis. Z Zellforsch, 98: 477-505.

66. Vitale-Calpe R (1970). Ultrastructural studies of spontaneous spermiation in the guinea pig. Z Zellforsch, 105: 222-223.

67. Kaur J, Ramakrishnan PR and Rajalakshmi M (1990). Inhibition of sperm maturation in rhesus monkey by cyproterone acetate. Contraception, 42: 349-359.

68. Perey B, Clermont Y and Le Blond CP (1961). The wave of the seminiferous epithelium in the rat. Am J Anat, 108: 47-77.

69. Heller CT and Clermont Y (1964). Kinetics of the germinal epithelium in man. Recent Progr. Horm. Res. 20: 545-571.

70. Parvinen M (1982). Regulation of the seminiferous epithelium. Endocr Reviews, 3: 404-417.

71. Zamudio NM, Chong S and O'Bryani MK (2008). Epigenetic regulation in male germ cells. Reproduction, May 30.

72. Bourc'his D and Bestor TH (2004). Meiotic catastrophe and retrotransposon reactivation in male germ cells lacking Dnmt3L. Nature, 431: 996-99.

73. Webster KE, O'Bryan MK, Fletcher S, Crewther PE, Aapola U, Craig J, Harrison DK, Aung H, Phutikanit N, Lyle R, Meachem SJ, Antonarakis SE, de Kretser DM, Hedger MP, Peterson P, Carroll BJ and Scott HS (2005). Meiotic and epigenetic defects in Dnmt3L knockout mouse spermatogenesis. Proc Natl Acad Sci USA, 102: 4068-4073.

74. Redon C, Pilch D, Rogakou E, Sedelnikova O, Newrock K and Bonner W (2002). Histone DNA variants H2AX and H2AZ. Curr Opin Genet Dev, 12: 162-169.

75. Handel M A (2004). The XY body: a specialized meiotic chromatin domain. Exp Cell Res, 296: 57-63.

76. Turner JM (2007). Meiotic sex chromosome inactivation. Development, 134: 1823-1831.

77. Namekawa SH., Park PJ, Zhang LF, Shima JE, McCarrey JR., Griswold MD and Lee JT (2006). Postmeiotic sex chromatin in the male germline of mice. Curr Biol, 16: 660-667.

78. Doenecke D, Drabent B, Bode C, Bramlage B, Franke K, Gavenis K, Kosciessa U and Witt O (1997). Histone gene expression and chromatin structure during spermatogenesis. Adv Exp Med Biol, 424: 37-48.

79. Govin J, Caron C, Lestrat C, Rousseaux S and Khochbin S (2004). The role of histones in chromatin remodeling during mammalian spermatogenesis. Eur J Biochem, 271: 3459-3469.

80. Sonnack V, Failing K, Bergmann M and Steger K (2002). Expression of hyperacetylated histone H4 during normal and impaired human spermatogenesis. Andrologia, 34: 384-390.

81. Wouters-Tyrou D, Martinage A, Chevaillier P and Sautiere P (1998). Nuclear basic proteins in spermatogenesis. Biochemie, 80: 117-128.

82. Martianov I., Brancorsini S, Catena R, Gansmuller A, Kotaja N, Parvinen M, Sassone-Corsi P and Davidson I (2005). Polar nuclear localization of H1T2, a histone H1 variant, required for spermatid elongation and DNA condensation during spermiogenesis. Proc Natl Acad Sci USA, 102: 2808-2813.

83. Tanaka H and Baba T (2005). Gene expression in spermiogenesis. Cell Mol Life Sci, 62: 344-354.

84. Chong S, Vickaryous N, Ashe A, Zamudio N, Youngson N, Hemley S, Stopka T, Skoultchi A, Matthews J, Scott HS, de Kretser D, O'Bryan M, Blewitt M and Whitelaw E (2007). Modifiers of epigenetic reprogramming show paternal effects in the mouse. Nature Genet, 39: 614-622.

85. von Ebner V (1871). Untersuchungen über den Bau der Samenkamälichen und die Entwicklung der Spermatozoiden bei den Säugenthieren und beim Menschen. Leipzig: Rollet's Untersuchungen aus dem Institut für Physiologie und Histologie in Graz, pp. 200.

86. von Ebner V (1888). Zur Spermatogenese bei den Säugenthieren. Arch Mikrobiol Anat, 31: 236-292.

87. Fawcett DW and Burgos MH (1956). The fine structure of the Sertoli cells in the human testis (Abstract). Anat Record, 124: 401.

88. Cavicchia JC and Dym M (1977). Relative volume of Sertoli cells in monkey seminiferous epithelium. Am J Anat, 150: 501-503.

89. Kerr JB, Mayberry RA and Irby DC (1984). Morphometric studies on lipid inclusions in Sertoli cells during the spermatogenic cycle in the rat. Cell Tissue Res, 236: 699-709.

90. Nagano T (1966). Some observations on the fine structure of the Sertoli cell in the human testis. Z Zellforsch, 73: 89-106.

91. Fawcett DW (1975). Ultrastructure and function of the Sertoli cells. In:. Hamilton DW and Greep RO (eds): Handbook of Physiology, Section 7, Endocrinology, Vol 5, Male Reproductive System, pp. 21-55, Williams and Wilkens, Baltimore.

92. Ribbert HC (1904). Die abscheidung intravenos injzierten gelosten Karmins in den Geweben. Z Allg Physiol, 4: 201-214.

93. Bouffard G (1906). Injection des couters de benzidine aux animaux nomaux. Annales de l'Institut Pasteur de Lille, 20: 539-546.

94. Pari G (1910). Uber die verwendharkeit vitaler Karmineinspritzungen fur dies pathologische Anatomie. Frank Z Pathol, 4: 1-29.

95. Waites GMH and Setchell BP (1966). Changes in blood flow and vascular permeability of the testis, epididymis and accessory reproductive organs of the rat after administration of cadmium chloride. J Endocrinol, 34: 329-342.

96. Setchell BP (1967). The blood-testicular fluid barrier in sheep. J Physiol (Lond), 189: 63P-65P.

97. Flickinger C and Fawcett DW (1967). Junctional specializations of the Sertoli cells in the seminiferous epithelium. Anat Record, 158: 207-222.

98. Millette CF and Bellve AR (1977). Temporal expansion of membrane antigens during mouse spermatogenesis. J Cell Biol, 74: 86-97.

99. Tung PS and Fritz IB (1978). Specific surface antigens on rat pachytene spermatocytes and successive classes of germ cells. Dev Biol, 64: 297-315.

100. Waites GMH and Gladwell RT (1982). Physiological significance of fluid secretion in the testis and blood testis barrier. Physiol Rev, 62: 624-671.

101. Franke WW, Grund C, Frink A, Weber K, Jokusch BM, Zentgraf H and Osborn M (1978). Location of actin in the microfilament bundles associated with the junctional specializations between Sertoli cells and spermatids. Biol Cellulaire, 31: 7-14.

102. Russel LD (1980). Sertoli-germ cell interactions: a review. Gamete Res, 3: 179-202.

103. Schulze C (1984). Sertoli cells and Leydig cells in men. Cell Tissue Res, 153: 339-355.

104. Bardin CW, Cheng CY, Musto NA and Gunsalus GL (1988). The Sertoli cell. In: Knobil E, Neill J (eds), The Physiology of Reproduction, 2nd ed. pp. 933-974, New York, Raven Press.

105. Josso N, Cate RL, Vigier JY, di Clemente N, Wilson C, Imbeaud S, Pepinsky RB, Guerrier D, Boussin *et al.* (1993). Anti-Müllerian hormone, the Jost factor. Rec Progr Horm Res, 48: 1-59.

106. Sivashanmugam P, Hall SH, Hamil KG, French FS, O'Rand MG and Richardson RT (2003). Characterization of mouse Eppin and a gene cluster of similar protease inhibitors on mouse chromosome 2. Gene, 17: 125-134.

107. Hansson V, Ritzen EM, French FS and Nayfeh SN (1975). Androgen transport and receptor mechsnism in testis and epididymis. In: Hamilton DW and Greep RO (eds) Handbook of Physiology, Section 7, Endocrinology, Vol 5, Male Reproductive System, pp. 173-201, Williams and Wilkens, Baltimore.

108. de Winter JP, Vanderstichele HM, Verhoeven G, Timmerman MA, Wesseling JG and de Jong FH (1994). Peritubular myoid cells from immature rat testes secrete activin-A and express activin receptor type II *in vitro*. Endocrinology, 135: 759-767.

109. Gnessi L, Emidi A, Jannini EA, Carosa E, Maroder M, Arizzi M, Ulisse S and Spera G (1995). Testicular development involves the spatiotemporal control of PDGFs and PDGF receptors gene expression and action. J Cell Biol, 131: 1105-1121.

110. Fawcett DW (1973). Observations on the organization of the interstitial tissue of the testis and on the occluding cell junctions in the seminiferous epithelium. Adv Bio Sci, 16: 83-99.

111. de Kretser DM (1967). The fine structure of the testicular interstitial cells in men of normal androgenic status. Z Zellforsch, 80: 594-609.

112. Christensen AK (1975). Leydig cells. In: Hamilton DW and Greep RO (eds), Handbook of Physiology, Section 7, Endocrinology, Vol 5, Male Reproductive System, pp. 21-55, Williams and Wilkens, Baltimore.

113. Ewing LL, Zirkin BR, Cochran RC, Kromann N, Peters C and Ruiz-Bravo N (1979). Testosterone secretion by rat, rabbit, guinea pig, dog and hamster testes perfused *in vitro*: correlation with Leydig cell mass. Endocrinology, 105: 1135-1142.

114. Kaler LW and Neaves WB (1978). Attrition of the human Leydig cell population with advancing age. Anat Record, 192: 513-518.

115. Hall PF (1985). Trophic stimulation of steroidogenesis. In: Greep RO (ed), Search of the Elusive Trigger, Laurentian Hormone Conf, pp. 41, Academic Press, New York.

116. Seedorf U, Ellinghaus P, Roch Nofer J (2000). Sterol carrier protein-2. Biochim Biophys Acta, 1486: 45-54.

117. Stocco DM (2001). Tracking the role of a star in the sky of the new millennium. Mol Endocrinol, 15: 1245-54.

118. Papadopoulos V, Amri H, Li H, Yao Z, Brown RC, Vidic B and Culty M (2001). Structure, function and regulation of the mitochondrial peripheral-type benzodiazepine receptor. Therapie, 56: 549-56.

Environmental & Occupational Exposures (2010) *Pages 44–53*
Editors: **Sunil Kumar & R.R. Tiwari**
Published by: **DAYA PUBLISHING HOUSE, NEW DELHI**

Chapter 2

Female Reproductive System

Tarala D. Nandedkar*

Ex-Deputy Director, Sr. Grade,
Emeritus Scientist–CSIR,
National Institute for Research in Reproductive Health,
ICMR, Parel, Mumbai – 400 012

ABSTRACT

The female genitals include: the ovaries, the accessory glands, the fallopian tubes, the uterus, the cervix and the vagina. The ovarian follicles synthesize androgens as well as estrogens. Fertilization occurs in the fallopian tube. A series of changes occur in the female reproductive system in the form of periodic events called "menstrual cycle", which on an average takes 28 days to complete. During the reproductive years, the monthly discharge of degenerated endometrium occurs at regular intervals with minimal variation. This chapter describes the female reproductive system with endocrinal changes occurring during menstruation.

The diploid fertilized egg is formed in fallopian tube by the union of the haploid female gamete, the oocyte and the haploid male gamete, spermatozoon. If X chromosome of the oocyte and X chromosome from a sperm unite, the embryo thus formed enters the

* E-mail: nandedkartarala@hotmail.com

uterus; it implants and develops into a female fetus. Although the sex of the fetus is decided after fertilization, the differentiation of the female gonads and accessory glands occurs only in the third trimester of pregnancy[1].

In the females, reproductive organs or genitals are inside the body in the pelvic region (Figure 2.1a). The female genitals include: the ovaries, the accessory glands, the fallopian tubes, the uterus, the cervix and the vagina (Figure 2.1b).

Ovaries (Figure 2.1c)

The ovaries, in females are located inside the body as opposed to the testes present outside the body in males. The ovaries produce eggs and secrete the female hormones, estrogen and progesterone. Oogonia are the fundamental reproductive units of the ovary and are formed in the human fetus between the sixth and the ninth months of gestation. A baby girl is born with a finite number of about 60,000 of germ cells contained in sac-like depressions in the

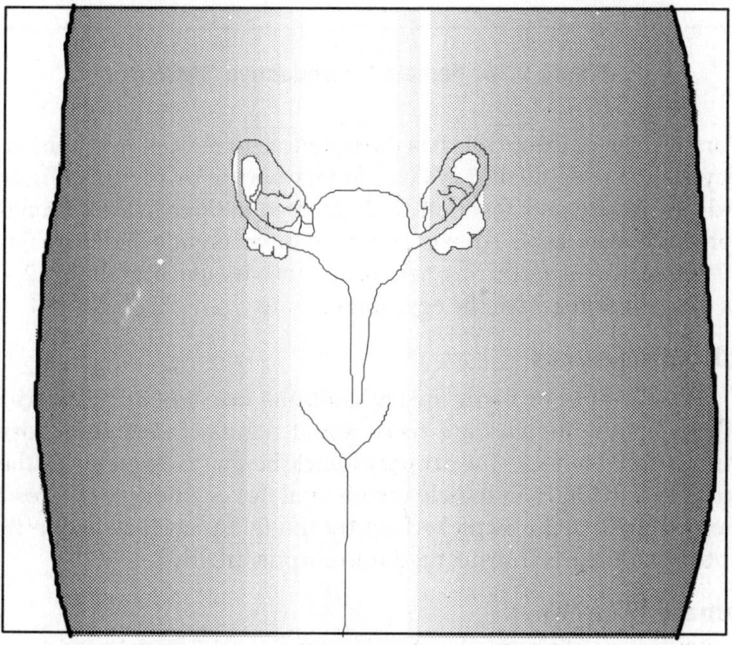

Figure 2.1a: Location in Pelvic Region

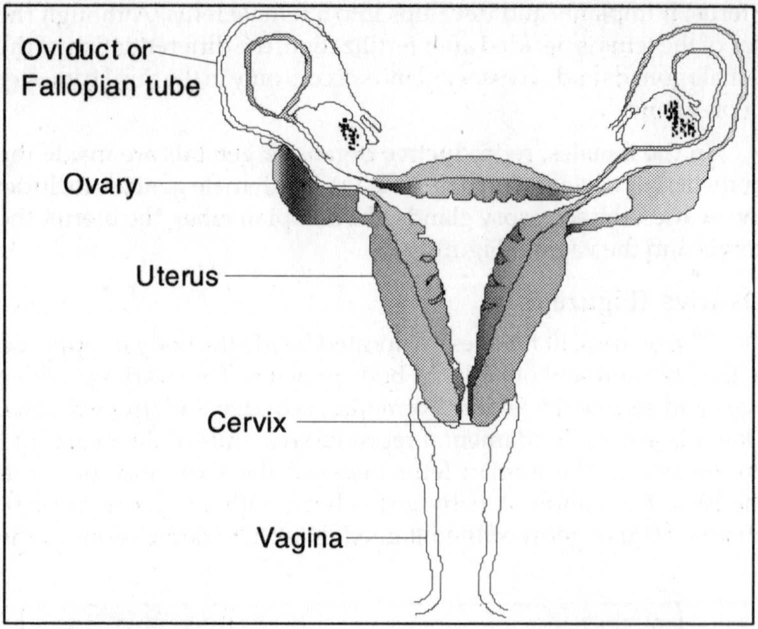

Figure 2.1b: Female Reproductive System

ovaries. Each of these cells has the potential to mature into primary oocyte and subsequently into secondary oocyte by meiosis (Figure 2.1d). However, only few hundreds succeed to ripen in the woman's reproductive life span. After puberty, a woman is endowed to ovulate 400-500 mature eggs during her entire reproductive life (about 12-47 yrs of age) while rest of the eggs degenerate.

Folliculogenesis

At the time of birth, ovary contains oocytes in primordial follicles. These follicles are recruited at regular intervals to form primary follicles. Once the primary follicle begins to develop, it either leads to form Graffian follicle which ovulates or undergoes atresia. The ovulated ovum is picked up by the fallopian tube while the ruptured follicle is transformed into corpus luteum[2].

Female Hormones

The ovarian follicles synthesize androgens as well as estrogens. Estrogen is involved in the development of female sexual features

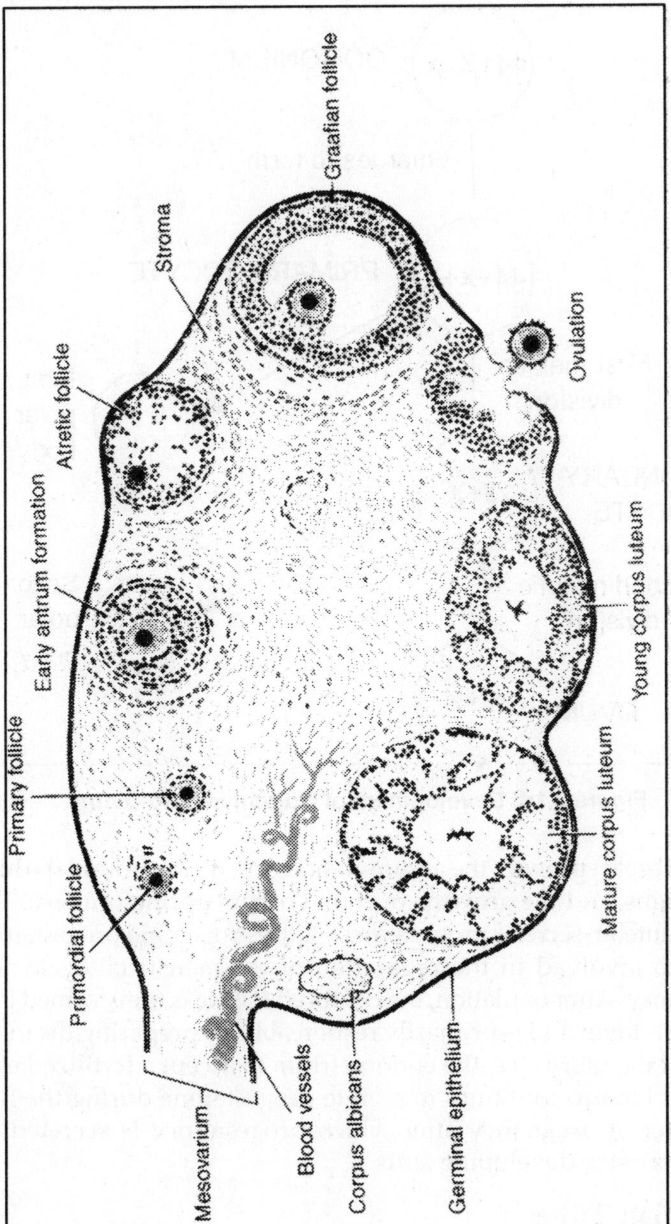

Figure 2.1c: Ovary: Follicular Development, Ovulation and Corpus Luteum (Reproduced from Juneja and Nandedkar, 2009)

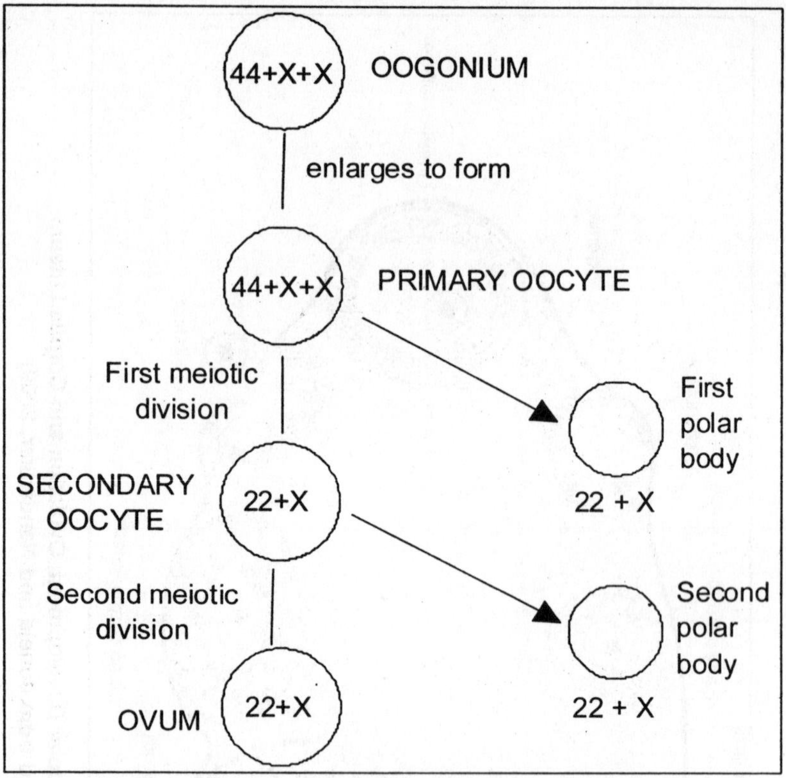

Figure 2.1d: Development of Oogonium into Ovum

such as breast growth, the accumulation of body fat around the hips and thighs, and the growth spurt that occurs during puberty. The corpus luteum secretes progesterone. Both estrogen and progesterone are also involved in the regulation of the menstrual cycle and pregnancy. After ovulation, the ruptured follicle is transformed into corpus luteum and is primarily responsible for preparing the inner layer of the uterus, *i.e.* the endometrium to accept a fertilized egg. Corpus luteum continues to secrete progesterone during the first trimester of pregnancy after which progesterone is secreted by placenta of the developing fetus.

Fallopian Tubes

The fallopian tubes are referred to as oviducts in species other than humans. These are tubular coiled structures extending from the ovary and joined to the uterus at both proximal ends. Fertilization occurs in the fallopian tube. The fimbrial end towards the ovary picks up the egg. The secretory cells provide nutrition to the gametes while the ciliary cells aid in the movement of the sperm towards the egg and in the migration of the zygote to the uterus.

Uterus

The uterus or "womb" is a hollow, muscular tube- like structure, in which the zygote develops into a blastocyst and burrows itself in the uterine endometrium. The embryo draws nourishment, develops and grows in the endometrium until birth. During pregnancy, the uterus stretches from three to four inches in length to a size, which will accommodate a growing baby. During this time, muscular walls increase in weight from two to three ounces to about two pounds, and these powerful muscles release the baby through the birth canal with great force. The womb then shrinks back to half its pregnant weight before the baby is a week old. By the time the baby is a month old, the uterus may be as small as that before pregnancy.

The Menstrual Cycle (Figures 2.2a/b)

A series of changes occur in the female reproductive system (Figure 2.2a) in the form of periodic events called "menstrual cycle", which on an average takes 28 days to complete (Figure 2.2b) although it can vary from 24-32 days. The uterus is lined with tissues, which change during the menstrual cycle and are under the influence of ovarian hormones, estrogen and progesterone. The menstrual cycle is divided into four stages *viz.* follicular phase, ovulatory phase, luteal phase and menstruation. All these stages are regulated by the hypothalamo-pituitary-ovarian axis. If there is no fertilization of the egg by the sperm, there is no embryo to implant in the endometrium. This results in the lack of stimulus for the production of estrogen and progesterone by the ovary. The decrease in the levels of estrogen and progesterone interrupt the blood supply to the uterine lining. As the cells of the uterine lining do not receive adequate blood supply they become necrotic and are shed from the uterus (Figure 2.2a). The mixture of blood and the cells that make up the lining of the uterus is called menstrual fluid. The passage of this fluid through the vagina and out of the body is called menstruation or menstrual period. It usually lasts from three to seven days. At the end of the period, a new cycle begins with the follicular phase[3].

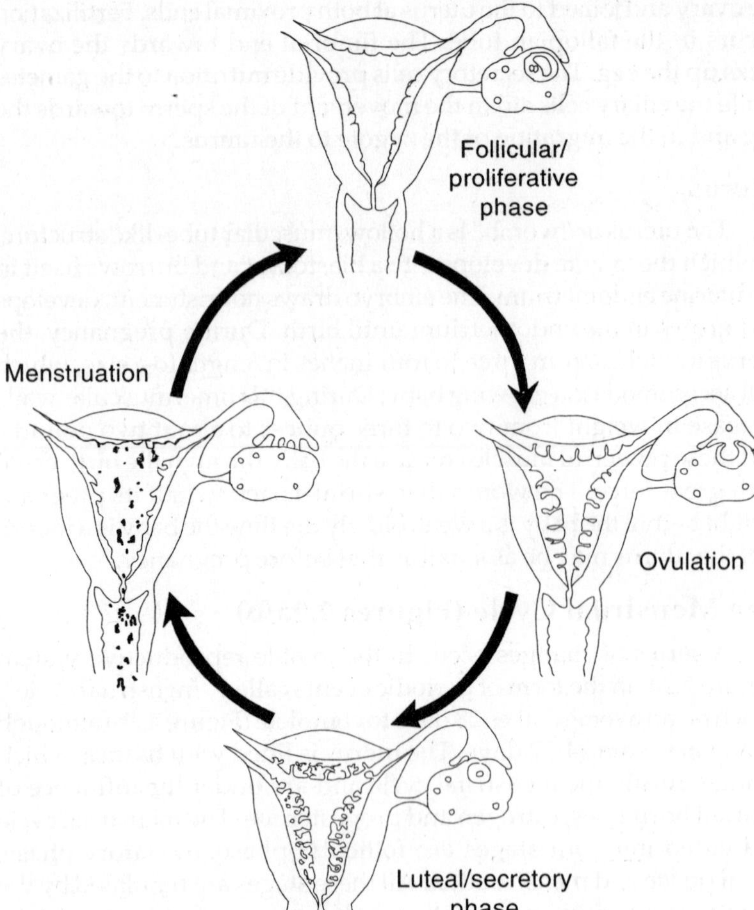

Figure 2.2a: Cyclic Changes in Female (Reproduced from Juneja and Nandedkar, 2009)

During the follicular phase, the egg matures, and the lining of the uterus grows thicker, many tiny blood vessels grow into the thickened lining, in preparation for receiving a fertilized egg. It takes 14 days for the egg to develop to this stage of the cycle. Ovulatory

Figure 2.2b: Changes in Uterus/Endometrium and Basal Body Temperature

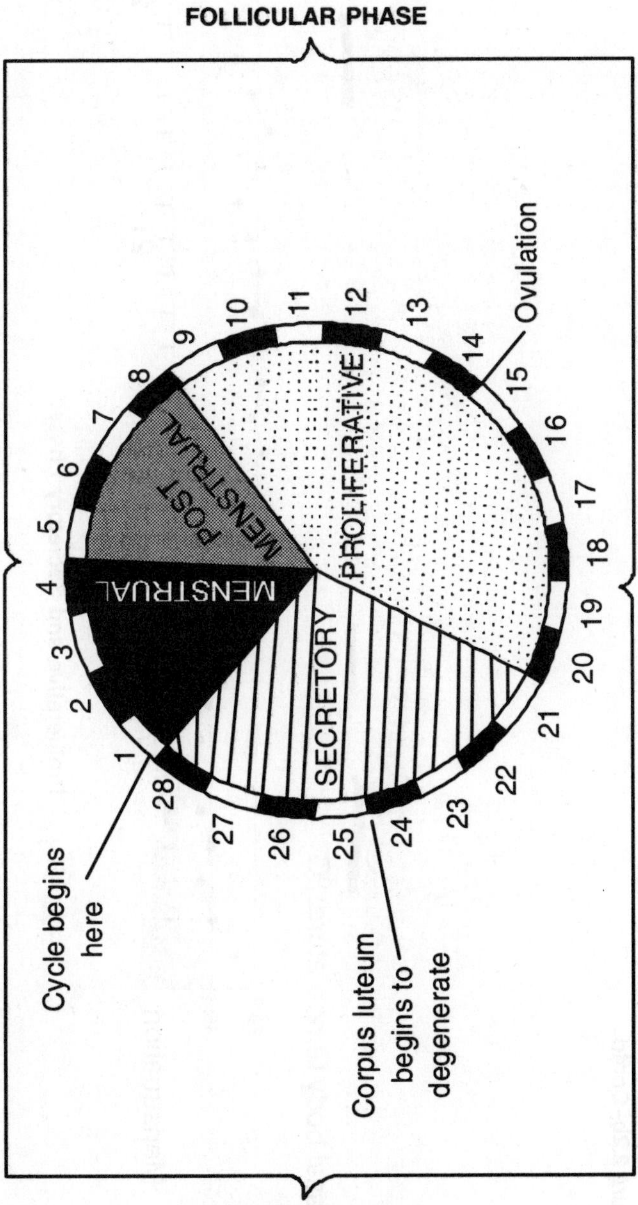

Contd...

Figure 2.2b–Contd...

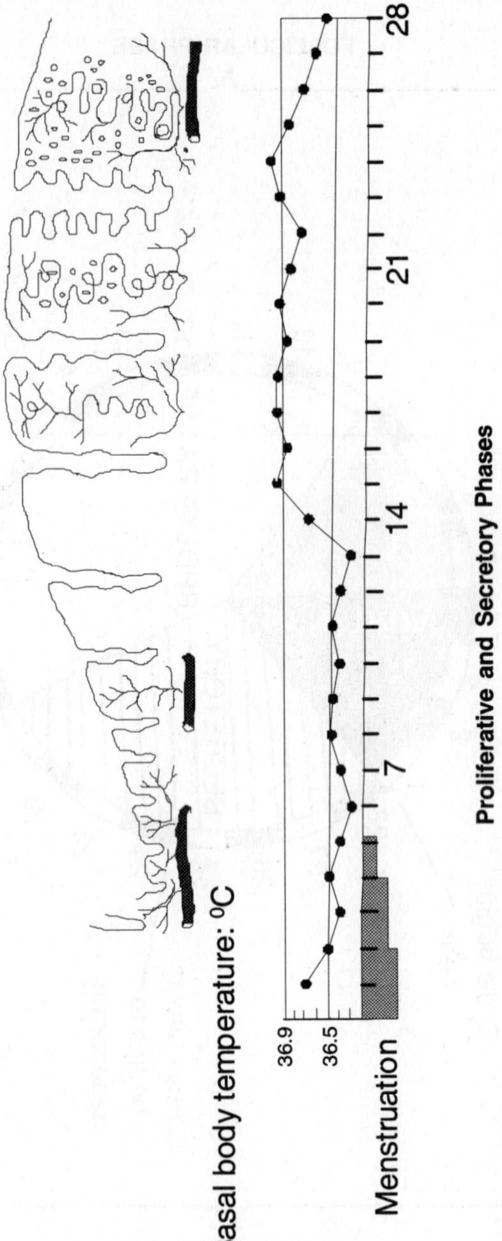

phase is the shortest phase in the cycle (2 days). Ovulation is the release of an egg from a ruptured follicle. Following ovulation, an egg is virtually swallowed into the fallopian tube, where it continues to travel towards the uterus to meet the sperm for fertilization. The egg has nutrients to survive for about 48 hours. Luteal phase lasts for about 14 days, the cells of the ruptured follicle grow larger and along with blood vessels fill the cavity, forming corpus luteum. The corpus luteum secretes progesterone which increases basal body temperature (Figure 2.2b). The increased levels of these hormones inhibit the secretion of LH and FSH from the pituitary gland. Progesterone thickens the lining of the uterus and prepares it to receive the embryo, four or five days after the egg is released from the ovary.

Menstruation is a mark of puberty in women. During the reproductive years, the monthly discharge of degenerated endometrium occurs at regular intervals with minimal variation. Regular menses document a normal female sex chromatin pattern, a mature hypothalamo-pituitary-ovarian axis, and a responsive end organ. The menstrual cycle is ordinarily judged by its periodicity, duration of blood flow, and amount of flow. Irregularities in menstrual cycle length can be caused by changes in diet, exercise, environment and serious emotional disturbance and hormonal imbalances which can lead to infertility.

References

1. Neil J D 2006 In 'Knobil and Neil's Physiology of Reproduction' Vol: 1. 385-423, Elsevier Academic Press, London, UK.
2. Hogarth PJ 1978 Biology of Reproduction pp: 116-131, Eds. John Wiley and Sons, NY.
3. Juneja H S and Nandedkar T D 2009 In 'Assisted Conception: A module for Infertility' pp: 11-12, Bhalani Publishing House, Mumbai.

Environmental & Occupational Exposures (2010) ***Pages 54–77***
Editors: **Sunil Kumar & R.R. Tiwari**
Published by: **DAYA PUBLISHING HOUSE, NEW DELHI**

Chapter 3

Reproductive Toxicity Testing under the REACH Legislation

Ulrike Bernauer and Barbara Heinrich-Hirsch

Federal Institute for Risk Assessment,
Thielallee 88–92, D-14195 Berlin

ABSTRACT

REACH is a new European Community Regulation on chemicals and their safe use. The aim of REACH is to improve the protection of human health through better and earlier identification of the intrinsic properties of chemical substances on one hand and to perform toxicological evaluation of a high number of chemicals within a short period of time in a most effective way by concomitant reduction of the use of laboratory animals.

Evaluation of the endpoints of reproductive and developmental toxicity under REACH is a big challenge because reproductive and developmental toxicities are very important and severe endpoints; among the toxicological endpoints concerning adverse health effects in humans, and testing for reproductive and developmental toxicity will most probably result in a high demand of investigations using experimental

* E-mail: ulrike.bernauer@bfr.bund.de

animals within the tonnage-triggered testing requirements. On the other hand, up to now the use of alternatives to experimental animals in order to investigate reproductive and developmental toxicity endpoints may be problematic.

In this chapter, several aspects concerning reproductive and developmental toxicity testing under REACH will be described. These aspects refer to the tonnage triggered testing requirements, waiving of testing, the use of all available information about a substance, alternatives to experimental animal studies and intelligent testing strategies.

Background

REACH is a new European Community Regulation on chemicals and their safe use[1] (EC 1907/2006). It deals with the Registration, Evaluation, Authorisation and Restriction of Chemical substances. The new law entered into force on 1 June, 2007. The aim of REACH is to improve the protection of human health and the environment through the better and earlier identification of the intrinsic properties of chemical substances. The REACH Regulation gives greater responsibility to industries, therefore manufacturers and importers are obliged to collect all available relevant information on the intrinsic properties of a substance and to register the information in a central database run by the European Chemicals Agency[2] (ECHA) in Helsinki. The type and quantity of information on the intrinsic properties of a given substance depends on the quantity of that substance that is manufactured or imported into the EU. The toxicological information requirements in the framework of the registration procedure for substances are laid down in the REACH Annexes VII–X, where information requirements for substances produced or imported in quantities of ≥ 1 tpa (tons per annum), ≥ 10 tpa, ≥ 100 tpa, and ≥ 1000 tpa are laid down. These information requirements may be adapted if appropriate and if plausibly justified. Exemption from conducting individual toxicity tests ("waiving") is possible in cases where testing is technically not feasible (*e.g.* in the case of explosive substances) or in cases where exposure is to be neglected (REACH Annexes VIII–XI). This consideration is based on the main aim of the legislation to regulate risk. Risk is defined by hazard on the one hand and exposure on the other hand. Hence, according to the regulation it is not required to identify specific inherent toxicological properties, the hazard, if there is no exposure. This is based on the consideration that without exposure there is no risk. On the other hand, in cases where exposure to a certain substance is given, knowledge on possible adverse effects on reproduction and development is of utmost importance, because the maintenance of the human species is dependent on the integrity of the reproductive cycle and because the occurrence of developmental disorders are self-evidently serious health conditions. Therefore it is important that the potential hazardous properties with respect to reproduction are established for chemicals with relevant human exposure that may be present in the environment, at the workplace and in consumer products.

The term *reproductive toxicity* is used to describe the adverse effects induced (by a substance) on sexual function and fertility in adult males and females, developmental toxicity in the offspring and effects on or mediated via lactation, as defined in Part 3 of the Globally Harmonised System of Classification and Labelling of Chemicals System (GHS)[3]. In practical terms, reproductive toxicity is characterised by multiple diverse endpoints, which relate to impairment of male and female reproductive functions or capacity (*fertility*) and the induction of non-heritable harmful effects on the progeny (*developmental toxicity*)[4]. Effects on male or female fertility include adverse effects on libido, sexual behaviour, any aspect of spermatogenesis or hormonal or physiological response, which would interfere with the capacity to fertilise, fertilisation itself or the development of the fertilised ovum up to and including implantation. Developmental toxicity includes any effect interfering with normal development, both before and after birth. It includes effects induced or manifested either pre- or post-natally. This includes embryotoxic/ fetotoxic effects such as reduced body weight, growth and developmental retardation, organ toxicity, death, abortion, structural defects (teratogenic effects), functional effects, peri- and post-natal defects, and impaired postnatal mental or physical development up to and including normal pubertal development. So it is easily understandable, that both reproductive and developmental toxicity are the consequence of disturbance of highly complex and interwoven processes, which can hardly be assessed by one single type of animal test. It is even more problematic to assess reproductive and developmental toxicity by using alternative (*e.g. in vitro*) tests avoiding vertebrate animal testing. Although REACH is very specific about the requirements for experimental animal test data, the law discourages testing in vertebrate animals. Article 13 of REACH states: "in particular for human toxicity, information shall be gathered, whenever possible by means other than vertebrate animal tests, through the use of alternative methods, for example *in vitro* methods or qualitative or quantitative structure-activity relationship models ((Q)SAR) or from information from structurally related substances (grouping or read-across)." Article 25 states: "in order to avoid animal testing, testing on vertebrate animals for the purposes of this Regulation shall be undertaken only as a last resort." However, the use of alternative tests in order to fulfil the REACH requirements (*i.e.* in order to come to a conclusion whether a substance is toxic to reproduction and development) is difficult, *e.g.* because a negative *in vitro* test cannot be interpreted as indicating the absence of a reproductive hazard (ECHA, 2008 a). Other methodologies such as considerations on the chemical structure (structure-activity relationships (SARs) or quantitative structure-activity relationships (QSARs) are also in most cases not applicable for the endpoints reproductive and developmental toxicities, because currently there are almost no available structural alerts for these two endpoints. These facts currently would make it inevitable to perform in vivo animal tests using vertebrate animals. The respective tests required under the specific information requirements under REACH usually consume large amounts of animals and thus are labour intensive and expensive.

Nevertheless, all available information on a substance (*i.e.* physico-chemical properties, chemical structure (and structural similarity to other substances), toxicological properties (from *in vitro* or in vivo tests, not necessarily focussed on reproductive toxicity testing) can either be used in order to develop testing strategies yielding the highest grade of information for the assessment of reproductive and developmental toxicity in connections with as lowest costs and vertebrate animal consumption as possible. Furthermore, the integrated use of all available information on a substance is essential for the Weight of Evidence (WoE) assessment of substances with the aim of deriving NOAEL (No-observed-adverse effect level) values and decisions on classification and labelling with respect to the endpoints reproductive toxicity and development. These possibilities for the assessment of reproductive toxicity under REACH will be described in detail in the subsequent section.

Assessment of Reproductive and Developmental Toxicity under REACH

Information Requirements for Reproductive Toxicity Testing under REACH

Tonnage Triggered Testing Requirements

The reproductive and developmental toxicity data requirements of REACH are presented in Table 3.1. Testing for reproductive toxicity is not relevant for tonnage levels < 10 t/y (tonnes per year). At tonnage levels above 10 t/y, the type and extent of testing requirements depends on tonnage. In all cases, however, some considerations have to be performed in order to decide whether testing for reproductive toxicity is required or not. These questions are addressed in Table 3.1 under "Specific rules for adaptation from standard information required".

In brief, testing for reproductive toxicity is not required, if (1) the substance is already classified for effects on fertility as Repr Cat. 1 or Cat. 2; R60 and/or for effects on development as Repr Cat 1 or Cat 2; R61 or (2) the substance is classified as a genotoxic carcinogen (Carc Cat. 1 and Mut Cat. 3 or Carc Cat. 2 and Mut Cat. 3) or as a germ cell mutagen (Mut Cat. 1 or Cat. 2) and appropriate risk management measures have been implemented or (3) the substance exhibits a low toxicological activity, negligible systemic absorption and no or no significant human exposure[1)] or (4) if an exposure-based information waiving provision is justified.[1)]

Tonnage Level ≥ 10 t/y

If sufficient data on the substance are available which allow a conclusion on the toxic potential adverse to reproduction and/or development (*e.g.* information on structurally related substances or *in vitro* methods), no further testing is required. Otherwise, a reproduction / developmental toxicity screening test according to OECD TG 421[6] or a combined repeat dose toxicity study with the reproduction / developmental toxicity screening test according to OECD TG 422[7] is the standard information requirement. Both of these tests may provide sufficient information on male and female

---

1) Up to now, a definition of what constitutes "no significant exposure" is not given. Attempts have been made to discuss this issue[5]).

Table 3.1: Tonnage-Rriggered Reproductive and Developmental Toxicity Data Requirements of REACH

Tonnage Level)*	*Relevant REACH Annex*	*Standard Information Required*	*Specific Rules for Adaptation from Standard Information Required*
10 tonnes or more	VIII	Screening for reproductive/ developmental toxicity, one species (OECD 421 or 422), if there is no evidence from available information on structurally related substances, from (Q)SAR estimates or from *in vitro* methods that the substance may be a developmental toxicant.	The study does not need to be conducted if: ✰ The substance is known to be a genotoxic carcinogen and appropriate risk management measures are implemented; or ✰ The substance is known to be a germ cell mutagen and appropriate risk management measures are implemented; or ✰ Relevant human exposure can be excluded in accordance with Annex XI section 3; or ✰ A pre-natal developmental toxicity study (Annex IX, 8.7.2) or a two-generation reproductive toxicity study (Annex IX, section 8.7.3) is available. If a substance is known to have an adverse effect on fertility, meeting the criteria for classification as Repr Cat 1 or 2: R62, and the available data are adequate to support a robust assessment, then no further testing for fertility will be necessary. However, testing for developmental toxicity must be considered. If a substance is known to cause developmental toxicity, meeting the criteria for classification as Repr Cat 1 or 2: R61, and the available data are adequate to support a robust risk assessment, then no further testing for developmental toxicity will be necessary, however, testing for effects on fertility must be considered.

Contd...

Table 3.1–Contd...

Tonnage Level*)	Relevant REACH Annex	Standard Information Required	Specific Rules for Adaptation from Standard Information Required
			In cases where there are serious concerns about the potential for adverse effects on fertility or development, either a pre-natal developmental toxicity study (Annex IX, section 8.7.2) or a two-generation reproductive toxicity study (Annex IX, section 8.7.3) may be proposed by the registrant instead of the screening study.
100 tonnes or more	IX	Pre-natal developmental toxicity study, one species, most appropriate route of administration, having regard to the likely route of human exposure (B.31 of the Commission Regulation on test methods as specified in Article 13 (3) or OECD 414). Two-generation reproductive toxicity study, one species, male and female, most appropriate route of administration, having regard to the likely route of human	The studies do not need to be conducted if: ☆ The substance is known to be a genotoxic carcinogen and appropriate risk management measures are implemented; or ☆ The substance is known to be a germ cell mutagen and appropriate risk management measures are implemented; or ☆ The substance is of low toxicological activity (no evidence of toxicity seen in any of the tests available), it can be proven from toxicokinetic data that no systemic absorption occurs via relevant routes of exposure (*e.g.* plasma/blood concentrations below detection limit using a sensitive method and absence of the substance and of metabolites of the substance in urine, bile or exhaled air) and there is no or no significant human exposure.

Contd...

Table 3.1–Contd...

*Tonnage Level**)	*Relevant REACH Annex*	*Standard Information Required*	*Specific Rules for Adaptation from Standard Information Required*
		exposure, if the 28-days or 90-days study indicates adverse effects on reproductive organs or tissues.	If a substance is known to have an adverse effect on fertility, meeting the criteria for classification as Repr Cat 1 or 2: R62, and the available data are adequate to support a robust assessment, then no further testing for fertility will be necessary. However, testing for developmental toxicity must be considered. If a substance is known to cause developmental toxicity, meeting the criteria for classification as Repr Cat 1 or 2: R61, and the available data are adequate to support a robust risk assessment, then no further testing for developmental toxicity will be necessary, however, testing for effects on fertility must be considered. The study shall be initially performed on one species. A decision on the need to perform a study at this tonnage level or the next on a second species should be based on the outcome of the first test and all other relevant available data. The study shall be initially performed on one species. A decision on the need to perform a study at this tonnage level or the next on a second species should be based on the outcome of the first test and all other relevant available data.

Contd...

Table 3.1–Contd...

Tonnage Level)*	*Relevant REACH Annex*	*Standard Information Required*	*Specific Rules for Adaptation from Standard Information Required*
1000 tonnes or more	Annex X	Developmental toxicity study, one species, most appropriate route of administration, having regard to the likely route of human esxposure (OECD 414). Two-generation reproductive toxicity study, one species, male and female, most appropriate route of administration, having regard to the likely route of human exposure, unless already provided as part of Annex IX requirements.	The studies need not be conducted if: ☆ The substance is known to be a genotoxic carcinogen and appropriate risk management measures are implemented; or ☆ The substance is known to be a germ cell mutagen and appropriate risk management measures are implemented; or ☆ The substance is of low toxicological activity (no evidence of toxicity seen in any of the tests available), it can be proven from toxicokinetic data that no systemic absorption occurs via relevant routes of exposure (*e.g.* plasma/blood concentrations below detection limit using a sensitive method and absence of the substance and of metabolites of the substance in urine, bile or exhaled air) and there is no or no significant human exposure. If a substance is known to have an adverse effect on fertility, meeting the criteria for classification as Repr Cat 1 or 2: R62, and the available data are adequate to support a robust assessment, then no further testing for fertility will be necessary. However, testing for developmental toxicity must be considered.

Contd...

Table 3.1–Contd...

*Tonnage Level**)	*Relevant REACH Annex*	*Standard Information Required*	*Specific Rules for Adaptation from Standard Information Required*
			If a substance is known to cause developmental toxicity, meeting the criteria for classification as Repr Cat 1 or 2: R61, and the available data are adequate to support a robust risk assessment, then no further testing for developmental toxicity will be necessary, however, testing for effects on fertility must be considered.

*) Standard information requirements for substances manufactured or imported in quantities of.

reproductive performance (*e.g.* gonadal function, mating behaviour, conception, development of the conceptus and parturition) to allow classification and risk assessment. However, the following caveats should be mentioned: the screening tests do not cover all aspects of reproduction and development (*e.g.* post-natal effects associated with prenatal exposure or effects resulting from post-natal or lactational exposure) and furthermore, the exposure duration and the limited animal number might narrow the significance of the results of these tests. Therefore, these tests cannot be regarded as an alternative or replacement of the definitive reproductive toxicity studies and their results should be interpreted with caution. However, these tests are useful for an initial hazard assessment and may help to develop further testing strategies (or: decide on further testing)[8,9]. If a 28-day study (EU B.7 or OECD TG 407[10]) is not available for the substance under consideration, it is recommended to perform a test according to OECD TG 422[7], because it also includes investigations of repeat-dose toxicity thus contributing to animal welfare. In case that the initial data review concerning the substance of interest already indicates alerts for reproductive toxicity, it might be more appropriate to perform a two-generation reproduction toxicity study (*e.g.* OECD TG 416[11]–see "Tonnage level ≥ 1000 t/y") or a prenatal developmental toxicity study (*e.g.* OECD TG 414[12]–see "Tonnage level ≥ 100 t/y") already at this tonnage level. In case that concerns arise concerning post-natal effects (*e.g.* reduced pup survival), a testing strategy allowing to investigate these effects (*e.g.* a two-generation study (*e.g.* OECD TG 416[11]) or a screening study (*e.g.* OECD TG 421/422[6,7]) with an extended postnatal observation period might be used. Usually (in case of negative findings) testing in a second species will not be required at this tonnage level.

Tonnage Level ≥ 100 t/y

At this tonnage level, a prenatal developmental toxicity study (OECD TG 414[12]) as well as a reproductive/developmental screening test (OECD TG 421/422 (OECD[6,7]) build the standard data requirements. The prenatal developmental toxicity study is used to evaluate the potential effects of a substance on prenatal development, *i.e.* effects induced *in utero* which are manifested before birth. Positive results in these tests can be used for hazard classification and human health risk assessment, unless there is sufficient evidence, that the effects seen in animals will not occur in humans. Further, the results of the prenatal development toxicity test form the basis for decisions on the necessity of further testing or the necessity of performing a developmental toxicity study in a second species.

In case that the prenatal developmental toxicity test of a substance results in an alert for reproductive toxicity, a two-generation reproduction toxicity study (EU B.35, OECD TG 416[11]– described under the ≥ 1000 t/y tonnage level) will be necessary. In case that a two-generation reproduction toxicity study is proposed at this tonnage level, then conduct of the screening tests (OECD TG 421/422[6,7]) won't be necessary. Further, the screening tests won't be necessary in case that adverse effects on reproductive organs have been detected in existing repeat-dose toxicity studies and these findings are sufficient for risk assessment and classification for fertility. It might also be advisable to perform a two-generation study in case that it is foreseen to produce or import higher tonnages. In certain cases (based on the outcome of the two-generation test (if performed at this tonnage level) and based on other probably available relevant data, it might be necessary to perform a two generation study (*e.g.* OECD TG 416[11], EU B. 35[13]) in a second species or to further include developmental neurotoxicity endpoints.

Tonnage Level ≥ 1000 t/y

A prenatal developmental toxicity study (EU B.31, OECD TG414[12]) and a two-generation reproduction toxicity study (EU B.35[13], OECD TG 416[11]) in the most relevant species form the standard data requirements for this tonnage level. The two-generation reproduction toxicity study is used to evaluate the effects of a substance on the complete reproductive cycle (*i.e.* libido, fertility, development of the conceptus, parturition, post natal effects in both dams and offspring and the reproductive capacity and capability of the offspring). If specific triggers are present, inclusion of optional developmental neurotoxicity endpoints should be considered for the two-generation reproduction toxicity study. In addition, the conduct of a developmental toxicity study in a second species might be necessary[14].

Other Sources of Information on Reproductive Toxicity

As stated in the REACH guidance documents[2], a detailed review and analysis of all existing data to identify any specific alerts and testing requirements concerning reproductive and developmental toxicity has to be performed. Information which can be utilized for these purposes might consist of non-testing data, arise from alternative or *in vitro* tests but also arise from animal testing (aside from the tests already described) or human data/ experience and will be discussed in the subsequent paragraph.

Non-testing Data

Non-testing data, such as the chemical structure, physico-chemical properties, read-across and (quantitative) structure-activity relationships ((Q)SARs) represent the most important basis for non-testing information. The chemical structure and physico-chemical properties (*e.g.* water solubility, vapour pressure, molecular weight, octanol-water partition coefficient) are helpful tools to estimate the possibility and the probable extent of the uptake of a substance by the different uptake routes (oral, dermal, inhalation) and may also allow to estimate probable pathways after uptake into an organism (*e.g.* metabolism, possibility to cross the placenta, to cross barriers such as the blood-brain or the blood-testes barrier, the possibility to occur in the milk).

Read-across is used to fill data gaps by grouping chemicals whose physico-chemical and human health-related toxicological properties are likely to be similar or follow a regular pattern as a result of structural similarity (or other similarity characteristic). Thus, the toxic potential of a substance might be extra- or interpolated across a homologous series or a category of substances. Further, read-across might also be performed by grouping chemicals with similar mechanisms.

QSARs are mathematical models (often statistical correlations) relating one or more quantitative parameters derived from chemical structure to a quantitative measure of a property or activity (*e.g.* a toxicological endpoint). In contrast to other toxicological endpoints (*e.g.* irritation, corrosivity, mutagenicity) for which structural alerts are already known, no structural alerts for reproductive toxicity have clearly been identified (groups of substances exhibiting reproductive toxic properties have been identified (*e.g.* phthalates), however, formal criteria to identify structural alerts for reproductive toxicity are still lacking). Further, up to now there are no validated QSAR approaches for reproductive toxicity, so at the current state, grouping approaches, SAR and QSAR methodologies require further progress until they might be utilized for risk assessment and classification with respect to reproductive toxicity. However, for the time being, these methodologies, in their progressing state, might be used as supportive instruments and as parts of a weight of evidence approach[15].

In vitro Data

Several promising *in vitro* approaches have been developed during the last years in order to cover certain endpoints and aspects of reproductive toxicity[16,17,18]. The most promising progress has been made concerning developmental toxicity (embryonic stem cell test[19], limb bud micromass culture[20], whole embryo culture[21]) and endocrine activity testing[22]. However, there are two major aspects which limit the use of these *in vitro* methodologies for risk assessment or classification purposes: (1) the mammalian reproductive cycle is very complex which–up to now–cannot be represented, even when a battery of *in vitro* tests is being applied and (2) most of the test systems used in *in vitro* assays do not adequately reflect or maintain the biotransformation capability as present in the intact organism[23], although great efforts have been undertaken to improve *in vitro* systems with respect to biotransformation performance[24].

Therefore, so far, *in vitro* assays can be used in order to establish structure-activity relationships and in a weight of evidence approach. It should be mentioned, that negative *in vitro* data cannot serve to claim absence of reproductive toxic properties of a substance or absence of the potential to interact with the endocrine system, whereas positive data might be the trigger for further testing. This may change in the future dependent on further progresses and developments of *in vitro* assays concerning reproductive toxicity and endocrine modulating properties.

In vivo Data

In vivo Data not Specifically Related to Reproductive Toxicity

Results from animal tests not specifically related to reproductive toxicity and results from further *in vivo* assays for endocrine activities or for reproductive toxicity, which do not belong to the information requirements under REACH might also contribute to estimate the toxic potential of a substance with respect to reproduction and development and to decide on the necessity of further testing or contribute to the development of testing strategies.

Effects on reproductive organs and on certain fertility parameters (*e.g.* sperm parameters) can be detected in repeat-dose toxicity studies (*e.g.* EU B.7, OECD TG 407[10] or OECD TG 408[25] or other repeat dose studies), which may allow the identification of a N(L)OAEL, which can be used in the risk assessment and a decision on classification and labelling. Besides, results from repeat-dose studies can be used as a trigger for further testing (*e.g.* in case that effects on the hormone system or on nervous system (triggering the inclusion of neuro-developmental endpoints in *e.g.* a two-generation study) have been observed.

In vivo Data Related to Reproductive Toxicity

In vivo Assays for Endocrine Activity

Furthermore, there are two *in vivo* tests for the detection of substances with oestrogenic or (anti) androgenic modes of action (the Uterotrophic bioassay in rodents OECD TG 440[26] and the Hershberger assay[27]). Further, new *in vivo* tests are under development allowing to assess hormonal activity, production of steroids and other parameters (*e.g.* pubertal assay, intact male assay) [28]. These *in vivo* tests may contribute to satisfy the data needs for risk assessment and for classification of effects on reproduction and may be also indicators or triggers to perform further testing. It should, however, be focussed here that substances being negative in the Hershberger or uterotrophic assays may nevertheless be endocrine active substances in case that their endocrine properties are different from estrogen- or (anti) androgen- dependent pathways.

Developmental Neurotoxicity Studies (*e.g.* OECD TG 426[29])

Tests on developmental neurotoxicity are used to investigate substance-induced changes in behaviour of the offspring due to effects on the central nervous system (but also due to effects on other organs such as liver, kidneys, and the endocrine system) arising from exposure of the mother during pregnancy and lactation.

One-Generation Reproduction Toxicity Study (*e.g.* EU B.34[13], OECD TG 415[30])

The one-generation reproduction toxicity study (EU B.34[13], OECD TG 415[30]), which does not belong to the standard information requirements under REACH, has been used in the past to assess effects on fertility, on growth, development and viability of the offspring and to assess weight and histopathology of reproductive organs, brain and other possible target organs. Under REACH, the one-generation reproduction toxicity study was discriminated compared to the two generation study, because it does not cover potential effects on all phases of the reproductive cycle such as post weaning development, maturation and the reproductive capacity of the offspring. However, in the recent past, the added value of producing a second generation has been questioned[31], and currently, there are ongoing activities concerning the development of an F1-extended one-generation assay, which includes further toxicological aspects and endpoints, and which might serve as an alternative to the requirement of a two generation study under REACH.

Further Assays

Further in vivo animal data, which might give information concerning reproductive toxicity, are the Chernoff/Kavlock tests[32], which is are further short-term in vivo screening tests for reproductive toxicity, the dominant-lethal assay, other mechanistic studies or studies on male and female fertility of no standard design.

Human Data

Epidemiological studies, clinical data, worker surveys and case reports may be the source for human data on reproductive toxicity. If properly performed sound epidemiological studies of high quality (with adequate controls, sound assessment of exposure, type, adequacy and relevance of health effects, bias and confounding factors), but also case reports and clinical data may be utilized for risk assessment and classification and labelling. However, the fact that humans are normally exposed to a variety of different substances limits the availability of such human studies. The methodological and statistical limitations of human data are the reason, why substances, which have been demonstrated to be reproductive toxicants in the animal model, cannot be exculpated from being reproductive toxicants in case of negative human data.

Integrated Testing Strategies (ITS)

Integrated testing strategies play an important role under REACH in order to ensure, that data adequate and sufficient for risk assessment and for classification and labelling will be utilized based on all available information and/or the most appropriate, most efficient ways of testing regarding also cost efficiency and animal welfare.

With respect to reproductive toxicity, ITS means, that all available (physico-chemical and toxicological) data of a substance, information resulting from other regulatory processes (*e.g.* the EU existing substances regulation), exposure information, as well as current risk management measures are taken into consideration before testing is considered.

In a first step (stage 1) certain issues are considered in order to decide, whether any testing for reproductive toxicity is necessary at all. The questions were described under section 1, "Tonnage triggered testing requirements". In case that stage 1 considerations result in the necessity of testing for reproductive toxicity, all available information (on the substance as well as on structurally related substances or substances probably exhibiting a comparable mode of action) has to be evaluated in a second step in order to identify alerts for reproductive toxicity and the degree of necessity of reproductive and developmental toxicity testing (Stage 2). The types of information that can be utilized for data review and evaluation is described in section 2, "Other sources of information on reproductive toxicity". As an outcome of the data review and evaluation, two options are possible, *i.e.* (i) there are sufficient data for classification and for risk assessment or (ii) further testing is necessary.

In case that testing is necessary, based on the tonnage level (but also based on future tonnage level), reproductive toxicity testing has to be performed as described under section 1, "Information Requirements for reproductive toxicity testing under REACH" and as presented in table 1. With careful attention, further issues have to be addressed, *i.e.* the selection of species, the necessity of testing in a second species at ≥ 100 and ≥ 1000 tonnage levels, the uptake pathway (which should be based on physico-chemical properties of the substance and the most likely human exposure pathway), consideration of the outcome of other toxicological tests (*in vivo* and *in vitro*, tests specifically addressing reproductive toxicity as well as tests not specifically addressing reproductive toxicity).

Discussion

Assessment of toxicity concerning reproduction and development is of very high concern, because it pertains to the perpetuation of the human species. Therefore, testing of chemicals for reproductive and developmental toxic properties is an important issue. Mammalian reproduction is very complex, thus, tests for evaluating reproductive and developmentally toxic properties have to regard this complexity.

Currently, neither any single *in vitro* tests nor any test battery of different *in vitro* test is enough robust and significant for risk assessment or for classification of substances with respect to reproductive toxicity. Therefore, in vivo animal tests belong to the standard information requirements in case that testing for reproductive toxicity is necessary.

On the other hand, under REACH, a large amount of substances has to be evaluated in relative short time and the number of tests with vertebrate animals should be as low as possible if needed at all.

With respect to reproductive toxicity, a compromise has to be found, which regards on one hand the fact that currently the complexity of reproductive toxicity can only be adequately addressed by (in most cases very labour intensive and time consuming) *in vivo* animal studies and on the other hand the fact that animal welfare and time- and cost efficiency have to be regarded under REACH.

Several strategies are currently applied under REACH in order to regard these different aspects, which fall under the term "Integrated testing strategies". This comprises the strategy, that all available information is utilised in order to decide, whether and to which extent testing is necessary and in order to develop testing strategies to perform the necessary tests as efficient meaningful as possible.

Currently, there are a lot of efforts and progresses underway with respect to refine and further develop *in vitro* and in vivo tests for developmental toxicity.

Concerning *in vivo* animal data, there are activities ongoing with the aim to update and improve current OECD test guidelines. The activity associated with the update of the repeated-dose oral 28 day (EU B.7, OECD TG 407[10]) study aims at integrating the identification of chemicals acting through (anti)estrogenic, (anti)androgenic and (anti)thyroid mechanisms into the guideline by regarding additional parameters based on male and female reproductive organs and the thyroid[33].

Another activity has been triggered because the value of producing a second generation in a two-generation reproduction toxicity study has been questioned[34] on one hand, and because the one-generation reproduction toxicity study (EU B.34[13], OECD TG 415[30]) does not address the issues of post-weaning development, maturation and reproductive capacity and capability of the offspring. Therefore, the ILSI Agricultural Chemical Safety Assessment Project has proposed an F1-extended one-generation study, which incorporates additional postnatal parameters, clinical pathology, a functional observational battery, optional immunotoxicity endpoints, oestrus cyclicity and semen analysis and optional endpoints addressing developmental neurotoxicity[35]. Development of a test guideline based on the ILSI/ACSA proposal is in progress. After adoption of this new OECD test guideline, it may be used as an alternative to or even replace the two-generation reproduction toxicity study (EU B.35[13], OECD 416[11]) which is currently used as the definitive test under the relevant tonnage level within the REACH legislation.

Far more activities and developments are currently ongoing with respect to *in vitro* assays. As far as *in vitro* and molecular toxicology further develop, non-animal tests might be developed and validated, which might come closer to the in vivo situation than currently possible.

Therefore, reproductive toxicity testing is a dynamic field and updated tests and new tests might be integrated in the future into the testing requirements and testing strategies of the REACH legislation concerning reproductive toxicity.

For the time being, the application of integrated testing strategies and Weight of Evidence Analyses represent important tools for the assessment of reproductive and developmental toxicity and contribute to making the assessment as efficient as possible.

References

1. European Commission (2006): Regulation (EC) No 1907/2006 of the European Parliament and of the council of 18 December 2006 concerning the Registration, Evaluation, Authorisation and Restriction of Chemicals (REACH), establishing a European Chemicals Agency, amending Directive 1999/45/EC and

repealing Council Regulation (EEC) No 793/93 and Commission Regulation (EC) No 1488/94 as well as Council Directive 76/769/EEC and Commission Directives 91/155/EEC, 93/67/EEC, 93/105/EC and 2000/21/EC, available at http://eur-lex.europa.eu/JOHtml.do?uri=OJ:L:2007:136:SOM:EN:HTML

2. ECHA (European Chemical Agency) (2008a): Guidance on information requirements and chemical safety assessment. Chapter R.7a: Endpoint specific guidance. Available at: http://reach.jrc.it/docs/guidance_document/information_requirements_r7a_en.pdf
3. United Nations (2005) Globally Harmonised System of Classification and Labelling of Chemicals (GHS). Part 3 Health Hazards, page 175. Available at http://www.unece.org/trans/danger/publi/ghs/ghs_rev01/01files_e.html
4. World Health Organization (WHO) (2001) Principles for evaluating health risks to reproduction associated with exposure to chemicals. Environmental Health Criteria 225. World Health Organization, Geneva
5. Bernauer U, Heinemeyer G, Heinrich-Hirsch B, Ulbrich B and Gundert-Remy, U. (2008): Exposure-triggered reproductive toxicity testing under the REACH legislation: A proposal to define significant/relevant exposure. Toxicol Lett 176: 68–76.
6. OECD (1995a): OECD Guideline for the testing of chemicals: 421 "Reproduction/Developmental Toxicity Screening Test" (Adopted 27 July 1995), OECD, Paris.
7. OECD (1996): OECD Guideline for the testing of chemicals: 422 „Combined Repeated Dose Toxicity Study with the Reproduction/Developmental Toxicity Screening Test" (Adopted 22 March 1996), OECD, Paris.
8. Reuter U, Heinrich-Hirsch B, Hellwig J, Holzum B and Welsch F (2003): Evaluation of OECD screening tests 421 (reproduction/developmental toxicity screening test) and 422 (combined repeated-dose toxicity study with the reproduction/developmental toxicity screening test). Reg Toxicol Pharm 38: 17-26.

9. Ulbrich B and Palmer AK (1995): Detection of effects on male reproduction- a literature survey. J Amer Coll Toxicol 14: 292-327.

10. OECD (1995b): OECD Guideline for the testing of chemicals: 407: „Repeated Dose 28-day Oral Toxicity Study in rodents (Adopted 27 July 1995), OECD, Paris.

11. OECD (2001b): OECD Guideline for the testing of chemicals: 416: „Two Generation Reproduction Toxicity Study" (Adopted 22 January 2001), OECD, Paris.

12. OECD (2001a): OECD Guideline for the testing of chemicals: 414 „Prenatal developmental toxicity study" (Adopted 22 January 2001), OECD, Paris.

13. EU B35: Annex V to Directive 67/548/EEC: Methods fort he determination of physico-chemical properties, toxicity and ecotoxicity, available at: http://ecb.jrc.it/testing-methods/

14. Janer G, Slob W, Hakkert BC, Vermeire T and Piersma AH (2008): A retrospective analysis of developmental toxicity studies in rat and rabbit: What is the added value of the rabbit as an additional test species? Regul Tox Pharmacol 50: 206-217.

15. ECHA (European Chemical Agency) (2008b): Guidance on information requirements and chemical safety assessment. Chapter R.6: QSARs and grouping of chemicals. Available at: http://reach.jrc.it/docs/guidance_document/information_requirements_r6_en.pdf

16. Genschow E, Spielmann H, Scholz G, Seiler A, Brown N, Piersma A, Brady M, Clemann N, Huuskonen H, Paillard F, Bremer S and Becker K (2002): The ECVAM international validation study on *in vitro* embryotoxicity tests: results of the definitive phase and evaluation of prediction models. ATLA 30: 151-176.

17. Piersma AH (2006): Alternatives to animal testing in developmental toxicity testing. Basic Clin Toxicol Pharmacol 98: 427-431.

18. Spielmann H, Seiler A, Bremer S, Hareng L, Hartung T, Ahr H, Faustman E, Haas U, Moffat GJ, Nau H, Vanparys P, Piersma A, Riego Sintes J and Stuart J (2006): The practical application of three validated *in vitro* embryotoxicity tests. The report and

recommendations of an ECVAM/ZEBET workshop (ECVAM workshop 57). ATLA 34: 527-538.

19. Genschow E, Spielmann H, Scholz G, Pohl I, Seiler A, Clemann N, Bremer S and Becker K (2004): Validation of the embryonic stem cell test in the international ECVAM validation study on three *in vitro* embryotoxicity tests. ATLA 32: 209-244.

20. Spielmann H, Genschow E, Brown NA, Piersma AH, Verhoef A, Spanjersberg MQ, Huuskonen H, Paillard F and Seiler A (2004): Validation of the rat limb bud micromass test in the international ECVAM validation study on three *in vitro* embryotoxicity tests. ATLA 32: 245-274.

21. Piersma AH, Genschow E, Verhoef A, Spanjersberg MQ, Brown NA, Brady M, Burns A, Clemann N, Seiler A and Spielmann H (2004): Validation of the postimplantation rat whole-embryo culture test in the International ECVAM validation study on three *in vitro* embryotoxicity tests. ATLA 32: 275-307.

22. Nordic Chemicals Group (2005) Information Strategy for Reproductive Toxicity. Nordic Project on Integrated Information Strategies. Step 2 project report (draft 5. April 2005)

23. Coecke S, Ahr H, Blaauboer BJ, Bremer S., Casati S., Castell J., Combes R., Corvi R., Crespi CL., Cunningham ML., Elaut G., Eletti B., Freidig A., Gennari A., Ghersi-Egea JF, Guillouzo A., Hartung T., Hoet T., Ingelman-Sundberg M., Munn S., Janssens W., Ladstetter B., Leahy D., Long A., Meneguz A., Monshouwer M., Morath S., Nagelkerke F., Pelkonen O., Ponti J., Prieto P., Richert L., Sabbioni E., Schaack B., Steiling W., Testai E., Vericat JA and Worth A. (2006): Metabolism: a bottleneck *in vitro* toxicological test development. The report and recommendations of ECVAM workshop 54. ATLA 34: 49-84.

24. Jacobs MN, Janssens W, Bernauer U, Brandon E, Coecke S, Combes R, Edwards P, Freidug A, Freyberger A, Kolanczyk R, McArdle C, Mekenyan O, Schmieder P, Schrader T, Takeyoshi M and van der Burg B (2008): The use of metabolising systems for *in vitro* testing of endocrine disruptors. Submitted to Drug Metabolism Reviews.

25. OECD (1998): OECD Guideline for the testing of chemicals: 408: Repeated Dose 90-day Oral Toxicity Study in rodents (Adopted 21 September 1998), OECD, Paris.

26. OECD (2007a): OECD Guideline for the testing of chemicals: 426: "Developmental neurotoxicity study" (Adopted 16 October 2007), OECD, Paris.

27. OECD (2003): OECD Draft report of the OECD validation of the rodent Hershberger bioassay: Phase 2. testing of androgen agonist, androgen antagonist and 5 alpha-reductase inhibitor in dose response studies by multiple laboratories. ENV/JM/TG/EDTA (2003) 5.

28. US-EPA (2002). Draft detailed review paper on steroidogenesis screening assays and endocrine disruptors. May 2002.

29. OECD (2007b): OECD Guideline for the testing of chemicals: 440: Uterotrophic bioassay in rodents: a short-term screening test in rodents for oestrogenic properties" (Adopted 16 October 2007), OECD, Paris.

30. OECD (1983): OECD Guideline for the testing of chemicals: 415 „One-Generation Reproduction Toxicity Study" (Adopted 26 May 1983), OECD, Paris.

31. Janer G, Hakkert BC, Slob W, Vermeire T and Piersma AH (2007b): A retrospective analysis of the two-generation study: What ist the added value of the second generation? Reprod Toxicol 24: 97-102.

32. Hardin BD, Becker RA, Kavlock RJ, Seidenberg JM and Chernoff N (1987): Workshop on the Chernoff / Kavlock preliminary developmental toxicity test. Teratog Carcinog Mutagen 7: 119-127.

33. Gelbke HP, Hofmann A, Owens JW, Freyberger A (2007): The enhancement of the subacute repeat dose toxicity test OECD TG 407 for the detection of endocrine active chemicals: comparison with toxicity tests of longer duration. Arch Toxicol 81, 227-250.

34. Janer G, Hakkert BC, Piersma AH, Vermeire T and Slob W (2007a): A retrospective analysis of the added value of the rat two-generation reproductive toxicity study versus the rat subchronic toxicity study. Reprod Toxicol 24: 103-113.

35. Cooper RL, Lamb IV JC, Barlow SM, Bentley K, Brady AM, Doerrer NG, Eisenbrandt DL, Fenner-Crisp PA, Hines RN, Irvine

LFH, Kimmel CA, Koeter H, Li AA and Makris SL (2006): A tiered approach to life stages testing for agricultural chemical safety assessment. Crit Rev Toxicol 36: 69-98.

36. EU B34: Annex V to Directive 67/548/EEC: Methods fort he determination of physico-chemical properties, toxicity and ecotoxicity, available at: http://ecb.jrc.it/testing-methods/

Environmental & Occupational Exposures (2010) *Pages 78–101*
Editors: **Sunil Kumar & R.R. Tiwari**
Published by: **DAYA PUBLISHING HOUSE, NEW DELHI**

Chapter 4

Role of Environment, Occupational Exposure, Life Style and Diet on Free Radical Induced Mitochondrial DNA Damage and Reproductive Failure

*S. Venkatesh[1], R. Kumar[1], D. Pathak[1], M.B. Shamsi[1], M. Tanwar[1], R. Deecaraman[2] and R. Dada**

[1]*Laboratory for Molecular Reproduction and Genetics, Department of Anatomy, All India Institute of Medical sciences, New Delhi – 110 029*

[2]*Dr. M.G.R. Educational and Research Institute, Maduravoyal, Chennai – 95*

ABSTRACT

Significant decrease in human fertility is the major concern for the last 50 years. Though role of ROS is well established in human reproduction, its pathological function is yet to be clearly defined. But OS is recently gained much importance as it is involved in conditions such as sperm DNA damage, lipid peroxidation, impaired sperm motility and viability to impair male fertility. Various chemicals, polluted soil, water and air

* Corresponding Author–E-mail: rima_dada@rediffmail.com

are believed to be the source of various xenobiotics. These major toxicants in the environment may affect different stages of germinal cell maturation and disrupt spermatogenesis and oogenesis. As environmental factors, occupational exposure, life style behaviour and nutrition are considered to play an important role in the human health; they may be responsible for unexplained cause of infertility.

Introduction

Every human being in the world live to reproduce their generation. Though overall the phenomenon of reproduction seems to be simple, it is a complex process of giving birth to a new life. When a married couple fails to reproduce, the consequences they face are numerous and the condition is called as infertility. Infertility is the major concern among the married couples when they fail to achieve pregnancy after one year of regular unprotected intercourse. Generally infertility affects 15 per cent of the married couples where in approximately 40 per cent of these cases male infertility is the major factor. Another 40 per cent of infertility problems are caused by abnormalities of the woman's reproductive system, and the remaining 20 per cent involve couples where both partners suffer reproductive problems. The cause of infertility includes chromosomal aberrations, mutation, varicocele, hypogonadism, cryptochidism, infection and recently azoospermia factor (AZF) deletion[1] in male, whereas in case of female it includes pelvic inflammatory diseases, blocked fallopian tubes, polycystic ovary, ovulatory disorder and menstrual disorder. Though the cause of infertility in human is multifactorial, 40-90 per cent of them are diagnosed with unexplained causes known as idiopathic infertility. Nowadays, idiopathic infertility among the married couple is suspected to increase in number. These unknown causes among the infertile patients may be due to sudden environmental changes, life style behaviour and occupational exposure that affect the normal production and physiological functions of the germ cell. The recent suspect in the idiopathic cases that could affect the normal fertilization is believed to be oxidative stress and mitochondrial DNA (mtDNA) mutations. Since humans live in aerobic environment and the cells require oxygen for their survival, oxidative metabolism is inevitable. Though it is normal process in every human being, the production of excess ROS in certain known and unknown condition affects the physiological function of the germ cells. Hence, this chapter deals with the role of environmental and occupational exposure, life style and nutrition in the production of ROS and associated mtDNA mutation in the pathogenesis of human infertility.

Reactive Oxygen Species (ROS) and Human Reproduction

A free radical is defined as "any atom or molecule that possesses one or more unpaired electrons". Reactive oxygen species are highly reactive oxidizing agents belonging to the class of free radicals that react with every biochemical substance like lipids, amino acids, carbohydrates, protein, and DNA they come in contact. Therefore ROS is considered as a causative factor of variety of diseases. It is well established that low levels of ROS are necessary for optimal functions of spermatozoa to achieve capacitation, hyperactivation, motility, acrosome reaction, oocyte fusion and fertilization[2,3]. Similarly ROS also play an important role in the regulation of oocyte maturation, folliculogenesis, ovarian steroidogenesiss, corpus luteal function and luteolysis[3] in female fertility. Though it is well demonstrated that generation of ROS in the human fertility is necessary for the normal fertilization, its excess production in some known and unknown pathological conditions have detrimental effects on both male and female fertility. The mechanism behind this effect in male infertility is ROS induced lipid peroxidation of sperm plasma membrane[4] and in addition ROS may also affect the sperm axoneme, inhibit mitochondrial function and affect the synthesis of DNA, RNA and proteins[5]. Excess ROS and associated mtDNA mutation may impair ATP production leading to abnormal cleavage[6] embryogenesis and thus has life long implications on health. Hence excess production of ROS may be one of the major factors leading to human infertility.

ROS Associated Oxidative Stress and mtDNA Mutation in Infertility

It is well established that ROS is one of the major group of free radicals, when produced in excess affects the normal mitochondrial function leading to infertility. A condition known as oxidative stress occurs when the production of reactive oxygen species (ROS) overwhelms the antioxidant defense produced against them. Hence, oxidative stress is suspected to be one of the major causes of many human diseases including infertility. The antioxidant system includes enzymatic and non-enzymatic substance. Superoxide dismutase (SOD), catalase and glutathione peroxidase/reductase (GPx/GRD)) are the most important enzymatic antioxidants that scavenges both intracellular and extracellular radicals, where non-enzymatic antioxidants such as vitamin C, vitamin E, glutathione, urate, ubiquinone, transferrin, pyruvate and carotenoids acts by chain breaking or preventive mechanism. These antioxidant system presents in both male and female reproductive system and comfortably balance the ROS produced under normal physiological conditions. It is also known that production of ROS is significantly increased in dysfunctional mitochondria, which inturn affect mitochondrial function. This process may be due to ROS induced damage to the mitochondrial genome, which is closely associated with oxidative phosphorylation (OXPHOS) system and the damaged mtDNA may function abnormally thus causing an further increased ROS production. Several studies have been reported that human cells harboring mutated mtDNA had lower respiratory function and showed increased production of superoxide anions, hydroxyl radicals and H_2O_2[7,8]. However, excess production of ROS further damages mtDNA, which are more susceptible than nuclear genome. As ROS are by product of OXPHOS pathway, mtDNA is the first site of ROS mediated damage. Hence, during course of evolution majority of genes have migrated from mitochondria to the nuclear genome. Ultimately, impairment of electron transport chain results in enhanced production of ROS in mitochondria due to incomplete reduction of oxygen[9,10]

Moreover, ROS induced chain-propagating reaction is responsible for overall increase in the steady state level of mtDNA damage and it is also believed that ROS mediated damage to mitochondria may inactivate electron transport chain, thus altering normal mitochondrial function[11] (Figure 4.1). *Yakes and Houten*[11] reported that exposure of human fibroblast cell line to H_2O_2 for 60 min resulted in non-repairable mtDNA damage, which supports the sensitivity of mtDNA to ROS. Thus mitochondria are not only the main producer of ATP but are also major intracellular source of ROS.

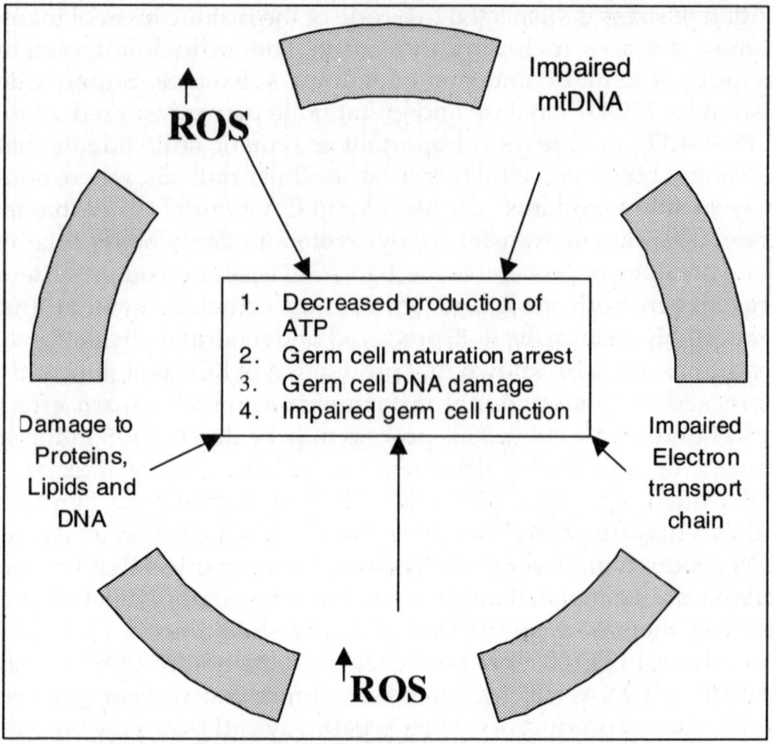

Figure 4.1: ROS Induced mtDNA Damage in Infertility

Environmental and Occupational Exposure

As reproduction of human is very closely associated with the environment, any change in the later could affect the human fertility. Not only change in the environment, but also exposure to various chemical substances, heat and radiation at working place may also suspected to be the major factors that influencing variety of human diseases including infertility. Industrialization, urbanization, rural to urban migration is the recent well known development that has brought sudden change in the environment, occupation, life style and food habits in the developing countries. Effect of these on reproduction is clear from the evidence of decrease in overall sperm quality over the past 50 years and increase in female fertility problems like polycystic ovary, abortions, endometriosis, early pregnancy loss

Table 4.1: Effect of Various Factors on Male and Female Fertility

Factors	*Effect on Men*	*Effect on Women*
Pollutants	☆ Decreased semen quality ☆ Oxidative DNA damage	☆ Decreased pregnancy rates ☆ Preterm birth ☆ Oxidative DNA damage
Pesticides	☆ Decreased semen quality ☆ Sperm DNA damage ☆ Cryptochidism ☆ Increased ROS ☆ Altered hormone levels (EDs) ☆ mtDNA damage	☆ Spontaneous abortion ☆ Increased ROS ☆ Altered hormone levels (EDs)
Metals	☆ Decreased semen quality ☆ Impaired testicular function and sperm production ☆ Altered antioxidant levels	☆ Miscarriage ☆ Altered antioxidant levels
Smoking	☆ Decreased sperm count and sperm motility ☆ Increased sperm abnormalities ☆ Increased ROS level ☆ Increased mtDNA damage ☆ Affected offspring ☆ Decreased rate of ART	☆ Impaired follicle development ovarian resume and early embryonic development ☆ Early menopause ☆ Delayed conception ☆ Affected offspring ☆ Decreased rate of ART
Alcohol	☆ Decreased semen quality ☆ Increased ROS level ☆ Increased DNA damage ☆ Altered antioxidant levels	☆ Miscarriage ☆ Extra uterine pregnancy ☆ Increased ROS level ☆ Increased mtDNA damage

Contd...

Table 4.1–Contd...

Factors	*Effect on Men*	*Effect on Women*
Chemicals	☆ Endocrine disruptors ☆ Altered mtDNA gene and copy ☆ Hypospadias ☆ Cryptochidism ☆ Decreased testosterone level ☆ Anti-androgenic	☆ Endocrine disruptors ☆ Spontaneous abortion ☆ Defective offspring
Temperature andradiation	☆ Suppression of spermatogenesis ☆ Increased scrotal temperature ☆ Impaired sperm motility	☆ Altered antioxidant levels
Malnutrition	☆ Decreased antioxidant enzymes level ☆ Impaired gonadal development ☆ Impaired germ cell multiplication	☆ Delayed ovulation and menstruation ☆ Decreased antioxidant enzymes level ☆ Impaired gonadal development
Obesity	☆ Altered spermatogenesis ☆ Altered hormone levels	☆ Impaired germ cell multiplication ☆ Miscarriage ☆ Altered hormone levels
Stress	☆ Impaired semen quality ☆ Altered hormone level	☆ Delayed fertility ☆ Altered hormone level
Clothing	☆ Increased scrotal temperature ☆ Decreased sperm production	

and pre-implantation failure. So the following factors (Table 4.1) cannot be underestimated in the pathogenesis of infertility.

Pollution

The recent rapid decline in male and female reproductive health is believed to be due to environmental factors like pollution. Recent report from Times of India[12] revealed that drinking water in a village near Amritsar, India has been highly polluted with heavy metals like mercury, copper, cadmium, chromium and lead along with the pesticides. Pesticides are also reportedly found in vegetables, human milk and in blood samples. The report also revealed the high incidence of DNA mutation, cancer, numbness, spontaneous abortions and reproductive toxicity. However, men exposed to traffic pollutants have been reported to have decreased semen quality than who are not exposed to pollutants[13]. Studies in females have also revealed that poor air quality positively correlated with reduced pregnancy rates and preterm birth. Some of the pollutants present in the air are bromine, vanadium, carbon monoxide, sulphur oxides and nitrogen oxides. Air pollutants emitted by diesel cars are 7.5 times more than the petrol cars. Benzene and other hydrocarbons from the automobile diesel exhaust are another widely distributed toxic air pollutants that may impair female fertility. There is also high probability for the production of ROS by the pollutants present in the environment. Moreover, particulate air pollution is believed to generate ROS from the surface of particles and alter the functions of mitochondria. These particulate matter induce oxidative DNA damage in *in vitro* systems. So oxidative stress induced DNA damage is considered to be an important mechanism in urban particulate air pollution[14]. Studies had also established a clear association between airborne concentration of pollutants and various disorders.

Pesticides

Pesticides are chemical substances used to destroy insects in order to protect variety of crops and foods. The production and use of pesticides have been increased in the recent years. Not only pesticides, many other groups of toxicants like fungicide and herbicide are also suspected to be reproductive disrupture, are still in commercial use and promote toxic effects to the workers. More commonly used pesticide DDT (dichloro diphenyl trichloroethane) and its metabolite DDE (dichloro diphenyldichloro ethylene) have been reportedly impair the quality of seminal parameters

DDT is weakly estrogenic but it is metabolized to DDE which is a strong and potent antiandrogen. They are absorbed in the body by multiple ways and undergo enterohepatic recirculation, bioaccumulate in the body and their effects are biomagnified. Recent studies have reported that there are over 20,000 deaths and one million cases annually of pesticide poisoning each year. Humans now live in a sea of estrogens. These agents may cause increase in blood levels of estrogen, which inhibit the hypothalamo-pituitary gonadal axis due to feedback inhibition. This results in decreased production of FSH and fixing of Sertoli cell number. Functional and fully differentiated Sertoli cells are essential for sexual differentiation and spermatogenesis. Any alteration of Sertoli cell number result in decreased production of Anti Mullerian Hormone (AMH), Mullerian Inhibiting Substance (MIS), Meiosis Preventing Substance (MPS) and decreased germ cell differentiation. Sertoli cells are known to play an important role in regulation of the testicular microenvironment in the seminiferous tubules and each Sertoli cell supports the development of a limited number of germ cells. In most mammals, Sertoli cell replication occurs only during fetal and post natal life. Sertoli cell number thus becomes fixed at a particular stage of development. In man the Sertoli cell number increases significantly between late fetal and prepubertal life and increases further during puberty. Hence, the window for adverse effect on Sertoli cells in man is longer than that known for other mammalian species. Any disturbance in the development of the reproductive system, which leads to decrease in number of Sertoli cells, reduces the individual's capacity for spermatogenic production in adult life. FSH is involved in determination of Sertoli cell number and estrogen produced by Sertoli cells keeps FSH level in check by feedback inhibition. Thus, exposure to environmental hormones or xenoestrogens or environmental endocrine disruptors accumulate in the body and their effects are biomagnified over a period of time. This elevation in maternal and fetal estrogens inhibit FSH secretion resulting in decreased Sertoli cell number and thus decreased production of AMH and MPS and decreased expression of genes expressed in the Sertoli cells which then results in abnormal sexual differentiation, decreased spermatogenesis, leading to cryptorchidism and hypospadias. It also eventually may lead to testicular cancer, which may be congenital or may manifest after puberty. The process whereby the environmental endocrine xenoestrogens lead to cancer is known as hormonal carcinogenesis. They also proposed that testicular cancers are associated with increased estrogenic activity in testicular tissue. The most common conditions associated with testicular cancer are cryptorchidism, infertility and over exposure to pesticides and radiation. Carcinoma *in situ* is associated with cryptorchidism (2-4 per cent), infertility (0-1 per cent), ambiguous genitalia (25 per cent). Skakkebaek *et al.* (2001) reported that poor semen quality; testicular cancer, undescended testis and hypospadias are symptoms of one underlying entity the Testicular Dysgenesis Syndrome (TDS). The rapid increase in the incidence of TDS suggests that environmental and lifestyle factors are major contributors to the decline in male reproductive health.

Workers exposed to fenvalerate, a synthetic pyrethroid insecticide used for fruits and vegetables protection has been reported to cause increased sperm DNA damage. Semen quality also tends to decrease in workers exposed to variety of pesticides. The decrease in quality and sperm DNA damage might be attributed to oxidative stress[16] produced by the toxicant pesticides and it is a well know fact that oxidative stress alters the genome of mitochondria, which are highly susceptible to free radicals. This alteration of mtDNA disrupts ATP production and thus leads to depressed gametogenesiss in both males and females that would bring the defects in the maturation and normal function of germ cells.

Pesticides are widely studied for their effect on human reproduction. Men exposed to certain pesticide have been found to be infertile[17]. Moreover, cryptochidism[18] has also been reported to be associated with pesticide exposure. It has been reported that females exposed to variety of pesticides are under risk of unexplained infertility. Commonly used pesticides such as organophosphate, organochlorine and bipyridyl herbicides are reported to establish oxidative stress through free radical stimulation, lipid peroxidation and alteration of antioxidant activities in the body. This may be one of the mechanisms lying in the impairment of human reproduction by the pesticides in the pathogenesis of human infertility. However, pesticides like endosulfan, lindane, aldicarb, carbaryl, chlordecone, dieldrin, p,p′-methoxychlor, toxaphene and organophosphate are reported to be endocrine disruptures. The effects of majority of these pesticides are biomagnified as they undergo enterohepatic recirculation and bioaccumulate in the body.

Metals

Metals are major category of widely occurring natural element that are potential toxicants even at low concentration in the tissues. Particularly heavy metals like lead, mercury, cadmium and arsenic are suspected to be major toxicants to many tissues. Though toxicity of metals are widely reported in various diseases involving brain, kidney and heart, its involvement in the pathogenesis of human infertility is not clearly established. However, Aluminum, a widely distributed pollutant has been reported to decrease the semen quality[20]. Studies have also been reported that lead exposure at low level affected sperm quality, testosterone, estrogen, prolactin and seminal plasma Zn levels[21]. Not only are lead, other heavy metals such as Cd, Al and Hg also considered harmful to testicular function and sperm production. Metals are also reported to decrease semen quality by disturbing the testicular function. Lead, Cadmium and Nickel are reported to induce oxidative stress by increasing malonaldehyde level, serum glutathione–S- transferase and catalase activity in diesel engine tunning workers[22]. In human reproduction, metals may induce the formation of free radicals and consequently modify DNA bases, enhances lipid peroxidation and alter the antioxidant enzymes[23]. Fe, Cu, Cr, V and Co are reported to undergo redox cycling where Hg, Cd and Ni bind to thiol (SH) group of protein and decreases the level of glutathione. Arsenic also binds to thiol and also tends to induce the formation of ROS such as H_2O_2, OH^-, $O_2^{\cdot -}$[24]. As it is well known fact that human spermatozoa and ovum is well protected with antioxidants, the above metal toxicant can undoubtedly establish OS in both male and female reproductive system that may lead to fertility impairment. As human are exposed to metals from various sources such as contaminated water, soil, air and food[25], it is necessary to find its pathological levels in the tissues to overcome the fertility impairment in human reproduction.

Smoking

Tobacco in all forms adversely affects various organ systems. Especially, gonads are vulnerable to several chemical components in tobacco. Smoking has been reported to have great impact on both male and female fertility. Cigarette smoking in man is associated with decreased sperm counts and sperm motility and also increased abnormalities in sperm morphology[25]. As more than 4000 chemicals are present in cigarette, it is suspected to generate free radicals and damages mitochondrial DNA[26]. Several components in tobacco induce inflammatory changes in various tissues. In testes of men who smoke there are increased ROS levels due to testicular inflammation and the infiltration of leukocytes in seminal plasma. In women, smoking has negative impact on follicle development, ovarian reserve and early embryo development as oxidative stress induced by smoking impairs folliculogenesis. Also smoking results in increased time to pregnancy (TTP) and smoking during pregnancy is believed to affect the offspring inspite of its sex, and smoking also delays conception, and increased risk of miscarriage in women. Numerous chemicals present in the tobacco generate free radicals that increase excess ROS production which may disrupt mitochondrial genome, impairs electron transport chain thus increase further ROS production and establishes oxidative stress.

Alcohol

Alcohol is the most consumed euphoric drink worldwide. Though its pathological effect in the human health is well studied, its role in the pathogenesis of human infertility is not completely understood. Alcohol consumption has been reported to have severe impact on the semen quality of male population. However, recent studies revealed that alcohol decreases sperm count, motility and sperm morphology[27] in man and it may also lead to miscarriage and extrauterine pregnancy in female[28]. The mechanism behind this may be due to the generation of ROS concurrently with many mechanisms to set up oxidative stress in the pathogenesis of infertility. Thus OS can damage essential complex molecules like protein, fatty acid, lipid and DNA of the germ cell. *Wu and Cederbaum*[29] proposed the other mechanism involved in the pathogenesis that includes a) production of acetaldehyde, which interacts with protein and lipids and further generates free radicals and cause cell damage, b) damage to mitochondrial DNA, c) increases free Fe in the cell that promotes ROS generation, and d) decreases the antioxidant activity. Chronic administration of alcohol has been reported to induce OS in the rat testes either due to increased lipid peroxidation or decreased antioxidant[30]. So, overall increase in OS and mtDNA mutation in the germ cell may cause DNA damage and maturation arrest of germ cells.

Chemicals and Solvents

Increase in chemical industries and wide use of chemicals may lead to suspect the increased exposure of different chemicals to workers and human population. Many of the chemicals are reported to impair the reproductive health and also reported as endocrine disruptors (ED). EDs mimic estrogen thereby block progesterone or alter testosterone levels and thus affects both male and female fertility. Many of the chemical substances such as cosmetics, detergents, pesticides, plastics and pollutants have been reported to be EDs These environmental endocrine disruptors also includes Atrazine (herbicide), Polyvinyl chloride (PVC) from plastics, dioxin an incinerated product of PVC, Bisphenol-A (BPA) a plasticizer and polystyrenes which have been exposed to the population through paints, waxes, solvents and many routinely used household chemicals and materials. Exposed to many potent oestrogens like diethyl stilboesterol or ethinyl oestradiol in pregnancy undoubtedly results in various reproductive disorders[31]. A widely used chemical N,N-Dimethyl formamide in industries has been reported to be male reproductive toxicant. Its effect on female reproduction is not clearly known. The mechanism behind its toxicity has been reported to be mtDNA common deletion and alteration in mtDNA copy number[32]. Moreover, toluene that is present in gums, ink, coatings, gasoline and cosmetics has been found to cause miscarriage and reduced fertility in women, whereas in men it caused decreased sperm count and hormonal changes. Exposure to certain environmental chemicals like polychlorinated biphenyl (PCB), phthalate esters (PE) may have deleterious effect in human reproductive function. Phthalate esters, a widely used chemical when exposed to pregnant mice, the male pups exhibit high frequency of hypospadias, abnormal testes, cryptochidism with suppressed testosterone levels [33,34,35]. Painters, dyers and people employed in paper industry are exposed to high levels of anti-androgenic compounds like alkyl phenol ethoxylates (APEs), Bisphenol-A (BPA), phthalates [Dibutyl phthalate (DBP), Diethyl hexyl phthalate (DEHP)] and gums, which mimic estrogen and cause negative feedback of hypothalamus pituitary gonadal axis. Women of reproductive age[36]are suspected to be the most affected for phthalate esters. This may ultimately setup an oxidative stress status and further damage the susceptible mitochondrial genome.

Radiation and Temperature

Global warming[37] or "heating" as it is now known has pushed India back in sectors like agriculture, forest including health. It affects large part of the world in all terms including human health. Radiation and temperature is believed to be a major physical factor that affects human reproductive health. Higher temperature also increases the concentration of ozone (O_3) at ground levels. Since there is a close association between local climate and body temperature, increase in temperature is reported to cause suppression of spermatogenesis[38]. Even an increase in temperature by 1°C causes decrease in the production of healthy sperm by 40 per cent [39]. Also, high temperature results in production of abnormal sperms with coiled tails and tapered head[40]. Pachytene spermatocytes are most temperature sensitive. High temperature causes activation of p53 and its translocation from nuclear membrane to nucleoplasm inhibits clonal proliferation of cell with damaged DNA.

Increased environmental temperature further increased scrotal temperature which results in elevation of testicular temperature. These changes also alter sexual behaviour and mood disorders. Increase in temperature can also increase air and water pollution, which further impairs human fertility. Studies have been reported that heat scrotal stress in mice affects genetic integrity of sperm, where DNA damage in spermatocytes is more than spermatid [41]. Studies also suggested that car drivers and laptop users have increased scrotal temperature. There are no studies revealed the effect of high temperature on the production of ROS, but the antioxidant enzyme activities may be impaired at elevated temperature. Moreover, the percentage of abnormal morphology and impaired motility has been reported to be more with the increase in frequency of using mobile phones[42]. Excess electromagnetic waves may also impair spermatogenesis by generating heat in the testicles.

Nutrition and Diet

It is a well-known fact that nutrition and diet is an important factor affecting the incidence of variety of diseases. Importantly, antioxidant substances in the diet protect protein, lipids and DNA by scavenging the free radicals that causes pathological damage. Thus the recent reports of having at least 4 to 5 serving of fruits and vegetables daily is considered good for health. These products are rich in antioxidants that could scavenge the free radicals. So diet with low antioxidants may increase the DNA damage[43] and oxidative stress, which further damage DNA of both nucleus and mitochondria. And studies have reported that lipid peroxidation and oxidation of DNA is decreased in vegetarian compared to non-vegetarians[44]. High intake of cottonseed oil, which contain pesticide residue and a chemical called gossypol are reported to interfere with spermatogenesis[45]. A normal calorie intake is also necessary for normal onset of menstruation and ovulation, where underweight women suffering from anorexia nervosa are reported to ovulate and menstruate rarely[46]. Even low concentration of circulating leptin are low in underweight women[47] may be another reason for the above. Increase in sedentary life style and improper diet is believed to be the reason for increase in obese population. Obesity in men has been reported to alter spermatogenesis due to hypoandrogenism and increased levels of estrogen[48]. Increase or decrease in Body mass index (BMI) range of 20-25 kg/m^2 have been reported to affect the sperm quality[49]. Not only in men, in women also has BMI been reported to affect fertility. BMI of women less than or greater than the range 19-30 kg/m^2 may adversely affect their reproductive health. This is due to increased estrogen level in severe obese subject. And also obese women are reported less likely to be ovulated and more likely to suffer from miscarriage[50,51]. Obesity is a major health problem today in India. With increasing incidence of diabetes mellitus (DM) there are associated microvasculature changes and associated subnormal testicular functions. Recent news published in Times of India[52], an Indian newspaper reported that obesity, poor diet and lack of exercise induced type–II diabetes also affects male fertility by damaging DNA of sperm cells. Malnutrition and improper diet during the time of gonadal development and germ cell multiplication could impair the fertility in both men and women. Excess of saturated fats consumed would change the fatty acid composition of the sperm membrane and decreases the fluidity, thus decreases sperm motility also.

Life Style

Tight clothing has been reported to increase the scrotal temperature by 1.5 to 2°C by bringing the scrotum close to the anterior abdominal wall. Tight fitting clothes like jeans, undertrousers[53] are believed to increase the scrotal and testicular temperature. Moreover, frequent sauna bath and thermal underwear also believed to adversely affect spermatogenesis. Prenatal maternal stress is anti-androgenic and male fetus conceived from mother with high stress levels may cause delayed and abnormal descent of testis. However, mental stress may also negatively affect the semen quality due to free radicals[54]. Use of marijuana has been suspected to suppress pituitary secretion in both male and female and thus alters the gonadal function. Increasing use of certain drugs and anabolic steroids has been reported to impair fertility by acting on testes and lower the testosterone production. Drug includes cimetidine, allopurinol, ketoconazole, spironoloctone, sulfasalazine and anti epileptics used in the treatment of respective disorders may also have negative effects on semen quality. Moreover, chemotherapeutic drugs for cancer treatment have been found to affect semen quality severely. Hence, depending on their dosage and duration patients undergoing such treatment are advised to undergo semen cryopreservation prior to the treatment. Lack of exercise, physical activity, and the fast food culture has increased higher obese population, which adversely affected reproductive health.

Assisted Reproduction Technique (ART) and its Environment

In this era of ART increasing number of infertile couples are opting for assisted conception. However, the early artificial environment of ova and sperm during *in vitro* procedures has life implications on health. Ovarian hyperstimulation and altered hormonal mileu can results in epimutations, which has transgenerational effects. Moreover, ultracentrifugation of sperms during its preparation for ART can result in increased ROS production and ROS induced sperm damage. Oxidative stress is a major factor, which negatively influences ART outcome. A data reports that only 35 per cent of the ART transfer procedures results in live birth delivery[55]. Men who drink alcohol frequently can have decreased rate of *in vitro* fertilization (IVF). Alcohol consumption by female can also affect pregnancy rate, miscarriage rate and egg retrieval in IVF and also they require higher doses of ovarian stimulation drugs for ART. Although small amount of ROS needed for fertilization and sperm binding to the zona pellucida, high levels of ROS negatively affect embryogenesis and gastrulation.

Genetic Factors

Genetic factors are another cause for idiopathic infertility. In male, Y chromosome is the only haploid complement of the human genome that does not undergo recombination repair and hence tends to accumulate mutation at a much higher rate than any autosomes. It has been suggested that environmental factors[56] also plays an important role in inducing Y chromosome mutations. Any genetic alterations in the germ cells are also believed to affect the reproductive system. Hence, Y- chromosome microdeletion and single nucleotide polymorphism has been reported to cause either azoospermia or oligozoospermia.

Conclusion

Significant decrease in human fertility is the major concern for the last 50 years. Though role of ROS is well established in húman reproduction, its pathological function is yet to be clearly defined. But OS is recently gained much importance as it is involved in conditions such as sperm DNA damage, lipid peroxidation, impaired sperm motility and viability to impair male fertility. But so far only few studies have reported mutation in mtDNA of the spermatozoa[57,58]. Similarly it is also involved in abortions, endometriosis, polycystic ovary, intrauterine growth retardation to impair female fertility. So it is very important to further elucidate the role of oxidative stress in unexplained infertility. Since industrialization and urbanization leads to accumulation of unfavorable environmental factors, occupational exposure and change in life style and diet, it can cause changes in human reproductive function. Various chemicals, polluted soil, water and air are believed to be the source of various xenobiotics. High temperature in the working place, radiation, and exposure to harmful substance like solvents, pesticides and EDs also has been shown to have negative influence on human fertility. In the last 10 years of an ongoing study in our laboratory, we found that about 8-10 per cent infertile oligozoospermic men and about 20 to 22 per cent azoospermic men with non-obstructive azoospermia harboured cytogenetic numerical or structural abnormalities[59]. In addition 9.83 per cent cytogenetically normal men harboured Yq microdeletion in AZF loci. Further in 33 OAT (Oligo-Astheno-Teratozoospermic) men a high frequency of mitochondrial mutation was detected in gene regulating oxidative phosphorylation (OXPHOS). In these men with

Table 4.2: Exposure to Various Reproductive Toxicants in Idiopathic Infertile Male Patients (Category-wise)

Category (Number of Sperms/ml)	*N*	*Smoking*	*Alcohol*	*Pesticide*	*Temp./Radiation*	*Chemicals*	*Smoking and Drink*	*More than Two Factors*	*Total*	*Cytogenetic Abnormalities*	*Yq-microdeletion*	*MtDNA Mutation*
Azoospermia (0 million/ml)	161	12	17	9	4	9	20	12	83	11	12	02
Oligozoospermia (<20million/ml)	116	14	14	4	6	11	15	9	73	6	12	31
Normozoospermia (>20million/ml)	43	3	8	0	3	11	5	3	33			
Total	320	29	39	13	13	31	40	24	189 (60%)	17	24	33

genetic abnormalities many had exposed to high temperature, chemicals, radiation and pesticides. An ongoing study (Table 4.2) in our lab revealed that 60 per cent of idiopathic infertile male patients are exposed to anyone or more reproductive toxicants continuously for certain period of time in their adult lifetime. These major toxicants in the environment may affect different stages of germinal cell maturation and disrupt spermatogenesis and oogenesis. As environmental factors, occupational exposure, life style behaviour and nutrition are considered to play an important role in the human health; they may be responsible for unexplained cause of infertility. Since, reproductive health depends on several confounding factors like environment, nutrition, genetic make up, life style and habit, it is very difficult to elucidate the role of a single agent in pathogenesis of reproductive ill health, subfertility and infertility. And there are many other factors, which are still not yet evaluated for their effect on human fertility. Hence as majority of the infertility cases are of unknown origin, the above factors must be evaluated with the detailed history of both the partners with respect to their nutrition, habits, disease and occupation and to better correlate them with their fertility status and also formulate programmes to minimize exposure.

References

1. Dada R, Kumar R, Kumar R, Sharma RK, Gupta NP, Gupta SK, *et al.*, AZF deletion in varicocele cases with oligospermia. *IJMS* 2007;*61*:505-10

2. Griveau JF, Le Lannou D. Reactive oxygen species and human spermatozoa: Physiology and pathology. *Int J Androl* 1997;20:61-9.

3. Agarwal A, Nallela KP, Allamaneni SSR, Said TM. Role of antioxidants in treatment of male infertility: an overview of the literature. *Reprod Biomed online* 2004;8:616-27.

4. Baker MA. Oxidative stress, sperm survival and fertility control. *Mol cell Endocrinol* 2006;250:66-9.

5. De Lamirande E, Gagnon C. Reactive oxygen species and human spermatozoa. II. Depletion of adenosine triphosphate plays an important role in the inhibition of sperm motility. *J Androl* 1992;13:379-86.

6. Nasr-Esfahani MH, Aitken R, Johnson MH. Hydrogen peroxide levels in mouse oocytes and early cleavage stage embryos developed *in vitro* or *in vivo*. *Development* 1990;109:501-7.
7. Liu CY, Lee CF, Hong CH, Wei YH. Mitochondrial DNA mutation and depletion increase the susceptibility of human cells to apoptosis. *Ann NY Acad Sci* 2004;1011:133-45.
8. Taylor RW, Tumbull DM. Mitochondrial DNA mutations in human disease. *Nat Rev Genet* 2005;6:389-402.
9. Suzuki H, Kumagai T, Goto A, Sugiura T. Increase in intracellular hydrogen peroxide and up regulation of nuclear respiratory gene evoked by impairment of mitochondrial electron transfer in human cells. *Biochem Biophys Res Commun* 1998;249:542-5.
10. Wallace DC. Mitochondrial disease in man and mouse. *Science* 1999;283:1482-8.
11. Yakes FM, Van Houten B. Mitochondrial DNA damage is more extensive and persists longer than nuclear DNA damage in human cells following oxidative stress. *Proc Natl Acad Sci USA* 1997;94:514-9.
12. Water turns poison in Punjab villages. Pesticides and toxic waste alter DNA. Times of India, Delhi edn. India 18th May, 2007. page.1
13. De Rosa M, Zarrilli S, Paesano L, Carbone U, Boggia B, Petretta M, *et al.*, Traffic pollutants affect fertility in men. *Hum Reprod* 2003;18:1055-61.
14. Risom L, Møller P, Loft S. Oxidative stress-induced DNA damage by particulate air pollution. *Mutat Res* 2005:592:119-37.
15. Aneck-Hahn NH, Schulenburg GW, Bornman MS, Farias P, de Jager C. Impaired semen quality associated with environmental DDT exposure in young men living in a malaria area in the Limpopo Province, South Africa. *J Androl* 2007; 8:423-3.
16. Lebailly P, Vigrenx C, Lechevrel C, *et al.*, DNA damage in mononuclear leucocytes of farmers measured using the alkaline Comet assay: modifications of DNA damage levels after a one day field spraying period with selected pesticides. *Cancer Epidemiol Biomarkers Prev* 1998;7:929-40.

17. Irvine DS. Epidemology and aetiology of male infertility. *Hum Reprod* Suppl 1998;1:33-44.

18. Weidner IS, Moller H, Jensen TK, Skakkebaek NE. Cryptorchidism and hypospadias in sons of gardeners and farmers. *Environ Health Perspect* 1998;106:793-796.

19. Greenlee A, Arbuckle T, Chyou P. Risk Factors for Female Infertility in an Agricultural Region. *Epidemiology* 2003;14:429-36.

20. Hovatta O, Venäläinen ER, Kuusimäki L, Heikkilä J, Hirvi T, Reima I. Aluminium, lead and cadmium concentrations in seminal plasma and spermatozoa, and semen quality in Finnish men. *Hum Reprod* 1998;13:115-9.

21. Telisman S, Colak B, Pizent A, Jurasoviæ J, Cvitkoviæ P. Reproductive toxicity of low-level lead exposure in men. *Environ Res* 2007;105:256-66.

22. Devi SS, Biswas AR, Biswas RA, Vinayagamoorthy N, Krishnamurthi K, Shinde VM, *et al.*, Heavy metal status and oxidative stress in diesel engine tuning workers of central Indian population. *J Occup Environ Med* 2007;49:1228-34.

23. Valko M, Morris H, Cronin MT. Metals, toxicity and oxidative stress. *Curr Med Chem* 2005;12:1161-208.

24. Ercal N, Gurer-Orhan H, Aykin-Burns N. Toxic metals and oxidative stress part I: mechanisms involved in metal-induced oxidative damage. *Curr Top Med Chem* 2001;1:529-39.

25. Sépaniak S, Forges T, Monnier-Barbarino P. Cigarette smoking and fertility in women and men. [Article in French] *Gynecol Obstet Fertil* 2006;34:945-9.

26. Knight-Lozano CA, Young CG, Burow DL, *et al.*, Cigarette smoke exposure and hypercholesterolemia increase mitochondrial damage in cardiovascular tissues. *Circulation* 2002;105:849-54.

27. Stutz G, Zamudio J, Santillán ME, Vincenti L, de Cuneo MF, Ruiz RD. The effect of alcohol, tobacco, and aspirin consumption on seminal quality among healthy young men. *Arch Environ Health* 2004;59:548-52.

28. Eggert J, Theobald H, Engfeldt P. Effects of alcohol consumption on female fertility during an 18-year period. *Fertil Steril* 2004;81:379-83.

29. Wu D, Cederbaum AI. Alcohol, oxidative stress, and free radical damage. *Alcohol Res Health* 2003;27:277-84.

30. Maneesh M, Jayalekshmi H, Sanjiba Dutta, Amit Chakrabarti, Vasudevan DM. Role of oxidative stress in ethanol induced germ cell apoptosis -an experimental study in rats. *Ind J Clin Biochem* 2005;20:62-67.

31. Sharpe RM, Franks S. Environment, lifestyle and infertility–an inter-generational issue. *Nat Cell Biol* 2002;4 Suppl:s33-s40.

32. Shieh DB, Chen CC, Shih TS, Tai HM, Wei YH, Chang HY. Mitochondrial DNA alterations in blood of the humans exposed to N,N-dimethylformamide. *Chem Biol Interact* 2007;165: 211-9.

33. Li LH, Jester WF Jr, Laslett AL, Orth JM. A single dose of Di-(2-ethylhexyl) phthalate in neonatal rats alters gonocytes, reduces Sertoli cell proliferation and decreases cyclin D2 expression. *Toxicol Appl Pharmacol* 2000;166:222-9.

34. Mylchreest E, Wallace DG, Cattley RC, Foster PM. Dose-dependent alterations in androgen-regulated male reproductive development in rats exposed to Di(*n*-butyl) phthalate during late gestation. *Toxicol Sci* 2000;55:143-51.

35. Parks LG, Ostby JS, Lambright CR, Abbott BD, Klinefelter GR, Barlow NJ, *et al.*, The plasticizer diethylhexyl phthalate induces malformations by decreasing fetal testosterone synthesis during sexual differentiation in the male rat. *Toxicol Sci* 2000;58:339-349.

36. Blount BC, Silva MJ, Caudill SP, Needham LL, Pirkle JL, Sampson EJ, *et al.*, Levels of seven urinary phthalate metabolites in a human reference population. *Environ Health Perspect* 2000;108:979-82.

37. The Times of India (Indian news paper). Health/Science. Global warming will push India back. 19 Nov 2007.

38. Wang C, Cui YG, Wang XH, Jia Y, Sinha Hikim A, Lue YH, *et al.*, transient scrotal hyperthermia and levonorgestrel enhance testosterone-induced spermatogenesis suppression in men through increased germ cell apoptosis. *J Clin Endocrinol Metab* 2007;92:3292-304.

39. http://natcure.blogspot.com/2007/07/laptop-and-sperm-counts.html.

40. Dada R, Gupta NP, Kucheria K. Spermatogenic arrest in men with testicular hyperthermia. *Teratog Carcinog Mutagen* 2003; Suppl 1:235-43.

41. Pérez-Crespo M, Pericuesta E, Rey R, Gutiérrez-Adán A. Scrotal Heat Stress in Mice Affects Viability and DNA Integrity of Sperm, and Sex Ratio of the Offspring. *Reprod Domest Anim* 2006;41:104.

42. Wdowiak A, Wdowiak L, Wiktor H. Evaluation of the effect of using mobile phones on male fertility. *Ann Agric Environ Med* 2007;14:169-72.

43. Kapiszewska M. A vegetable to meat consumption ratio as a relevant factor determining cancer preventive diet. The Mediterranean versus other European countries. *Forum Nutr* 2006;59:130-153.

44. Krajèovièová-Kudláèková M, Duš inská M. Oxidative DNA damage in relation to nutrition. *Neoplasma* 2004;51:30-33.

45. Weller DP, Zaneweld JD, Farnsworth NR. Gossypol: pharmacology and current status as a male contraceptive. *Econ Med Plant Res* 1985;1:87-112.

46. Franks S, Robinson S, Willis D. Nutrition, insulin and polycystic ovary syndrome. *Rev Reprod* 1996;1:47-53.

47. Grinspoon S, Gulick T, Askari H. Serum leptin levels in women with anorexia nervosa. *J Clin Endocrinol Metab* 1996;8:3861-3.

48. Hammoud AO, Gibson M, Peterson CM, Hamilton BD, Carrell DT. Obesity and male reproductive potential. *J Androl* 2006;27:619-2.

49. Jensen TK, Andersson AM, Jørgensen N, Andersen AG, Carlsen E, Petersen JH, *et al.*, Body mass index in relation to semen quality and reproductive hormones among 1,558 Danish men. *Fertil Steril* 2004;82:863-70.

50. Sebire NJ, Jolly M, Harris JP, Wadsworth J, Joffe M, Beard RW, *et al.*, Maternal obesity and pregnancy outcome: a study of 287, 213 pregnancies in London. *Int J Obes Relat Disord* 2001;25:1175-82.

51. Hamilton-Fairley D, Kiddy D, Watson H, Paterson C, Franks S. Association of moderate obesity with a poor pregnancy outcome in women with polycystic ovary syndrome treated with low dose gonadotrophin. *Br J Obstet Gynaecol* 1992;99:128-131.

52. Diabetes may hit male fertility. Times of India, Delhi edn. India 4th May, 2007. page.21.

53. Jung A, Leonhardt F, Schill WB, Schuppe HC. Influence of the type of undertrousers and physical activity on scrotal temperature *Hum Reprod* 2005;20:1022-7.

54. Eskiocak S, Gozen AS, Kilic AS, Molla S. Association between mental stress and some antioxidant enzymes of seminal plasma. *Indian J Med Res* 2005;122:491-6.

55. Mayne ST, Wright ME, Cartmel B. Assessment of antioxidant nutrient intake and status of epidemiologic research. *J Nutr* 2004;134:3199S-200S.

56. Edwards RG, Bishop CE. On the origin and frequency of Y chromosome deletions responsible for severe male infertility. *Mol Human Reprod* 1997;3:549-54.

57. Kumar R, Bhat A, Bamezai RNK, Shamsi MB, Kumar R, Gupta N P, *et al.*, Necessity of nuclear and mitochondrial genome analysis prior to ART/ICSI. *Ind J of Biochem Biophys*. In press.

58. Kumar R, Bhat A, Sharma RK, Bamezai RNK, Dada R. Mitochondrial DNA mutations and polymorphism in idiopathic asthenozoospermic men of Indian origin. Proceedings of the 57th annual meeting of American Society of Human Genetics; 2007 Oct 23-27; San Diego: California.

59. Dada R, Gupta NP, Kucheria K. Cytogenetic and molecular analysis of male infertility: Y chromosome deletion during nonobstructive azoospermia and severe oligozoospermia. *Cell Biochem Biophys* 2006;44:171-7

Environmental & Occupational Exposures (2010) ***Pages 102–141***
Editors: **Sunil Kumar & R.R. Tiwari**
Published by: **DAYA PUBLISHING HOUSE, NEW DELHI**

Chapter 5

Environmental Factors on Semen Quality

Satish Kumar Adiga* and Guruprasad Kalthur

Clinical Embryology Laboratory,
Division of Reproductive Medicine
Kasturba Medical College, Manipal – 576 104

Semen quality is an ill-defined term that refers to one or more of several semen characteristics that can be measured in a fresh ejaculate. Seminal volume, sperm concentration, viability, percentage of motile spermatozoa and percentage of sperm with normal morphology are the most important factors for male fecundity. The main advantages of semen analysis are the possibility to examine men independently of marriage, the possibility to find changes across exposure conditions within the same person, and the possibility to detect adverse effects at an early stage when no alteration of fertility is yet present[1]. Male reproductive toxicity is often associated with diminished libido or impotence in which case it may be impossible to obtain the semen sample from the men. However, many factors which influence the semen quality have to be taken into account when analyzing the data. Semen quality can be affected by sexual activity and period of abstinence, occupation, age, medication and diseases, nutrition, alcohol and smoking habits and stress. Several

* E-mail: satish.adiga@manipal.edu

confounding factors influencing the semen quality are listed in Table 5.1.

Table 5.1: Confounding Factors of Semen Analysis[1]

Characteristic	*Effect*
Sexual abstinence	Semen volume and sperm density increases with abstinence period
High fever (>38°C)	Temporary suppression of spermatogenesis
Age	Decline in sperm production with increase in age
Season	Semen volume, sperm density high in winter than in summer
Smoking	Smokers have 10-15 per cent lower sperm count than non-smokers
Alcohol intake	Interference with spermatogenesis and sexual function through inhibition of testosterone synthesis
Radiant heat	Short term exposure can cause a reversible decrease in sperm count with a delay of 5 weeks
Sexually transmitted diseases	Epididymal infection causing obstruction of the genital duct system
Urogenital disorders	Testicular maldescent, cancer, hypospadia, varicocele, testicular torsion, mumps and orchitis are associated with reduced sperm quality
Cytotoxic drugs and radiation	Dose dependent effect on spermatogenesis
Medication	Sulphasalazine, colchicine, niradozole, nitrofurantoin cimetidine, spironolactone, anabolic steriods, antiandrogens, progestagens, oestrogens and LHRH agonists suppress spermatogenesis
General anesthesia	Temporary depression of fertility
Surgery in urogenital region	Disorders of ejaculation following prostatectomy, bladder neck incision, treatment of urethral valves and strictures
Hernia surgical repair	Damage of vas deferens
Retroperitoneal surgery	Ejaculatory problem due to sympathetectomy
Geographical distribution	Environmental temperature, sunlight, environmental toxicants, regional difference in diet and life style can influence the spermatogenesis
Measurement error	Specimen spillage during collection

Biomarkers of Semen Quality

Spermatozoa are the primary focus of reproductive toxicologists since the male reproductive potential is based on his ability to deliver spermatozoa to the fertilization site in the female genital tract. Critical functions of the male reproductive tract such as sperm production and epididymal sperm maturation can be affected by the toxic agents, life style and occupation, which in turn can lead to infertility. Therefore, spermatozoa have the potential to become multipurpose biomarkers that provide a critical link between exposure-mediated damage to target organs and changes in fertility and other reproductive end points.

Sperm Count

A large number of studies conducted on semen donors and infertile men have suggested that sperm count has dropped significantly over the years[2–7]. A systematic review of the International literature on semen analysis performed in 14,947 normal men in 61 publications revealed a highly significant drop in mean sperm counts from 113 million/ml in 1938 to 66 million/ml in 1990. In addition, the number of men with oligozoospermia (<20 million/ml) and men with sperm counts in the lower end of the normal range (20-40 million/ml) had increased; whereas the percentage of those with high sperm counts (>100 million/ml) had decreased[8]. Several studies have shown a decrease in sperm count in men exposed to various environmental toxicants like pesticides, heavy metals, heat, radiation, and organic solvents.

Seminal sperm concentration may not be a sensitive and specific measure of male fertility. Human sperm production in healthy men is inherently influenced by its high inter individual and intra-individual variability[9]. Even though the cutoff point set by WHO[10] for normal sperm count is 40×10^6 per ejaculate, men with sperm concentrations well below this value have been shown to be fertile[11].

Sperm Morphology

Sperm morphological defect due to environmental and lifestyle factors is a subject of controversy. Exposure to toxic agents may affect the segregation of the chromosomes during spermatogenesis production of spermatozoa but also affect the production of morphologically and functionally competent spermatozoa by interfering with normal spermiogenesis or maturation process. There has also been speculation that the observed variations could be due to exposure to environmental chemicals acting as endocrine disrupters[12].

Sperm Motility

The fertilizing potential of spermatozoa is directly related to its motility. Measurement of sperm motility could be a sensitive method to evaluate the male reproductive toxicity. Toth *et al.*[13] have observed that reproductive toxicants at low doses can affect the motility of sperm even when other semen parameters are normal. Several conditions are known to impair human sperm motility, such as antisperm antibodies, infections of genital tract, anatomical pathologies, metabolic defects and structural phenotypic and genotypic defects[14]. The environmental toxicants may have a major role in affecting the sperm motility. Carbon disulfide and lead were found to damage the density, morphology, and motility of sperm[15]. Methyl mercury has been reported to affect sperm motility[16], and impairment of sperm motility after exposure to lead has been reported in rats[17].

Sperm DNA Integrity

Although the analysis of semen parameters may provide some indication of the function of the testis and sperm, it does not provide information on the condition of the male genome contained in sperm heads[18]. The integrity of sperm DNA is central to the transmission of genetic information during reproduction and chromatin abnormalities or DNA damage can result in paternal fertility problems[19]. Therefore, the assessment of genetic damage in gametes has become promising and sensitive approach in correlating the abnormal reproductive function.

Chromosomal abnormalities, such as aneuploidy in spermatozoa can lead to congenital birth defects, loss of pregnancy, genetic diseases in the offspring and perinatal death. Based on conservative estimates, aneuploidy in the general population could be around 7 per cent [20]. Recent studies have shown that smoking and alcohol consumption are associated with an increased risk of sperm aneuploidy[21,22]. Persons exposed to heavy air pollution have an elevated level of sperm with an extra Y-chromosome, although other seminal parameters such as sperm density remained unchanged[23]. Reproductive toxicants such as pesticides may affect the normal disjunction of chromosomes during meiosis altering the number of chromosomes in sperm nuclei. Such spermatozoa upon fertilization can yield embryo with chromosomal abnormality, which may be a cause for recurrent pregnancy loss. Other factors, which are associated with sperm aneuploidy, are listed in Table 5.2.

Table 5.2: Possible Environmental Factors Associated with Sperm Aneuploidy Risk in Human

Factor	*Example*	*Reference*
Smoking	Disomy of chromosome 13	Shi *et al.*, 2001[22]
Alcohol	XX18 aneuploidy, XY 18-18 diploidy	Robbins 2003[24]
Radiation	Numerical and structural chromosomal aberrations	Martin *et al.*, 1986[25]
Chemotherapeutic agents	Sex chromosomal and autosomal aneuploidy	Robbins *et al.*, 1997[24]
Pesticides	Sex chromosome disomy	Padungtod *et al.*, 1999[26]

The chromatin in mammalian spermatozoa is extremely compact and stable and, differs substantially from the chromatin of somatic cells. A substantial number of studies have been conducted to analyze the integrity of DNA in human sperm and have yielded important information on the possible relationship of sperm DNA damage with defective sperm function and male infertility[27]. Reactive oxygen species (ROS) are the major cause for sperm DNA damage[28] which can lead to the functional and/or structural alteration of DNA[29]. High sperm DNA damage and increased level of ROS has been detected in the seminal plasma of men occupationally exposed to pesticides, organic solvents, radiation, heat and heavy metals.

DNA fragmentation is an excellent marker for exposure to potential reproductive toxicants and a diagnostic/prognostic tool for potential male infertility. The most popular assays to detect DNA fragmentation are single cell gel electrophoresis (SCGE or comet assay), terminal deoxynucleotidyl transferase (TdT) nick end-labeling assay (TUNEL) and sperm chromatin structure assay (SCSA)[30,31]. Relationship between the DNA damage assessment using above methods and defective fertilizing ability have been demonstrated[18].

Seminal Plasma

Toxic agents can reach the ejaculate via testicular plasma, epididymal plasma, secretions of vas deferens and ampullary secretions and secretory fluids of seminal vesicles and other accessory glands. Toxic metals like Pb and Cd, chlorinated pesticides like DDT, DDE, endosulfan, and aldrin are detected in human semen. High level of Cd, nicotin and several polycyclic aromatic hydrocarbons are identified in semen of heavy smokers. The level of these toxic agents in semen had inverse relationship with semen quality.

Occupational Exposures

Pesticides

Pesticide exposure has been associated with considerable changes in semen parameters suggesting that the testicle is one of the most vulnerable organs to pesticides. Much of the research about reproductive health among occupationally exposed workers was prompted by the discovery of the testicular toxicity of dibromochloropropane (DBCP) among agricultural workers or workers in a pesticide factory. Among this population, a wide range of negative reproductive effect ranging from azoospermia and oligospermia, damage of germinal epithelium, genetic alterations in the sperm, reduced fertility and increased risk of spontaneous abortions among wives[32, 33] was observed. The reproductive toxicity of BDCP is mainly due to altered androgen production in Leydig cells. A large number of subsequent studies on men exposed to different pesticides like Ethylene dibromide (EDB), carbaryl, DDT, chlordecone, endosulfan etc. further confirmed its negative influence on semen quality. Carbaryl is a broad spectrum insecticide which can be readily absorbed through the human skin, especially scrotum. Human studies among exposed workers have shown inconsistent results. Some studies have shown that carbaryl exposure does not have any influence on testicular function[34]. However, increased level of morphologically abnormal sperm was observed in workers of Carbaryl production area by Wyrobek *et al.*[35] which may be due to the genetic damage caused by the insecticide. A reduction in sperm motility and count was observed in fertile men from agrarian area compared to fertile men from urban area[36] suggesting the possible effect of pesticides.

Many pesticides, such as DDT and chlordecone, are persistent in the environment and/or bioaccumulate in the food chain. DDT, its metabolite Dichlorodiphenyl-dichloroethylene (DDE) and chlordecone act as endocrine disruptors. DDT is a well-known pesticide widely used to control insects on agricultural crops, to control head lice and to kill insects carrying diseases such as typhus and malaria. The presence of DDE in the environment is primarily the consequence of the breakdown of DDT. The two most recent studies carried out in Mexico and South Africa enrolled men with high environmental exposures and both demonstrated strong associations between serum concentrations of *p,p*2 -DDE and various measures of sperm motility[37,38]. Men who are chronically exposed to chlordecone havebeen found to have decreased sperm motility[39] but no effect on fertility was observed[40]. These persistent pesticides have an effect on chromatin integrity of spermatozoa. In European men exposed to PCB and DDE, a negative correlation between their blood level and sperm chromatin was noted[41].

Exposure to multiple pesticides is common among farmers who mix and spray the pesticides to improve their crop. A decrease in sperm concentration, motility, and altered morphology is observed in most of the studies conducted on men exposed to multiple herbicides, insecticides or fungicides[42–44]. In male cotton filed workers exposed to mixture of pesticides such as endosulfan, organophosphorous pesticides (malathion, methyl-parathion), DDT, BHC, synthetic pyrethroids (fenvelarate, cypermethrin) a high abortion rate, congenital anomalies and still births were observed[45]. A non-significant change in sperm morphology, motility and vitality was observed in Danish pesticide spraying farmers[46]. However, in another study conducted on Danish ornamental flower greenhouse workers, sperm density and motility was found to decrease with increasing duration of work in the greenhouses[43]. It is difficult to identify the causative agent for reproductive disorder in case of multiple pesticide exposure. Prenatal exposure to pesticide may have an adverse effect on male reproductive function. Female greenhouse workers with confirmed pesticide exposure during pregnancy gave birth to boys with smaller penises and testicles, lower serum concentrations of testosterone and inhibin B, higher serum concentrations of SHBG and FSH, and higher LH:testosterone ratio than unexposed workers suggesting an adverse effect of pesticides on Leydig cells and Sertoli cells[47].

Assessment of occupational or environmental exposure to pesticides is extremely complicated, as a large number of chemicals and circumstances are involved. The majority of semen quality studies use a cross-sectional design that has several severe limitations such as selection bias due to differential participation and lack of information about the time dimension of the cause–effect relation. Therefore, it is no surprise that the results from recent studies are inconsistent concerning the effects of pesticide exposure on semen quality (Table 5.3).

Metals

Effect of metals on the reproductive function has been studied extensively. The reproductive toxicity of few metals such as lead, mercury and cadmium has been studied extensively. However, the reports on toxic effects of manganese, chromium, nickel, magnesium etc. are scanty (Table 5.4).

Lead

Lead is a highly toxic heavy metal which has an adverse effect on both male and female reproductive system. Exposure to a concentration in the range of 40- 60mg/dl of blood was considered safe by occupational health standards[61]. However, few studies have shown that there is an increased risk of finding decrease in semen quality[62] and reduced fertility[63]. A study performed in Yugoslavia observed that semen quality deteriorates even when the PbB level is in the range of 30-40pg/dl[64]. Decrease in seminal volume, sperm density, motility, viability and morphology, and increased frequency of spontaneous abortion is commonly observed in men exposed to lead[65–67].

Plausible mechanisms for impaired spermatogenesis are a direct effect on testicular function or an effect mediated by hormonal imbalances. A decreased testosterone and increased FSH and LH levels were observed in men occupationally exposed to lead[63]. Increased lipid peroxidation in seminal plasma was observed in men with >40mg/dl of lead[66]. Lead either affects DNA synthesis in precursors of the spermatozoa or interferes with the normal replacement of nuclear histones by cysteine rich protamines during sperm chromatin condensation. Lead has been shown to bind firmly with thiol groups present on cysteine residues in protamines in competition with zinc[68]. Moreover, in humans zinc contributes to

Table 5.3: Semen Quality in Men Exposed to Pesticides

Pesticide	*Semen Quality*	*Reference*
DDT	Negative association between serum DDT and sperm count	Dalvie *et al.*, 2004[48]
	Oligospermia and asthenospermia	Aneck-Hahn *et al.*, 2007[37]
	Abnormal sperm motion, tail defect	de Jager *et al.*, 2006[38]
Fenvalerate	Reduction in sperm count	
	Increased liquefaction time, abnormal sperm motion pattern	Lifeng *et al.*, 2006[49]
	Abnormal morphology, sperm chromosomal aberrations	Xia *et al.*, 2004[50]
	Low count, abnormal sperm motion pattern	Tan *et al.*, 2002[51]
	High sperm DNA damage	Bian *et al.*, 2004[52]
Carbaryl	Abnormal sperm morphology	Wyrobek *et al.*, 1981[35]
	Abnormal morphology, sperm DNA damage, sperm chromosomal aberration	Xia *et al.*, 2005[53]
	Low seminal volume, abnormal sperm motion pattern, abnormal morphology	Tan *et al.*, 2005[54]
Organophosphate	Low seminal volume, low motility and abnormal morphology	Yucra *et al.*, 2006[44]
	No association	Sanchez-Pena *et al.*, 2004[55]
	Sperm aneuploidy	Recio *et al.*, 2001[56]
DBCP	Oligospermia	Whorton *et al.*, 1977[57]
	Atrophy of seminiferous epithelium	Potashnik *et al.*, 1979[58]
	Elevated levels of FSH, LH, low sperm count	Mattison *et al.*, 1990[59]
Multiple pesticide exposure	Reduced sperm count, low testosterone level	Abell *et al.*, 2000[43]
	Reduced semen volume, high abnormal sperm morphology	Bigelow *et al.*, 1998[42]
	No significant change	Larsen *et al.*, 1998[46], Tielemans *et al.*, 1999[60]

Table 5.4: Effect of Different Metal Exposure on Semen Quality[85]

Metal	*Industry*	*Semen Quality*	*Reference*
Cadmium	Battery, electrical and metallic industries	Decrease in sperm motility	Dawson *et al.*, 1998[86]
		Asthenoteratozoospermia, decrease in fertilizing ability	Omu *et al.*, 1995[77]
Chromium	Metallurgical industries	Change in reproductive hormone, reduced sperm morphology	Li *et al.*, 1999[87]
		Decrease in sperm count, motility, morphology	Danadevi *et al.*, 2003[81]
Lead	Battery, electrical and metallic industries	Reduced sperm count	Chowdhury *et al.*, 1986[88]
		Reduced count, motility and morphology	Lancranjan *et al.*, 1975[67]
		Decrease in sperm count, no alteration in motility, morphology and hormones	Alexander *et al.*, 1996[89]
		Decreased seminal and prostatic function, decrease sperm chromatin stability	Wildt *et al.*, 1983[65]
		Decrease in sperm count, low protamine level	Quintanilla-Vega *et al.*, 2000[69]
Manganese	Foundries	Reduction in sperm motility, concentration	Wirth *et al.*, 2007[90]
		Longer liquefaction time, reduction in seminal volume, sperm count and viability	Wu *et al.*, 1996[91]
Mercury	Chemical industries	Tubular atrophy, sertoli cell only syndrome	Keck *et al.*, 1993[92]
		Abnormal sperm morphology, decrease in sperm motility	Choy *et al.*, 2002[73]
		No association	Rignell-Hydbom *et al.*, 2007[74]
Nickel	Welders	Sperm tail defect	Danadevi *et al.*, 2003[81]

sperm chromatin stability and binds to protamine P2. It has recently been shown that lead competes with zinc and binds human protamine 2 causing conformational changes in the protein[69]. This decreases the concentration of DNA protamine 2 binding which probably results in alterations in sperm chromatin condensation.

Mercury

Studies in humans have reported a negative influence of MeHg on human male reproduction. Infertile[70] and subfertile[71] men have been found to have higher MeHg levels than fertile men. Sertoli cell only syndrome and tubular atrophy has been observed among infertile patients with MeHg exposure[72]. Moreover, mercury seminal fluid levels have been found to correlate with abnormal sperm morphology and abnormal sperm motility[73]. However, Rignell-Hydbom *et al.*[74] did not find any associations between MeHg exposure and semen quality or quantity in Swedish fishermen exposed to methyl mercury.

Cadmium

Cadmium is a non-essential toxic element. It has toxic effect on many enzymes dependent on iron as a co-factor, one of these being cytochrome P450[75]. Leydig cells have ten times higher level of P450 than Sertoli cells, hence are more sensitive to increased Cd level[76]. Since cytochrome P450 is required for the functioning of 17-α-hydroxylase and 17-20 lyase, its disruption may well interfere with testicular steroidogenesis. Major changes in the levels of toxic elements in seminal fluid have been related to abnormal spermatozoa function and fertilizing capacity[77]. Exposure of men to even a moderate level of Cd (<10mg/L in blood) can lead to increase in abnormal sperm morphology[78]. Both cadmium and lead induce male reproductive toxicity through their interaction with Zn. Omu *et al.*[77] detected a significantly high level of Cd in serum of men who were smokers and implicated this metal as one of the causes of asthenoteratozoospermia.

Chromium

Studies suggesting the effect of chromium on semen quality are very scanty. The people working in metallurgic industries and welders are exposed to high levels of chromium along with the fumes from other metals, solvents, and heat. Adverse effect on sperm quality and fertility was observed in welders[79, 80]. Decline in sperm count, motility and increased percentage of morphologically abnormal sperm were observed in Indian welders exposed to chromium and nickel[81]. An increased risk of early abortion was observed in wives of stainless steel welders[82]. On the contrary, few studies fail to find any association between chromium level in blood and sperm quality[83]. Prolonged exposure to chromium can cause genomic instability in peripheral lymphocytes of stainless steel welders[84].

Solvents

Organic solvents have a wide range of applications in industry and are one of the most common occupational chemical toxicants. Because of the high volatility of the organic hydrocarbons, people who work in the industry are more prone to get exposed to these solvents either through breathe or through skin. Adverse reproductive outcomes such as spontaneous abortions in wives and congenital defects and childhood cancers were reported in children of men exposed to organic solvents. Occupational exposure to solvents involves several compounds, which makes it difficult to study the effect of a single compound. The available data suggest that a number of solvents used in industries can affect male reproductive function (2-EE, 2-ME, 2-bromopropane, carbon disulphide), while the evidence for others is more limited (Table 5.5).

Glycol ethers are an important group of organic solvents widely used as constituents of paint, glue, dyes, thinners and printing ink. The semen quality of painters, chemical industry workers, metal casters and semiconductor industry workers was found to be poor[92]. Carbon disulphide, which is mainly used in the manufacture of viscose rayon fibres, in the production of carbon tetrachloride and in analytical chemistry has been reported to cause decreased libido and loss of potency[93] and poor semen quality[94]. Men working in plastic production plant are prone to acetone and styrene exposure and exhibit altered sperm morphology and reduced sperm motility[95]. However, a European multi-centre study did not find any deterioration in semen quality and time to pregnancy (TTP) in men exposed to styrene in various industries in several European countries [96].

Exposure to degreasers such as trichloroethylene and tetrachloroethylene causes a reduction in sperm motility,

Table 5.5: Semen Findings of Men Exposed to Solvents

Solvent	*Semen Quality*	*Reference*
2- deoxy ethanol	Oligospermia	Welch *et al.*, 1988[92]
Ethylene dibromide	Decreased semen volume, high pH, decrease in motility and viability	Schrader *et al.*, 1988[101]
	Decrease in sperm count, motility, viability and morphology	Ratcliffe *et al.*, 1987[8]
Carbon disulfide	Oligo, astheno, teratospermia	Lancranjan 1972[7]
	Decreased libido, no change in semen quality and fertility	Vanhoorne *et al.*, 1994[102]
2-bromopropane	Reduced sperm count and motility	Kim *et al.*, 1996[99]
Styrene	Reduced sperm count	Kolstad *et al.*, 1999[96]
	High sperm DNA damage	Migliore *et al.*, 2002[103]
	Sperm chromosomal aberration	Naccarati *et al.*, 2003[104]

morphology[97] and prolonged TTP[98]. The effect of some compounds has only received limited interest; 2-bromopropane used as a substitute for Freon decreased semen quality among six out of eight male South Korean workers[99]. Likewise, trinitrotoluene is used in production of explosives and workers have been found to have decreased sperm motility and morphology[100].

Endocrine Disruptors and Semen Quality

Endocrine disrupting chemicals are synthetic and naturally occurring chemicals characterized by their ability to mimic the effects of endogenous hormones. Exposure to endocrine-disrupting chemicals may occur through environmental routes (air, soil, water, food) or via occupational exposures. Reported decrease in sperm concentration in the overall population and deterioration of sperm motility and morphology in patients seeking infertility treatment led to the hypothesis that "xeno-estrogens" in the environment are negative factors for male fertility[105]. The adverse effect of these agents may be due to their hormone mimicking action, antagonistic effect on endogenous hormones, effect on steroidogenic enzyme expression and/or activity and alteration of circulating hormone levels.

Pesticides

As pesticides comprise a large number of different substances with dissimilar structures and diverse toxicity, some pesticides may directly affect spermatogenesis, for instance, by changing the structure or motility of spermatozoa, damaging the spermatogonia, or destructing Sertoli cells, whereas most other pesticides act indirectly through endocrine disruption. In the literature, several mechanisms are discussed, but interference with hormone receptor recognition and binding is most often mentioned. Through this mechanism, pesticides may interact with the steroid hormone family of nuclear estrogen receptors and androgen receptors, which are both widely distributed in male reproductive tissues. Nevertheless, endocrine disruption by pesticides may also occur in other stages of hormonal regulation involving mechanisms such as hormone synthesis, transport, and clearance, post-receptor activation, thyroid function, and central nervous system (Table 5.6).

Phthalates

Phthalate esters are abundant industrial chemicals used in the production of plastics and are present in many personal care

Table 5.6: Endocrine Disruptors and Semen Quality

Endocrine Disruptor	*Semen Quality*	*Reference*
PCB	No associationIncreased sperm	Hauser *et al.*, 2003[126], Rignell-Hydbom *et al.*, 2007[74]
	DNA fragmentation index	Spano *et al.*, 2005[41]
	Decreased sperm count, low progressive motility	Dallinga *et al.*, 2002[127]
	Reduced sperm motility	Toft *et al.*, 2006[128]
Phthalate	Sperm DNA fragmentation, mitochondrial depolarization, increased ROS	Pant *et al.*, 2008[129]
	Delayed liquefaction time, normal sperm count, motility, viability	Zhang *et al.*, 2006[130]
	Decrease in sperm motility	Hauser *et al.*, 2005[111]
Phytoestrogens	Oligospermia	West *et al.*, 2005[131]
	High sperm DNA damage	West 2007[132]
	Early acrosomal loss	Fraser *et al.*, 2006[133]
Tobacco smoke	High sperm DNA damage	Shen *et al.*, 1997[134]
	Smoking related adducts in sperm DNA	Fraga *et al.*, 1996[135]

products including cosmetics[106]. Exposure to diethyl hexyl and dibutyl phthalates is associated with adverse effects on sperm motility[107]. Animal studies consistently demonstrated that phthalate esters are male reproductive toxicants[108, 109], with exposure associated with testicular atrophy, spermatogenetic cell loss, and damage to the Sertoli cell population. Phthalate monoesters target Sertoli cell functions in supporting the spermatogenesis process[110]. This may be due to the effect of phthalates in reducing the ability of Sertoli cells to respond to FSH[111]. A randomized controlled study of men with unexplained infertility reported a negative correlation between seminal plasma phthalate ester concentration and sperm morphology[112]. Environmental phthalate levels (range 9.8 to 5396.2 [ng/ml] ppb), measured by urinary metabolite MEP concentrations, were reported to be associated with increased DNA damage in sperm[113]. Similarly, reductions in sperm motility and morphology exhibited a dose-dependence on urinary MBP levels and MBzP levels in infertility patients. Urinary levels of monomethyl phthalate (MMP; 7.5 ng/ml) were weakly associated with poor sperm morphology[114]. In contrast, another study examining urinary phthalate metabolites in 234 young Swedish men demonstrated no association with decreased semen parameters for MEHP, MBP, and MBzP levels.

Polychlorinated Biphenyls

Polychlorinated biphenyls are members of a large family of widely used chemicals that have become ubiquitous environmental contaminants. Commercial production of PCBs commenced in 1929 in the United States, and the resulting products were marketed according to their chlorine content (Aroclor 1221, 1252, and 1260, for example). They have been used in a wide variety of applications including plasticizers, pesticide extenders, adhesives, cutting oils, and flame retardants. They are perhaps best known for their use in heat transfer fluids and dielectric fluids for transformers and capacitors. PCBs are very stable compounds that resist degradation and are lipophilic; thus they bioaccumulate in the food chain. They were first identified as a potential environmental hazard in 1966 by Jensen[115] and were subsequently shown to cause complete reproductive failure in mink. A significant decrease in progressive sperm motility, with increase in blood PCB level has been observed by several workers[116, 117] (Guo *et al.*, 2000, Bonde *et al.*, 2008). Rignell and Hydbom *et al.*[118] observed a slight negative impact of PCB and DDE on sperm chromatin integrity in Swedish fishermen.

Phytoestrogens

Phytoestrogens are nonsteroidal plant-derived compounds with potent estrogenic activity. Human exposure to phytoestrogens includes consumption of soy and soy products and diets high in farmed fish, as soy byproducts high in genistein are a major component of commercial fish diets[119]. Phytoestrogens exert their action by interacting with Estrogen receptor (ER) and progesterone receptor (PR), thereby inducing weak estrogenic and antiestrogenic actions[120, 121]. Isoflavonoids and lignans exert an inhibitory action on steroidogenic enzymes such as 5a-reductase, thereby reducing the conversion of testosterone to the active form DHT[122]. A number of phytoestrogens, including lignans, isoflavonoids daidzein and equol, enterolactone, and genistein, were found to induce SHBG production in the liver[123, 124].

The effects of short-term phytoestrogen supplementation on semen quality and endocrine function were examined in a group of young, healthy males by Mitchell *et al.*[121]. There was no significant difference in testicular volume, testosterone, FSH, LH or E2 compared to the control group. However, Chavarro *et al.*[125] observed that soy food and isoflavone intake has a negative correlation with semen quality in men attending the infertility clinic. To date, evidence linking dietary consumption of phytoestrogens and reduced semen quality is insufficient and requires further study.

Radiation

Testicular tissue is highly sensitive to ionizing radiation. Individuals at increased risk include workers in nuclear power stations, radiation health workers, military personnel and radioactive disposal units. There is also risk to the patients overexposed to the therapeutic dose or repeated diagnostic radiological investigations. A radiation dose in the range of 0.15 Gy may temporarily reduce the sperm counts, while 2 Gy may result in long-lasting or permanent azoospermia[136]. Clifton and Bremner[137] conducted a study on prisoners who volunteered for testicular X-irradiation. Decrease in sperm count was evident in men exposed to a dose of 0.11Gy and permanent sterility was observed in men exposed to a dose of 3 to 5 Gy. A study conducted on Japanese

Table 5.6: Semen Quality and Exposure to Physical Factors

Subjects	*Semen Quality*	*Reference*
Exposure to computers	No association	Sun *et al.*, 2005[142]
Radiofrequency heater operators	Non-significant change in semen quality and hormone level	Grajewski *et al.*, 2000[143]
Radar operators	Low sperm count	Weyandt *et al.*, 1996[144]
	Non-significant reduction in sperm count	Hjollund *et al.*, 1997[145]
	No change in semen quality	Schrader *et al.*, 1997[146]
	Reduced sperm motility, abnormal morphology	Ye *et al.*, 2007[147]
Microwave operators	Reduction in sperm count, motility and morphology	Lancranjan *et al.*, 1975[141]
Salvage workers in nuclear reactor	Altered sperm morphology, decrease in motility, impaired fertility potential	Bartoov *et al.*, 1997[139], Fischbein *et al.*, 1997[148]
Cell phone	Decrease in progressively motile sperm	Fejes *et al.*, 2005[149]
	Decrease in count, motility, viability and morphology	Agarwal *et al.*, 2008[150]
Ozone	Decrease in sperm count	Sokol *et al.*, 2005[151]

fishermen exposed to radioactive fallout (dose of 1.4 to 6 Gy for 14 days) in 1954 observed a severe depletion in sperm count, which reversed 2 years after the exposure[138].

An occupational exposure limit of 15 mSv/year has been adopted in several countries, and if this limit is not exceeded, testicular effects are unlikely. Apparent testicular effects of high-frequency electromagnetic radiation (HHF, 300 kHz–300 000 MHz including radar exposure and microwaves) that have been observed in earlier studies may result from testicular heating. So far, no consistent evidence indicates that non-ionizing radiation interferes with male reproductive function unless the amount of energy is sufficient to disrupt testicular temperature regulation. The salvage workers who had worked at the Chernobyl nuclear reactor accident site or in the vicinity thereof were found to manifest ultra-morphologic abnormalities in the sperm nucleus and to have impaired fertility potential seven years after the radiation exposure[139]. A significant reduction in sperm count was observed in military radar operators exposed to high frequency electromagnetic radiation[140] and men exposed to microwave[141].

Smoking

The effect of smoking on semen quality has been investigated in a number of cross-sectional studies, most of which have included infertility patients and are conflicting[152–154]. Lower semen quality in terms of the conventional semen characteristics was observed in normal, healthy smokers compared to non-smokers. Among the infertile men who visited IVF clinic smokers had 15 per cent lower sperm concentration and 18 per cent lower total sperm count than non-smokers[152]. However, a study conducted by Jensen *et al.*[154] on young men from 5 different European countries did not observe any association between smoking and semen quality. Several studies suggested that semen quality had a negative correlation with the number of cigarettes smoked per day[155–158].

An inverse relationship between cotinine (the major nicotine metabolite) in seminal plasma and sperm concentration, motility, morphology or total sperm count has been demonstrated[159–160]. The effect of prenatal exposure to tobacco smoke on male reproductive development and semen quality is still clearly not understood. Jensen *et al.*[154] hypothesized that there is a stronger association of prenatal exposure and poor semen quality than current smoking and that the association between current smoking and decreased semen quality may be confounded by the prenatal exposure. Among 1770 young men from five European countries, current smoking had no independent effect on semen quality, whereas prenatally exposed men had 20 per cent lower sperm concentration and a 25 per cent lower total sperm count compared with prenatally unexposed men[154].

Tobacco smoke can cause DNA damage or chromosomal damage in human germinal cells and spermatozoa[161]. Cigarette smoke constituents and their DNA reactive intermediates react directly with spermatozoa. High concentration of 8-OHdG, an oxidative lesion of Guanine, is found in seminal plasma of smokers with a concomitant increase in cotinine level[134,135]. Smoking related adducts in spermatozoa arise from oxidative DNA damage. Sun *et al.*[162] observed a high proportion of spermatozoa with DNA damage in male smokers recruited for assisted conception compared to non-smokers. DNA adducts in spermatozoa are potential source of transmissible prezygotic damage. A 3.7 fold increase in Benzo[a]pyrene concentration was observed in blastomeres of embryos derived from men who were smokers[163]. Paternal transmission of altered DNA can compromise the embryo development *in utero* resulting in failed implantation.

Alcohol

Impotence, testicular atrophy, gynecomastia, loss of sexual interest and erectile dysfunction are often associated with chronic alcoholism in men. Structural changes in the testicular tissue and decrease in the testicular and serum levels of testosterone is a common feature in alcoholic men. It increases the metabolic clearance rate of testosterone concomitant with an increase in hepatic 5a-reductase activity and increases conversion of androgens into estrogens. Ethanol and its metabolite acetaldehyde acts as Leydig cell toxin[164] and inhibit LH binding to Leydig cells, an inhibition of the enzymes responsible for the formation of sex hormones[165, 166]. Van Thiel *et al.*[164] demonstrated that ethanol acts as a Leydig cell toxin.

In chronic alcohol consumers a reduction in seminal volume, sperm concentration a decrease in percentage of spermatozoa with normal morphology has been observed[167, 168]. Goverde *et al.*[169] observed that daily consumption of alcohol decreases normal sperm morphology, irreversible tail defect and a significant decrease in the percentage of motility[170]. A recent study found an association between maternal alcohol consumption and risk of cryptorchidism[171]. Smoking plus alcohol may further deteriorate the semen quality.

Heat

The testes are located outside the body to keep temperature 2-4°C below the core temperature, and it is well known that internal heating as in fever and external heating for short periods of time may result in a dramatic but temporary decrease of sperm count and other aspects of semen quality after a delay of some 6–8 weeks[172]. Several studies observed a reduced sperm count among foundry workers, ceramics workers, bakers[173] welders[174], and increased morphological defects in male taxi drivers[175]. It is now well documented that the sedentary work position is associated with an increased scrotal temperature. Men sitting at work for 8 h a day have on average 0.7°C increased scrotal temperature during the day in comparison with employees with <8 h in the sedentary body position[176]. Although an increase of scrotal temperature of this order of magnitude might be sufficient to impair spermatogenesis, reduced sperm count seems not related to sedentary work[177,178]. Wearing tight underwear and trousers could increase testicular temperature. However, there are no convincing data to prove this.

Stress

Occupational stress and burn-out have been related to impotence, sham ejaculation, retrograde ejaculation, and reduced semen quality[179,180]. Physical stress leads to low testosterone level probably due to a reduction in LH pulse frequency. Studies have shown higher stress levels among infertile men than among fertile controls[181]. A study conducted by Giblin *et al.*[182] on healthy volunteers found that stress was negatively correlated with the proportion of normal sperm. However few other studies fail to draw any association between stress and semen quality[183,184].

Geographical Variation in Semen Quality

Geographical variation in semen quality is reported in many regions including France[185], the Nordic countries[186], the United States[187], and Canada[188]. Semen parameters are demonstrated to fluctuate with the environmental temperature and/or season, geographical and circannual variation[189]. Observed geographic variation in semen quality may be representative of differential exposures to environmental factors, including climate (temperature, sunlight), endocrine disrupters and other environmental chemicals, and regional differences in lifestyle (diet, exercise, alcohol/drug use).

References

1. Bonde JP, Giwercman A, Ernst E. Identifying environmental risk to male reproductive function by occupational sperm studies: logistics and design options. Occup Environ Med 1996; 53:511-9.
2. Nelson CMK, Bunge RG. Semen analysis: evidence for changing parameters of male fertility potential. Fertil Steril 1974; 25:503-7.
3. Leto S, Frensilli FJ. Changing parameters of donor semen. Fertil Steril 1981; 36:766-70.
4. Bostofte E, Serup J, Rebbe H. Has the fertility of Danish men declined through the years in terms of semen quality? A comparison of semen qualities between 1952 and 1972. Int J Fertil 1983; 28:91-5.
5. Osser S, Liedholm P, Ranstam J. Depressed semen quality: a study over two decades. Arch Androl 1984; 12:113-6.
6. Menkveld R, Van Zyl JA, Kotze TJW, Joubert G. Possible changes in male fertility over a 15-year period. Arch Androl 1986; 17:43-4.
7. Bendvold E. Semen quality in Norwegian men over a 20-year period. Int J Fertil 1989; 34:401-4.
8. Carlsen E, Giwercman A, Keiding N, Skakkebaek NE. Evidence for decreasing quality of semen during past 50 years. British Med J 1992; 305:609-13.
9. Jouannet P, Wang C, Eustache F, Kold-Jensen T, Auger J. Semen quality and male reproductive health: The controversy about human sperm concentration decline. Acta Pathologica, Microbiologica et Immunologica Scandinavica 2001; 109: 333-344.
10. World Health Organization. WHO laboratory manual. 4th ed. Cambridge, UK: Cambridge University Press, 1999.

11. Chia SE, Lim ST, Tay SK, Lim ST. Factors associated with male infertility a case-control study of 218 infertile and 240 fertile men. British J Obs and Gyne 2000; 107:55–61.

12. Jensen TK, Toppari J, Keiding N, Skakkebaek NE. Do environmental estrogens contribute to the decline in male reproductive health? Clin Chem 1995; 41: 1896–1901.

13. Toth GP, Wang SR, McCarthy H, Tocco DR, Smith MK. Effects of three male reproductive toxicants on rat cauda epididymal sperm motion. Reprod Toxicol 1992; 6: 507-15.

14. Baccetti B, Capitani S, Collodel G, Di Cairano G, Gambera L, Moretti E, Piomboni P. Genetic sperm defects and consanguinity. Hum Reprod 2001; 16: 1365- 71.

15. Letz G. Male reproductive toxicology. In: Occupational Medicine (LaDou J, ed). Norwalk, CT:Appleton and Lange Publisher, 1990;288–96.

16. Mohamed MK, Burbacher TM, Mottet NK. Effects of methyl mercury on testicular functions in Macaca fascicularis monkeys. Pharmacol Toxicol 1987; 60:29–36.

17. Hilderbrand DC, Der R, Griffin WT, Fahim MS. Effect of lead acetate on reproduction. Am J Obstet Gynecol 1973; 115:1058–1065.

18. Morris ID, Ilott S, Dixon L, Brison DR. The spectrum of DNA damage in human sperm assessed by single cell gel electrophoresis (Comet assay) and its relationship to fertilization and embryo development. Hum Reprod 2002; 17:990-8.

19. Larson KL, DeJonge CJ, Barnes AM, Jost LK, Evenson DP. Sperm chromatin structure assay parameters as predictors of failed pregnancy following assisted reproductive techniques. Hum Reprod 2000; 15:1717-22.

20. Vidal F, Blanco J, Egozcue J. Chromosomal abnormalities in sperm. Mol Cell Endocrinol 2001; 22 (Suppl 1): S51–S54.

21. Robbins WA, Vine MF, Truany KY, Everson RB. Use of fluorescence *in situ* hybridization (FISH) to assess effects of smoking, caffeine, and alcholol and aneuploidy load in sperm of healthy men. Environ. Mol Mutagens 1997; 30:175–83.

22. Shi Q, Ko E, Barclay L, Hoang T, Rademaker A, Martin R. Cigarette smoking and aneuploidy in human sperm. Mol Reprod Dev 2001; 59:417–21.

23. Selevan SG, Borkovec L, Slott VL, Zudova Z, Rubes J, Evenson DP, Perreault SD. Semen quality and reproductive health of young Czech men exposed to seasonal air pollution. Environ Health Perspect 2000; 108:887–94.

24. Robbins WA. FISH (fluorescence *in situ* hybridization) to detect effects of smoking, caffeine, and alcohol on human sperm chromosomes. Adv Exp Med Biol. 2003; 518:59-72.

25. Martin RH, Hildebrand K, Yamamoto J, Rademaker A, Barnes M, Douglas G, Arthur K, Ringrose T, Brown IS. An increased frequency of human sperm chromosomal abnormalities after radiotherapy. Mutat Res 1986; 174:219-25.

26. Padungtod C, Hassold TJ, Millie E, Ryan LM, Savitz DA, Christiani DC, Xu X. Sperm aneuploidy among Chinese pesticide factory workers: scoring by the FISH method. Am J Ind Med 1999; 36:230-8.

27. Shen HM, Ong CN. Detection of oxidative DNA damage in human sperm and its association with sperm function and male infertility. Free Radic Biol Med 2000; 28:529-36.

28. Griveau JF, Le Lannou D. Reactive oxygen species and human spermatozoa: physiology and pathology. Int J Androl 1997; 20:61–9.

29. Ames BN, Shigenaga MK, Hagen TM. Oxidants, antioxidants and the degenerative disease and aging. Proc Natl Acad Sci USA 1993; 90:7915–22.

30. Sailer BL, Jost LK, Evenson DP. Mammalian sperm DNA susceptibility to in situ denaturation associated with the presence of DNA strand breaks as measured by the terminal deoxynucleotidyl transferase assay. J Androl 1995; 16:80–7.

31. Hughes CM, Lewis SEM, McKelvey-Martin VJ, Thompson WA. Comparison of baseline and induced DNA damage in human spermatozoa from fertile and infertile men, using a modified comet assay. Mol Hum Reprod 1996; 2:613–19.

32. Goldsmith JR, Potashnik G, Israeli R. Reproductive outcomes in families of DBCP-exposed men. Arch Environ Health 1984; 39:85–9.

33. Potashnik G, Yanai-Inbar I. Dibromochloropropane (DBCP): an 8-year reevaluation of testicular function and reproductive performance. Fertil Steril 1987; 47:317–23.

34. Whorton MD, Milby TH, Stubbs HA, Avashia BH, Hull EQ. Testicular function among carbaryl-exposed exployees. J Toxicol Environ Health 1979; 5:929–41.

35. Wyrobek AJ, Watchmaker G, Gordon L, Wong K, Moore D, Whorton D. Sperm shape abnormalities in carbaryl-exposed employees. Environ Health Perspect 1981; 40:255–65.

36. Swan SH, Kruse RL, Liu F, Barr DB, Drobnis EZ, Redmon JB, Wang C, Brazil C, Overstreet JW; Study for Future Families Research Group. Semen quality in relation to biomarkers of pesticide exposure. Environ Health Perspect 2003; 111:1478–84.

37. Aneck-Hahn NH, Schulenburg GW, Bornman MS, Farias P, de Jager C. Impaired semen quality associated with environmental DDT exposure in young men living in a malaria area in the Limpopo Province, South Africa. J Androl 2007; 28:423-34.

38. de Jager C, Farias P, Barraza-Villarreal A, Avila MH, Ayotte P, Dewailly E, Dombrowski C, Rousseau F, Sanchez VD, Bailey JL. Reduced seminal parameters associated with environmental DDT exposure and p,p'-DDE concentrations in men in Chiapas, Mexico: a cross-sectional study. J Androl 2006; 27:16-27.

39. Cannon SB, Veazey JM Jr, Jackson RS, Burse VW, Hayes C, Straub WE, Landrigan PJ, Liddle JA. Epidemic kepone poisoning in chemical workers. Am J Epidemiol 1978; 107:529–37.

40. Taylor JR. Neurological manifestations in humans exposed to chlordecone: follow-up results. Neurotoxicol 1985; 6:231–36.

41. Spano M, Toft G, Hagmar L, Eleuteri P, Rescia M, Rignell-Hydbom A, Tyrkiel E, Zvyezday V, Bonde JP; INUENDO. Exposure to PCB and p,p'-DDE in European and Inuit populations: impact on human sperm chromatin integrity. Hum Reprod 2005; 12:3488–99.

42. Bigelow PL, Jarrell J, Young MR, Keefe TJ, Love EJ. Association of semen quality and occupational factors: comparison of case-control analysis and analysis of continuous variables. Fertil Steril 1998; 69:11–8.

43. Abell A, Ernst E, Bonde JP. Semen quality and sexual hormones in greenhouse workers. Scand J Work Environ Health 2000; 26:492–500.

44. Yucra S, Rubio J, Gasco M, Gonzales C, Steenland K, Gonzales G. Semen quality and reproductive sex hormone levels in Peruvian pesticide sprayers. Int J Occup Environ Health 2006; 12:355–61.

45. Rupa DS, ReddyPP, Reddy OS. Reproductive performance in population exposed to pesticides in cotton fields in India. Environ Res 1991; 55:123–28.

46. Larsen SB, Joffe M, Bonde JP. Time to pregnancy and exposure to pesticides in Danish farmers. Asclepios Study Group. Occup Environ Med 1998; 55:278–83.

47. Andersen HR, Schmidt IM, Grandjean P, Jensen TK, Budtz-Jørgensen E, Kjærstad MB, Bælum J, Nielsen JB, Skakkebæk NE, Main KM. Impaired Reproductive Development in Sons of Women Occupationally Exposed to Pesticides during Pregnancy. Environ Health Perspect. 2008; 116:566-72.

48. Dalvie MA, Myers JE, Thompson ML, Robins TG, Dyer S, Riebow J, Molekwa J, Jeebhay M, Millar R, Kruger P. The long-term effects of DDT exposure on semen, fertility, and sexual function of malaria vector-control workers in Limpopo Province, South Africa. Environ Res 2004; 96:1-8.

49. Lifeng T, Shoulin W, Junmin J, Xuezhao S, Yannan L, Qianli W, Longsheng C. Effects of fenvalerate exposure on semen quality among occupational workers. Contraception 2006; 73:92-6.

50. Xia Y, Bian Q, Xu L, Cheng S, Song L, Liu J, Wu W, Wang S, Wang X. Genotoxic effects on human spermatozoa among pesticide factory workers exposed to fenvalerate. Toxicol 2004; 203:49-60.

51. Tan LF, Wang SL, Sun XZ, Li YN, Wang QL, Ji JM, Chen LS, Wang XR. Effects of fenvalerate exposure on the semen quality

of occupational workers. Zhonghua Nan Ke Xue. 2002; 8:273-6.

52. Bian Q, Xu LC, Wang SL, Xia YK, Tan LF, Chen JF, Song L, Chang HC, Wang XR. Study on the relation between occupational fenvalerate exposure and spermatozoa DNA damage of pesticide factory workers. Occup Environ Med 2004; 61:999-1005.

53. Xia Y, Cheng S, Bian Q, Xu L, Collins MD, Chang HC, Song L, Liu J, Wang S, Wang X. Genotoxic effects on spermatozoa of carbaryl-exposed workers. Toxicol Sci 2005; 85:615-23.

54. Tan LF, Sun XZ, Li YN, Ji JM, Wang QL, Chen LS, Bian Q, Wang SL. Effects of carbaryl production exposure on the sperm and semen quality of occupational male workers. Zhonghua Lao Dong Wei Sheng Zhi Ye Bing Za Zhi 2005; 23:87-90.

55. Sanchez-Peña LC, Reyes BE, Lopez-Carrillo R, Moran-Martinez J, Cebrian ME, Quintanilla-Vega B. Organophosphorus pesticide exposure alters sperm chromatin structure in Mexican agricultural workers. Toxicol Appl Pharmacol 2004; 196:108-13.

56. Recio R, Robbins WA, Borja-Aburto V, Morán-Martínez J, Froines JR, Hernández RM, Cebrián ME. Organophosphorous pesticide exposure increases the frequency of sperm sex null aneuploidy. Environ Health Perspect 2001; 109:1237-40.

57. Whorton D, Krauss RM, Marshall S, Milby TH. Infertility in male pesticide workers. Lancet 1977; 11:1259–61.

58. Potashnik G, Yanai-Inbar I, Sacks MI, Israeli R. Effect of dibromochloropropane on human testicular function. Israel J Med Sci 1979; 15:438-42.

59. DR Mattison, DR Plowchlk, MJ Meadows, AZ Aljuburi, J Gandy, A Malek: Reproductive toxicity: Male and female reproductive systems as target for chemical injury. Med Clin N Am 1990; 74:391–411.

60. E Tielemans, Velde ER Burdorf, RF Weber, RJ VanKooij, H Veulemans, DJ Heedorik: Occupationally related exposures and reduced semen quality: A case control study. Fertil Steril 1999; 71:690–96.

61. Centers for Disease Control. Surveillance for occupational lead exposure-United States, 1987. Morbidity and Mortality Weekly Report 1989; 38:687-94.

62. Lerda D. Study of sperm characteristics in persons occupationally exposed to lead. Am J Ind Med 1992; 22:567-71.

63. Gennart JP, Buchet JP, Roels H, Ghyselen P, Ceulemans E, Lauwerys R. Fertility of male workers exposed to cadmium, lead, or manganese. Am J Epidemiol 1992; 135:1208-19.

64. Telisman, S., Cvitkovic, P., Gavella, M., and Pongracic, J. Semen quality in men with respect to blood lead and cadmium levels. In: International Symposium on Lead and Cadmium Toxicology. Peking, People's Republic of China, August 18-21, 1990, pp. 29-32.

65. Wildt K, Eliasson R, Berlin M. Effect of occupational exposure to lead on sperm and semen. In: Reproductive and Developmental Toxicity of Metals. 1983; 279–300.

66. Kasperczyk A, Kasperczyk S, Horak S, Osta³owska A, Grucka-Mamczar E, Romuk E, Olejek A, Birkner E. Assessment of semen function and lipid peroxidation among lead exposed men. Toxicol Appl Pharmacol 2008; 228:378-84.

67. Lancranjan I, Popescu HI, GAvãnescu O, Klepsch I, Serbãnescu M. Reproductive ability of workmen occupationally exposed to lead. Arch Environ Health 1975; 30:396-401.

68. Foster WG, McMahon A, Rice DC. Sperm chromatin structure is altered in cynomolgus monkeys with environmentally relevant blood lead levels. Toxicol Ind Health 1996; 12:723–35.

69. Quintanilla-Vega B, Hoover DJ, Bal W, Silbergeld EK, Waalkes MP, Anderson LD. Lead interaction with human protamin (HP2) as a mechanism of male reproductive toxicity. Chem Res Toxicol 2000; 13:594–600.

70. Choy CM, Lam CW, Cheung LT, Briton-Jones CM, Cheung LP, Haines CJ. Infertility, blood mercury concentrations and dietary seafood consumption: a case-control study. British J Obs and Gyne 2002; 109:1121–25.

71. Dickman MD, Leung CK, Leong MK. Hong Kong male subfertility links to mercury in human hair and fish. Sci Total Environ 1998; 214:165–74.

72. Keck C, Bergmann M, Ernst E, Muller C, Kliesch S, Nieschlag E. Autometallographic detection of mercury in testicular tissue of an infertile man exposed to mercury vapor. Reprod Toxicol 1993; 7:469–75.

73. Choy CM, Yeung QS, Briton-Jones CM, Cheung CK, Lam CW, Haines CJ. Relationship between semen parameters and mercury concentrations in blood and in seminal fluid from subfertile males in Hong Kong. Fertil Steril 2002; 78:426–28.

74. Rignell-Hydbom A, Axmon A, Lundh T, Jönsson BA, Tiido T, Spano M. Dietary exposure to methyl mercury and PCB and the associations with semen parameters among Swedish fishermen. Environ Health 2007; 6:14.

75. Maines MD. Characterization of hame oxygenase activity in Leydig and Sertoli cells of the rat testes: differential distribution of activity and response to cadmium. Biochemical Pharmacology 1984; 33:1493-502.

76. Abroushakra FR, Ward NI, Everand DM. The role of trace elements in male infertility. Fertil Steril 1989; 52:307-10.

77. Omu AE, Dashtu H, Mohammed AT, Mattappallil AB. Significance of trace elements in seminal plasma of infertile men. Nutrition 1995; 11 (suppl 5):502-05.

78. Telisman S, Cvitkovic P, Jurasovic J, Pizent A, Gavella M, Rocic B. Semen quality and reproductive endocrine function in relation to biomarkers of lead, cadmium, zinc and copper in men. Environ Health Perspect 2000; 108: 45–53.

79. Bonde JP. Semen quality and sex hormones among mild steel and stainless steel welders: A cross sectional study. Br J Ind Med 1990; 47:508–14.

80. Bonde JP, Hansen KS, Levine RJ. Fertility among Danish male welders. Scand J Work Environ Health 1990; 16:15–22.

81. Danadevi K, Rozati R, Reddy PP, Grover P. Semen quality of Indian welders occupationally exposed to nickel and chromium. Reprod Toxicol 2003; 17:451-6.

82. Hjollund NH, Bonde JP, Jensen TK, Henriksen TB, Andersson AM, Kolstad HA, Ernst E, Giwercman A, Skakkebaek NE, Olsen J. Male-mediated spontaneous abortion among spouses of

stainless steel welders. Scand J Work Environ Health 2000; 26:187-92.

83. Bonde JP, Ernst E. Sex hormones and semen quality in welders exposed to hexavalent chromium. Hum Exp Toxicol 1992: 11:259–63.

84. Knudsen LE, Boisen T, Christensen JM, Jelnes JE, Jensen GE, Jensen JC, Lundgren K, Lundsteen C, Pedersen B, Wassermann K, *et al.*, Biomonitoring of genotoxic exposure among stainless steel welders. Mutat Res. 1992; 279:129-43.

85. Ong CN, Shen HM, Chia SE. Biomarkers for male reproductive health hazards: are they available? Toxicol Lett 2002; 134:17-30.

86. Dawson EB, Ritter S, Harris WA, Evans DR Powell LC. Comparison of sperm viability with seminal plasma metal levels. Biol Trace Element Res 1998; 64, 215–19.

87. Li H, Chen Q, Li S, Xu Y, Yao W, Chen C. Studies on male reproductive toxicity caused by hexavalent Chromium. Zhonghua Yu Fang Xue Za Zhi 1999; 33:351–53.

88. Chowdhury AR, Chinoy NJ, Gautam AK, Rao RV, Parikh DJ, Shah GM, Highland HM, Patel KG, Chatterjee BB. Effect of lead on human sperm. Adv Contra Deliv Syst 1986; 11:208–10.

89. Alexander BH, Chckoway H, Van Netten C, Muller CH, Ewers TG, Kaufman JD, Mueller BA, Vaughan TL, Faustman EM. Semen quality of men employed at a lead smelter. Occup Environ Med 1996; 53:411–16.

90. Wirth JJ, Rossano MG, Daly DC, Paneth N, Puscheck E, Potter RC, Diamond MP. Ambient manganese exposure is negatively associated with human sperm motility and concentration. Epidemiology. 2007;18:270-3.

91. Wu W, Zhang Y, Zhang F. Studies on semen quality in workers exposed to manganese and electric welding. Zhonghua Yu Fang Yi Xue Za Zhi 1996; 30:266-8.

92. Welch LS, Schrader SM, Turner TW, Cullen MR. Effects of exposure to ethylene glycol ethers on shipyard painters: II. Male reproduction. Am J Ind Med 1988; 14:509–26.

93. Lancranjan I, Popescu HI, Klepsch I. Changes of the gonadic function in chronic carbon disulphide poisoning. Med Lav 1969; 60:566–71.

94. Meyer CR. Semen quality in workers exposed to carbon disulfide compared to a control group from the same plant. J Occup Med 1981; 23:435–39.

95. Jelnes JE. Semen quality in workers producing reinforced plastic. Reprod Toxicol 1988; 2:209–12.

96. Kolstad HA, Bisanti L, Roeleveld N, Bonde JP, Joffe M. Time to pregnancy for men occupationally exposed to styrene in several European reinforced plastics companies. Asclepios. Scand J Work Environ Health 1999; 25(Suppl. 1):66–9.

97. Eskenazi B, Fenster L, Hudes M, Wyrobek AJ, Katz DF, Gerson J, Rempel DM. A study of the effect of perchloroethylene exposure on semen quality in dry cleaning workers. Am J Ind Med 1991; 20:575–91.

98. Tola S, Vilhunen R, Jarvinen E, Korkala ML. A cohort study on workers exposed to trichloroethylene. J Occup Med 1980; 22:737–40.

99. Kim Y, Jung K, Hwang T, Jung G, Kim H, Park J, Kim J, Park J, Park D, Park S, Choi K, Moon Y. Hematopoietic and reproductive hazards of Korean electronic workers exposed to solvents containing 2-bromopropane. Scand J Work Environ Health 1996; 22:387–91.

100. Liu HX, Qin WH, Wang GR, Yang ZZ, Chang YX, Jiang QG. Some altered concentrations of elements in semen of workers exposed to trinitrotoluene. Occup Environ Med 1995; 52:842–45.

101. Schrader SM, Turner TW, Ratcliffe JM. The effects of ethylene dibromide on semen quality: a comparison of short-term and chronic exposure. Reprod Toxicol 1988; 2:191-8.

102. Vanhoorne M, Comhaire F, De Bacquer D. Epidemiological study of the effects of carbon disulfide on male sexuality and reproduction. Arch Environ Health 1994; 49:273–78.

103. Migliore L, Naccarati A, Zanello A, Scarpato R, Bramanti L, Mariani M. Assessment of sperm DNA integrity in workers exposed to styrene. Hum Reprod 2002;17:2912-8.

104. Naccarati A, Zanello A, Landi S, Consigli R, Migliore L. Sperm-FISH analysis and human monitoring: a study on workers occupationally exposed to styrene. Mutat Res 2003; 537:131-40.

105. Tas S, Lauwerys R, Lison D. Occupational hazards for the male reproductive system. Crit Rev Toxicol 1996; 26:261–307.

106. Koo HJ, Lee BM. Estimated exposure to phthalates in cosmetics and risk assessment. J Toxicol Environ Health A 2004; 67:1901–14.

107. Fredricsson B, Moller L, Pousette A, Westerholm R. Human sperm motility is affected by plasticizers and diesel particle extracts. Pharmacol Toxicol 1993; 72:128–33.

108. Park JD, Habeebu SS, Klaassen CD. Testicular toxicity of di-(2-ethylhexyl)phthalate in young Sprague-Dawley rats. Toxicol 2002; 171:105–15.

109. Kang KS, Lee YS, Kim HS, Kim SH. Di-(2-ethylhexyl) phthalate-induced cell proliferation is involved in the inhibition of gap junctional intercellular communication and blockage of apoptosis in mouse Sertoli cells. J Toxicol Environ Health A 2002; 65: 447–59.

110. Williams J, Foster PM. The production of lactate and pyruvate as sensitive indices of altered rat Sertoli cell function *in vitro* following the addition of various testicular toxicants. Toxicol Appl Pharmacol 1988; 94:160–70.

111. Hauser R, Williams P, Altshul L, Calafat AM. Evidence of interaction between polychlorinated biphenyls and phthalates in relation to human sperm motility. Environ. Health Perspect 2005; 113:425–30.

112. Rozati R, Reddy PP, Reddanna P, Mujtaba R. Role of environmental estrogens in the deterioration of male factor fertility. Fertil Steril 2002; 78:1187–94.

113. Duty SM, Singh NP, Silva MJ, Barr DB, Brock JW, Ryan L, Herrick RF, Christiani DC, Hauser R. The relationship between environmental exposures to phthalates and DNA damage in human sperm using the neutral comet assay. Environ. Health Perspect 2003; 111:1164–69.

114. Duty SM, Silva MJ, Barr DB, Brock JW, Ryan L, Chen Z, Herrick RF, Christiani DC, Hauser R. Phthalate exposure and human semen parameters. Epidemiology 2003; 14:269–77.

115. Jensen AA. Melanoma, fluorescent lights, and polychlorinated biphenyls. Lancet 1982; 2:935.

116. Guo YL, Hsu PC, Hsu CC, Lambert GH. Semen quality after prenatal exposure to polychlorinated biphenyls and dibenzofurans. Lancet. 2000; 356:1240–41.

117. Bonde JP, Toft G, Rylander L, Rignell-Hydbom A, Giwercman A, Spano M, Manicardi GC, Bizzaro D, Ludwicki JK, Zvyezday V, Bonefeld-Jørgensen EC, Pedersen HS, Jönsson BA, Thulstrup AM; INUENDO. Fertility and markers of male reproductive function in Inuit and European populations spanning large contrasts in blood levels of persistent organochlorines. Environ Health Perspect 2008; 116:269-77.

118. Rignell-Hydbom A, Rylander L, Giwercman A, Jönsson BA, Lindh C, Eleuteri P, Rescia M, Leter G, Cordelli E, Spano M, Hagmar L. Exposure to PCBs and p,p'-DDE and human sperm chromatin integrity. Environ Health Perspect 2005; 113:175-9.

119. Gontier-Latonnelle K, Cravedi JP, Laurentie M, Perdu E, Lamothe V, Le Menn F, Bennetau-Pelissero C. Disposition of genistein in rainbow trout (Oncorhynchus mykiss) and siberian sturgeon (Acipenser baeri). Gen Comp Endocrinol 2007; 150:298–308.

120. Kuiper GG, Lemmen JG, Carlsson B, Corton JC, Safe SH, van der Saag PT, van der Burg B, Gustafsson JA. Interaction of estrogenic chemicals and phytoestrogens with estrogen receptor beta. Endocrinology 1998; 139:4252–63.

121. Mitchell JH, Cawood E, Kinniburgh D, Provan A, Collins AR, Irvine DS. Effect of a phytoestrogen food supplement on reproductive health. in normal males. Clin Sci (Lond.) 2001; 100:613–18.

122. Evans BA, Griffiths K, Morton MS. Inhibition of 5 alpha-reductase in genital skin fibroblasts and prostate tissue by dietary lignans and isoflavonoids. J Endocrinol 1995; 147:295–302.

123. Adlercreutz H, Mousavi Y, Clark J, Höckerstedt K, Hämäläinen E, Wähälä K, Mäkelä T, Hase T. Dietary phytoestrogens and cancer: *in vitro* and in vivo studies. J Steroid Biochem Mol Biol 1992; 41:331–37.

124. Adlercreutz H, Höckerstedt K, Bannwart C, Bloigu S, Hämäläinen E, Fotsis T, Ollus A. Effect of dietary components, including lignans and phytoestrogens, on enterohepatic circulation and liver metabolism of estrogens and on sex hormone binding globulin (SHBG). J Steroid Biochem 1987; 27:1135–44.

125. Chavarro JE, Toth TL, Sadio SM, Hauser R. Soy food and isoflavone intake in relation to semen quality parameters among men from an infertility clinic. Hum Reprod 2008. Epub ahead of print.

126. Hauser R, Singh NP, Chen Z, Pothier L, Altshul L. Lack of an association between environmental exposure to polychlorinated biphenyls and p,p'-DDE and DNA damage in human sperm measured using the neutral comet assay. Hum Reprod 2003; 18:2525-33.

127. Dallinga, JW, Moonen EJ, Dumoulin JC, Evers JL, Geraedts JP, Kleinjans JC. Decreased human semen quality and organochlorine compounds in blood. Hum Reprod 2002; 17:1973–79.

128. Toft G, Rignell-Hydbom A, Tyrkiel E, Shvets M, Giwercman A, Lindh C H, Pedersen HS, Ludwicki JK, Lesovoy V, Hagmar L, Spano M, Manicardi GC, Bonefeld-Jorgensen EC, Thulstrup AM, Bonde JP. Semen quality and exposure to persistent organochlorine pollutants. Epidemiolology 2006; 17:450–58.

129. Pant N, Shukla M, Kumar Patel D, Shukla Y, Mathur N, Kumar Gupta Y, Saxena DK. Correlation of phthalate exposures with semen quality. Toxicol Appl Pharmacol 2008; 231:112-6.

130. Zhang YH, Zheng LX, Chen BH. Phthalate exposure and human semen quality in Shanghai: a cross-sectional study. Biomed Environ Sci 2006;19:205-9.

131. West MC, Anderson L, McClure N, Lewis SE. Dietary oestrogens and male fertility potential. Hum Fertil (Camb). 2005; 8:197-207.

132. West MC. The impact of dietary oestrogens on male and female fertility. Curr Opin Obstet Gynecol 2007; 19:215-21.

133. Fraser LR, Beyret E, Milligan SR, Adeoya-Osiguwa SA. Effects of estrogenic xenobiotics on human and mouse spermatozoa. Hum Reprod 2006; 21:1184-93.

134. Shen HM, Chia SE, Ni ZY, New AL, Lee BL, Ong CN. Detection of oxidative DNA damage in human sperm and the association with cigarette smoking. Reprod Toxicol 1997; 11:675–80.

135. Fraga CG, Motchnik PA, Wyrobek AJ, Rempel DM, Ames BN. Smoking and low antioxidant levels increase oxidative damage to sperm DNA. Mutat Res 1996; 351:199-203.

136. Rowley MJ, Leach DR, Warner GA, Heller CG. Effect of graded doses of ionizing radiation on the human testis. Radiat Res 1974; 59:665-78.

137. Clifton DK, Bremner WJ. The effects of testicular X-irradiation on spermatogenesis in men: A comparison with mouse. J Androl 1983; 4:387–92.

138. Kumatori T, Ishihara T, Hirashima K *et al.*: Follow up studies over a 25 year period on the Japanese fishermen exposed to radioactive fallout in 1954. In: KF, Hubner and SA Fry, eds. The medical basis for radiation accidents preparedness. North Holland, Amsterdam: Elsevier, 1980: 33–54

139. Bartoov B, Zabludovsky N, Eltes F, Smirnov VV, Grischenko VI VI, Fischbein A. Semen Quality of Workers Exposed to Ionizing Radiation in Decontamination Work after the Chernobyl Nuclear Reactor Accident. Int J Occup Environ Health 1997; 3:198-203.

140. Weyandt TB, Schrader SM, Turner TW. Semen analysis of samples from military personnel associated with military duty assignments. J Androl 1991; 13:1–29.

141. Lancranjan I, Maicanescu M, Rafila E, Klepsch I Popescu HI. Gonadic function in workmen with longterm exposure to microwave. Health Physics 1975; 29:381–83.

142. Sun YL, Zhou WJ, Wu JQ, Gao ES. Does exposure to computers affect the routine parameters of semen quality? Asian J Androl 2005; 7:263-6.

143. Grajewski B, Cox C, Schrader SM, Murray WE, Edwards RM, Turner TW, Smith JM, Shekar SS, Evenson DP, Simon SD, Conover DL. Semen quality and hormone levels among radiofrequency heater operators. J Occup Environ Med 2000; 42:993-1005.

144. Weyandt TB, Schrader ŞM, Turner TW, Simon SD. Semen analysis of military personnel associated with military duty assignments. Reprod Toxicol 1996; 10:521-8.

145. Hjollund NH, Bonde JP, Skotte J. Semen analysis of personnel operating military radar equipment. Reprod Toxicol 1997; 11:897.

146. Schrader SM, Langford RE, Turner TW, Breitenstein MJ, Clark JC, Jenkins BL, Lundy DO, Simon SD, Weyandt TB. Reproductive function in relation to duty assignments among military personnel. Reprod Toxicol 1998; 12:465-8.

147. Ye LL, Suo YS, Cao WL, Chen M. Radar radiation damages sperm quality. Zhonghua Nan Ke Xue 2007; 13:801-3.

148. Fischbein A, Zabludovsky N, Eltes F, Grischenko V, Bartoov B. Ultramorphological sperm characteristics in the risk assessment of health effects after radiation exposure among salvage workers in Chernobyl. Environ Health Perspect 1997;105 (Suppl 6):1445-9.

149. Fejes I, Závaczki Z, Szöllosi J, Koloszár S, Daru J, Kovács L, Pál A. Is there a relationship between cell phone use and semen quality? Arch Androl 2005; 51:385-93.

150. Agarwal A, Deepinder F, Sharma RK, Ranga G, Li J. Effect of cell phone usage on semen analysis in men attending infertility clinic: an observational study. Fertil Steril 2008; 89:124-8.

151. Sokol RZ, Kraft P, Fowler IM, Mamet R, Kim E, Berhane KT. Exposure to environmental ozone alters semen quality. Environmental Health Perspec 2005; 114, 360-65.

152. Kunzle R, Mueller MD, Hanggi W, Birkhauser MH, Drescher H, Bersinger NA. Semen quality of male smokers and nonsmokers in infertile couples. Fertil Steril 2003; 79:287–91.

153. Marinelli D, Gaspari L, Pedotti P, Taioli E. Mini-review of studies on the effect of smoking and drinking habits on semen parameters. Int J Hyg Environ Health 2004; 207:185–92.

154. Jensen TK, Jorgensen N, Punab M, Haugen TB, Suominen J, Zilaitiene B, Horte A, Andersen AG, Carlsen E, Magnus O, Matulevicius V, Nermoen I, Vierula M, Keiding N, Toppari J, Skakkebaek NE. Association of in utero exposure to maternal smoking with reduced semen quality and testis size in adulthood: a cross-sectional study of 1,770 young men from the general population in five European countries. Am J Epidemiol 2004; 159:49–58.

155. Saaranen M, Suonio S, Kauhanen O, Saarikoski S. Cigarette smoking and semen quality in men of reproductive age. Andrologia 1987; 19:670–76.

156. Vine MF, Margolin BH, Morrison HI, Hulka BS. Cigarette smoking and sperm density: a meta-analysis. Fertil Steril 1994; 61:35–43.

157. Vine MF, Tse CK, Hu P, Truong KY. Cigarette smoking and semen quality. Fertil Steril 1996; 65:835–42.

158. Pasqualotto FF, Sobreiro BP, Hallak J, Pasqualotto EB, Lucon AM. Cigarette smoking is related to a decrease in semen volume in a population of fertile men. BJU Int 2006; 97:324–26.

159. Sofikitis N, Takenaka M, Kanakas N, Papadopoulos H, Yamamoto Y, Drakakis P, Miyagawa I. Effects of cotinine on sperm motility, membrane function, and fertilizing capacity *in vitro*. Urol Res 2000; 28:370–75.

160. Wong WY, Thomas CM, Merkus HM, Zielhuis GA, Doesburg WH, Steegers-Theunissen RP. Cigarette smoking and the risk of male factor subfertility: minor association between cotinine in seminal plasma and semen morphology. Fertil Steril 2000; 74:930–35.

161. Rubes J, Lowe X, Moore D II, Perreault S, Slott V, Evenson D, Selevan SG, Wyrobek AJ. Smoking cigarettes is associated with increased sperm disomy in teenage men. Fertil Steril 1998; 70:715-23.

162. Sun JG, Jurisicova A, Casper RF. Detection of deoxyribonucleic acid fragmentation in human sperm: correlation with fertilization *in vitro*. Biol Reprod 1997; 56:602-7.

163. Zenzes MT, Puy LA, Bielecki R, Reed TE. Detection of benzo[a]pyrene diol epoxide-DNA adducts in embryos from

smoking couples: evidence for transmission by spermatozoa. Mol Hum Reprod 1999; 5:125-31.

164. Van Thiel DH, Galaver PK, Cobb CF, Santucci L, Graham TO. Ethanol, a Leydig cell toxin: evidence obtained *in vivo* and *in vitro*. Pharmacol Biochem Behav 1983; 18:317–23.

165. Bannister P, Losowsky MS. Ethanol and hypogonadism. Alcohol Alcohol 1987; 22:213–7.

166. Adler RA. Clinically important effects of alcohol on endocrine function. Clinical review 33. J Clin Endcrinol Metab 1992; 74:957–60.

167. Kucheria K, Saxena R, Mohan D. Semen analysis in alcohol dependence syndrome. Andrologia 1985; 17:558–63.

168. Brzek A. Alcohol and male fertility (preliminary report). Andrologia 1987; 19:32–6.

169. Goverde HJ, Dekker HS, Janssen HJ, Bastiaans BA, Rolland R, Zielhuis GA. Semen quality and frequency of smoking and alcohol consumption. An explorative study. Int J Fertil Menopausal Stud 1995; 40:135–8.

170. Donnelly GP, McClure N, Kennedy MS, Lewis SE. Direct effect of alcohol on the motility and morphology of human spermatozoa. Andrologia 1999; 31:43–7.

171. Damgaard IN, Jensen TK, Petersen JH, Skakkebaek NE, Toppari J, Main KM. Cryptorchidism and maternal alcohol consumption during pregnancy. Environ Health Perspect 2007; 115:272-7.

172. Mieusset R, Bujan L. Testicular heating and its possible contributions to male infertility: a review. Int J Androl 1995; 18:169–84.

173. Thonneau P, Bujan L, Multigner L, Mieusset R. Occupational heat exposure and male fertility: a review. Hum Reprod 1998; 13:2122–25.

174. Bonde JP. Semen quality in welders exposed to radiant heat. Br J Ind Med 1993; 50:1055–60.

175. Figa-Talamanca I, Cini C, Varricchio GC, Dondero F, Gandini L, Lenzi A, Lombardo F, Angelucci L, Di Grezia R, Patacchioli FR. Effects of prolonged autovehicle driving on male

reproduction function: a study among taxi drivers. Am J Ind Med 1996; 30:750–58.

176. Hjollund NH, Storgaard L, Ernst E, Bonde JP, Olsen J. The relation between daily activities and scrotal temperature. Reprod Toxicol 2002; 16:209–14.

177. Hjollund NH, Storgaard L, Ernst E, Bonde JP, Olsen J. Impact of diurnal scrotal temperature on semen quality. Reprod Toxicol 2002; 16:215–21.

178. Stoy J, Hjollund NH, Mortensen JT, Burr H, Bonde JP. Semen quality and sedentary work position. Int J Androl 2004; 27:5–11.

179. Clarke RN, Klock SC, Geoghegan A, Travassos DE. Relationship between psychological stress and semen quality among in-vitro fertilization patients. Hum Reprod 1999; 14:753–58.

180. Sheiner EK, Sheiner E, Carel R, Potashnik G, Shoham-Vardi I. Potential association between male infertility and occupational psychological stress. J Occup Environ Med 2002; 44:1093–99.

181. Harrison KL, Callan VJ, Hennessey JF. Stress and semen quality in an *in vitro* fertilization program. Fertil Steril 1987; 48:633–36.

182. Giblin PT, Poland ML, Moghissi KS, Ager JW, Olson JM. Effects of stress and characteristic adaptability on semen quality in healthy men. Fertil Steril 1988; 49:127–32.

183. Fenster L, Katz DF, Wyrobek AJ, Pieper C, Rempel DM, Oman D, Swan SH. Effects of psychological stress on human semen quality. J Androl 1997; 18:194–202.

184. Hjollund NH, Bonde JP, Henriksen TB, Giwercman A, Olsen J. Reproductive effects of male psychologic stress. Epidemiol 2004; 15:21–7.

185. Auger J, Jouannet P. Evidence for regional differences of semen quality among fertile French men. Hum Reprod 1997; 12: 740–45.

186. Jensen TK, Vierula M, Hjollund NH, Saaranen M, Scheike T, Saarikoski S, Suominen J, Keiski A, Toppari J, Skakkebaek NE. Semen quality among Danish and Finnish men attempting to conceive. The Danish First Pregnancy Planner Study Team. Eur J Endocrinol 2000; 142:47–52.

187. Saidi JA, Chang DT, Goluboff ET, Bagiella E, Olsen G, Fisch H. Declining sperm counts in the United States? A critical review. J Urol 1999; 161:460–62.

188. Younglai EV, Collins JA, Foster WG. Canadian semen quality: An analysis of sperm density among eleven academic fertility centers. Fertil Steril 1998; 70:76–80.

189. Chen Z, Toth T, Godfrey-Bailey L, Mercedat N, Schiff I, Hauser R. Seasonal variation and age-related changes in human semen parameters. J Androl 2003; 24:226–31.

Environmental & Occupational Exposures (2010) ***Pages 142–151***
Editors: **Sunil Kumar & R.R. Tiwari**
Published by: **DAYA PUBLISHING HOUSE, NEW DELHI**

Chapter 6

Testicular Hyperthermia and its Effect on Male Reproductive Health

S. Venkatesh[1], *R. Deecaraman*[2] *and R. Dada*[1]*

[1]*Laboratory for Molecular Reproduction and Genetics, Department of Anatomy, All India Institute of Medical sciences, New Delhi – 110 029*

[2]*Dr. M.G.R. Educational and Research Institute, Maduravoyal, Chennai – 95*

ABSTRACT

It is clear that various occupations, sedentary life style, posture, hot bath, increasing and prolonged use of laptop computers raises testicular temperature and adversely affects male reproductive health leading to sub fecundity in male population. Hence, in idiopathic infertile cases testicular hyperthermia and its causative factors should be evaluated for a better understanding of etiopathogenesis of infertility. Though infertility is a heterogeneous trait and several factors like occupation, environmental xenoestrogen, genetic factors, drug, endocrinal factors, alcohol intake and smoking can affect testicular function, however the role of high occupational environmental temperature cannot be ignored. In idiopathic cases where there are no other underlying causes of infertility,

* Corresponding Author–E-mail: rima_dada@rediffmail.com

it is important to take a detailed history of occupational, environmental and lifestyle factors in terms of period, duration of exposure and the type of exposure. Avoiding such exposure during the reproductive period can improve the fertility and chance of conception. This chapter suggests the inclusion of questionnaire with respect to occupation, life style and environment for the better evaluation of idiopathic male infertility cases associated with testicular hyperthermia. Thus, the testes are remarkable as a biological system for its functional regulation by temperature.

Introduction

Temperature is considered to be the most important factor in regulating the metabolism of human body through thermoregulatory system of the hypothalamus. Though normal body temperature of human body is 37°C, the testes are intrascrotal in position outside the abdomen with the testicular temperature being 2-3°C lower than the rectal or body temperature. It is well established that optimal spermatogenesis in man takes place at 2-3°C lower than internal body temperature. It has been proposed that spermatogenic DNA polymerase and recombination activities are optimum only at a testicular temperature (35°C). Also absence of subcutaneous fat in the scrotum, presence of hair, sweat glands and Dartos in the scrotum are the supportive mechanism to keep the scrotal temperature lower than the body temperature, which is optimum for spermatogenesis. Hence, elevation in testicular temperature may result in impaired spermatogenesis leading to poor sperm quality. Testicular hyperthermia results in qualitative or quantitative defect in sperm production. The elevation of testicular temperature may occur exogenously or endogenously. Endogenous conditions like cryptorchidism (intra abdominal testis) and Varicocele (dilation of pampiform plexus of vein) produces mild scrotal warming that can be detrimental to sperm production. Varicoceloctomy may reverse the condition and restore the fertility[1]. Decrease in the semen quality and increase in male infertility cases over the past 50 years may be due to changes in life style, environment polluation, occupational factors, sedentary lifestyle and exposure to a variety of gonadotoxins. Since spermatogenesis in men takes place at 2-3°C lower than the core body temperature, role of temperature in the production of spermatozoa and male fertility has been the focus of several studies and discussed in male reproduction recently. This chapter deals with the role of various factors that results in the elevation of testicular temperature and adversely affects semeniferous tubular function and male reproductive health.

Clothing

Modern lifestyle -like sedentary life, decreased outdoor activity, increasing use of laptop computers and tight clothing results in scrotal hyperthermia. Clothes like tight jeans, thermal underwear and synthetic fabrics result in significant elevation of testicular temperature. Clothing like tight jeans and underwear approximate the testes to the abdomen and increases the testicular temperature to near the internal body temperature. Consequently the functions of testes get disturbed and impair the production of mature spermatozoa. It has been reported that men wearing tight underwear for 3 months had a decreased sperm quality and sperm quality improved after wearing loose underwear[2]. Similar study was also reported by Jung *et al.*[3]. A recent study on fertile men reveled that clothing increased the scrotal temperature by 1.5°C to 2°C that may suppress the spermatogenesis[4]. This elevated scrotal temperature is due to increase in the temperature of air space between the scrotum and the clothes. Polyester pants have been reported to cause deleterious effect on spermatogenesis in dogs though there was no significant elevation in the testicular temperature[5]. This tight fitting clothing, thermal underwear, prolonged approximation of thighs cause elevation of testicular temperature and thus adversely affect spermatogenesis. These are short-term exposure and thus these testicular changes are reversible.

Modern lifestyle has lead to a large population of people opting for frequent hot baths and saunas. Increase in temperature (43-120°C) and humidity (3-50 per cent) in the enclosed environment of sauna is usually taken to relive pain and aches. Exposure of testes to frequent sauna (80-90°C) for 30mins/day for 2 weeks resulted in increased scrotal temperature from 35.2 to 37.6°C that reversibly affected sperm motility parameters[6]. Similarly recent study revealed the effects of hot bath on semen quality in infertile men. In this study[7] the infertile men were exposed to hot bath for > 30 min/week of >3 months showed increased in total motile sperm count > 200 per cent after discontinuation of high temperature exposure. Avoiding frequent hot/sauna bath during reproductive age can be advised to male population especially those trying to have offspring. Though these changes even a short period (~ 3 months) are reversible and lead to partial spermatogenic arrest and oligospermia however long term exposure can result in irreversible semeniferous tubular damage and permanent total spermatogenic arrest and result in azoospermia (Dada *et al*[8]. 2000)

Posture

Posture of the body also plays an important role in the regulation of testicular and scrotal temperature. Prolonged sittings are believed to increase the testicular temperature, as the testes are closer to the anterior abdominal wall. Previous study[9] has been reported that scrotal temperature was higher in the supine or seated position than in the standing position. A recent study also revealed that scrotal temperature were significantly higher (1.4 to 2.1°C) in the seated with leg crossed position when compared to the supine, standing and seated with leg apart position. With increasing uses of computer people are sitting for prolonged periods and with use of laptops the thighs are closely approximated resulting in testicular hyperthermia and also there is increased risk of testicular damage due to increased exposure to radiation. Thus cumulative effect of both the posture and clothing also results in elevated scrotal temperature. Thus the overall mechanisms behind this elevation in a scrotal temperature is association of the scrotum with the near body temperature as it make contact with the thighs and also reduction in scrotum and environment air exchange.

Occupation

Generally exposure to various chemicals, radiation and heat are believed to affect the men's reproductive health. It is well known that increase in body temperature results in various health problems. One of the most important factors which has adversely affected spermatogenesis (oligospermia, increased male genitourinary abnormalities and increased incidence of testicular cancer) is exposure to environmental pollutants. One of the major etiological factors that has resulted in recent marked decline in male reproductive health is elevation of environmental temperature both due to global warming "heating" as now its is called and occupational exposure to high environmental temperature. Testes is located outside the abdomen as spermatogenesis occurs optimally at 35-36°C. Recent study in our laboratory (*Dada et al*[8]) identified idiopathic infertile men engaged in jobs where there was occupational exposure to high temperature. These men worked in blast furnace (n-14), cement (n-6), brick (n-7), glass (n-3), dyeing (n-6), welding (n-4), melting tar (n-7) and plywood preparation factory (n-7). These men had no exposure to any other aetiological factors. On cytogenetic analysis these men had normal 46,XY chromosome complement and did not harbour Yq microdeletion in the azoospermic factor (AZF) loci. These men were either azoospermic (n=30) and 24 men were oligozoospermic with mean sperm count of 12.6±4.3 million/ml. Of these 24 men 18 men had oligoasthenoteratozoospermia. These men had increased percentage sperms morphological abnormalities (80 per cent) and impaired linear progressive motility (grade A+B< 25 per cent). The predominant morphological abnormalities were- thick-coiled tails (35.4 per cent), amorphous head (28.8 per cent), and tapered heads (23 per cent). The mean percentage of sperms with linear progressive motility in these men was only about 17 per cent. On taking a detailed history we found that men who were engaged in these occupation for very long periods (12-15 years) developed azoospermia and men with 5-7 year exposure had developed oligozoospermia.

Office jobs which involve sitting and working continuously for more than six hours/day has been reported to adversely affect optimal spermatogenesis. This study[10] also revealed that sedentary work position for more than 6 hrs /day significantly showed a difference of 2°C testicular temperature compared with that those sat for less than on hour. During sedentary work in these men, increase in the median average temperature of 0.7°C was observed by *Hjollund et al.*, [11] and scrotal temperature was observed to be higher in the daytime, in summer, and in leisure time when compared with working hours. An elevation of testicular temperature by 1°C cause depression of spermatogenesis by 14 per cent. These early changes are reversible and lead to partial spermatogenesis arrest and oligospermia. However long term continuous exposure results in complete and total spermatogenic arrest leading to azoospermia. Thus there is a need to increase awareness that occupational exposure has severe marked effect on testicular function so that strategies be developed to circumvent or minimize exposure. This could be by decreasing exposure by changing duties within the same job so that there are periods of restoration of semeniferous epithelium and spermatogenesis. It has also been reported that sedentary position elevated scrotal skin temperature and resulted in decreased sperm concentration. Similar decreased sperm quality has also been observed in vehicle drivers. It has been also suspected that numbers of infertility cases are increasing among software employers[12] due to their long night shift and sedentary position. And working night shifts might lead to stress and tension in men, which increases their scrotal temperature. Sudden rise and fall in temperature of important sexual organs may also impair the fertility of men.

Fever

It is well known that increase in body temperature or pyrexia affects the health including semen quality. An earlier study[13] reported that an oligospermic man developed azoospermia on prolonged pyrexia due to typhoid. It has been reported that fever has adverse effect of on sperm concentration, sperm morphology and motility[14]. The study also revealed that the meiotic phase and the post meiotic phase of spermiogenesis (early primary spermatocytes to early spermatids) are more susceptible to high temperature exposure. Another study also reported that short duration pyrexia (~ 2 days) of 39°–40°C decreased semen quality and increased sperm DNA fragmentation[15]. So it is necessary to evaluate the history of febrile illness during diagnostic evaluation of infertility.

Laptops

Increasing use of portable computers like laptops has been observed over the past few years among the adult population. Laptop generates heat and radiation and works internally at a temperature more than 70°C[16]. Moreover operating Laptops requires unique position where they are placed on the lap by approximating the thighs. This position also holds the scrotum closer to the thighs and increases the scrotal temperature. A study on scrotal temperature in Laptop computer users revealed that using such device for 60 min increased the scrotal temperature significantly. Mobile phones were also reported to affect semen quality but its effect on scrotal temperature is yet to be evaluated. Mobile phone use and increased DNA fragmentation is due to prolonged exposure to radiofrequency waves. Hence it is always advisable to sustain the use of such heat generating electronic systems by young men or to work by keeping them as far from body and not close to the testes.

Clinical Conditions

Varicocele

Varicocele is the pathological dilation of pampiniform plexus of veins. It is one of the leading causes of male infertility. The incidence of varicocele in the general population is about 15 per cent, while in infertile men the incidence is between 19 to 41 per cent. In men with secondary infertility the incidence is as high as 70-80 per cent. Thus varicocele is the most frequently identifiable and surgically correctable cause of male infertility. The aetiology and pathophysiology of varicocele is multifactorial. When low sperm counts are associated with varicocele, varicocelectomy can partially restore spermatogenesis and fertility. Though the etiology of varicocele is multifactorial and the cause of disruption of spermatogenesis in such cases may be many but one of the predominant and well documented cause of spermatogenetic arrest in these men is raised intratesticular temperature. In a study in men with varicocele we found that that 9.7 per cent men with varicocele harboured Yq microdeletions and such men had much more severe disruption of spermatogenesis and also did not show any improvment post varicocelectomy. Thus though the effect of high temperature is reversible following surgery but men who harbour genetic abnormalities have a poor prognosis.

High Temperature: Mechanisms of Action

Optimal spermatogenesis in man takes place at scrotal temperature, which is 2-3°C lower than the body temperature. Increase in scrotal temperature affects spermatogenesis and also decreases sperm quality. Increased scrotal heat in mice has been reported to damage DNA and decreases the viability of sperm. Increased temperature has also been reported to denature sperm proteins[17]. Moreover, generally germ cells and sertoli cells are very sensitive to high temperature[18], which is directly proportional to duration of exposure[9]. Short temperature exposure leads to reversible change in semeniferous epithelium and long-term exposure leads to permanent and total damage to semeniferous epithelium leading to azoospermia. Change in protein composition of cauda epididimyis fluid and sperm plasma membrane coating protein due to increased testicular temperature also impairs sperm quality[19]. Activation of a tumor suppressor gene p53 in cases with raised testicular temperature may also lead to spermatogenic impairment[20]. p53 translocates from nuclear membrane to nucleoplasm in cases with high testicular temperature and induces germ cell apoptosis[21] and prevents clonal proliferation of germ cells with damaged DNA. Another interesting study revealed the modification of sperm plasma membrane properties in men with elevated testicular temperature[22].

Acute or chronic exposure of the testes is also suspected to reduce the testicular weight. 70 per cent reduction of testis weight was observed in ram when they were exposed to a hot environment for 14 days[22]. Studies also revealed the increased numbers of abnormal pachytene spermatocytes after the testes of rat had been exposed to 43°C for 15 min. Heat exposure not only affects the germ cells but also have negative effects on Sertoli cells, which nourishes spermatogonial cells. High temperature also affects duration of spermatogeneic cycles. Though increase in temperature decreases the amplitude and increases the frequency of rhythmic blood flow (vasomotion), its effects on the testes function is not clear, but it is believed to alter the fluid filtration and reabsorbtion in the testes[23]. Moreover, various enzymes and expression of mRNA in testes are believed to get affected by heat.

References

1. Daitch J, Bedaiwy MA, Pasqualotto EB, Hendin BN, Hallak J, Falcone T, *et al.*, Varicocelectomy improves intrauterine insemination success rates among men with varicoceles. J Urol 2001; 165:1510-1513.
2. Sanger WG, Friman PC. Fit of underwear and male spermatogenesis: a pilot investigation. Reprod Toxicol 1990; 4:229-32.
3. Jung A, Leonhardt F, Schill WB, Schuppe HC. Influence of the type of undertrousers and physical activity on scrotal temperature Hum Reprod 2005; 20:1022-7.
4. Mieusset R, Bengoudifa B, Bujan L. Effect of posture and clothing on scrotal temperature in fertile men. J Androl 2007; 28:170-5.
5. Shafik A. Effect of different types of textile fabric on spermatogenesis: an experimental study. Urol Res 1993; 21:367-70.

6. Saikhun J, Kitiyanant Y, Vanadurongwan V, Pavasuthipaisit K. Effects of sauna on sperm movement characteristics of normal men measured by computer-assisted sperm analysis. Int J Androl 1998; 21:358-63.

7. Shefi S, Tarapore PE, Walsh TJ, Croughan M, Turek PJ. Wet heat exposure: a potentially reversible cause of low semen quality in infertile men. Int Braz J Urol 2007; 33:50-6.2007,33,50.

8. Dada R, Gupta NP, Kucheria K. Spermatogenic arrest in men with testicular hyperthermia. Teratog Carcinog Mutagen 2003;Suppl 1:235-43

9. Rock J, Robinson D. Effect of induced intrascrotal hyperthermia on testicular function in man. Am J Obstet Gynecol 1965; 93:793-801.

10. Roger Dobson. Office jobs 'can make men infertile'. The Independent. London Aug 21, 2002.

11. Hjollund NH, Bonde JP, Jensen TK, Olsen J. Diurnal scrotal skin temperature and semen quality. The Danish First Pregnancy Planner Study Team. Int J Androl 2000; 23:309-18.

12. http://sify.com/news/fullstory.php? id=14578808.

13. Koentjoro-Soehadi L Azoospermia caused by typhoid fever. A case report. Andrologia 1982; 14:31-2, 34.

14. Carlsen E, Andersson AM, Petersen JH, Skakkebaek NE. History of febrile illness and variation in semen quality. Hum Reprod 2003; 18:2089-92.

15. Sergerie M, Mieusset R, Croute F, Daudin M, Bujan L. High risk of temporary alteration of semen parameters after recent acute febrile illness. Fertil Steril 2007; 88:970.e1-7.

16. Sheynkin Y, Jung M, Yoo P, Schulsinger D, Komaroff E. Increase in scrotal temperature in laptop computer users. Hum Reprod 2005; 20:452-5.

17. Jiang MX, Zhu Y, Zhu ZY, Sun QY, Chen DY. Effects of cooling, cryopreservation and heating on sperm proteins, nuclear DNA, and fertilization capability in mouse. Mol Reprod Dev 2005; 72:129-34.

18. Martin-du Pan RC, Campana A. Physiopathology of spermatogenic arrest. Fertil Steril 1993; 60:937-46. Review.

19. Bedford JM. Effects of elevated temperature on the epididymis and testis: experimental studies. Adv Exp Med Biol 1991; 286:19-32. Review.

20. Yin Y, DeWolf WC, Morgentaler A. Experimental cryptorchidism induces testicular germ cell apoptosis by p53-dependent and -independent pathways in mice. Biol Reprod 1998; 58:492-6.

21. Yin Y, DeWolf WC, Morgentaler A. p53 is associated with the nuclear envelope in mouse testis. Biochem Biophys Res Commun 1997; 235:689-94.

22. Holt WV, North RD. Thermotropic phase transitions in the plasma membrane of ram spermatozoa. J Reprod Fertil 1986; 78:447-57.

23. Gomes WR, Butler WR, Johnson AD. Effect of elevated ambient temperature on testis and blood levels and *in vitro* biosynthesis of testosterone in the ram. J Anim Sci 1971; 33:804-7.

24. Setchell BP. The Parkes Lecture. Heat and the testis. J Reprod Fertil 1998; 114:179-94. Review.

Environmental & Occupational Exposures (2010) *Pages 152–159*
Editors: **Sunil Kumar & R.R. Tiwari**
Published by: **DAYA PUBLISHING HOUSE, NEW DELHI**

Chapter 7

The Impact of Air Pollution on Reproductive Health

Rajvi H. Mehta*

Hope Infertility Clinic, Bangalore

ABSTRACT

Several studies in the last decade have clearly shown that exposure of young men and women to air pollutants have a detrimental effect on their fertility. Most of the studies on fertility have been restricted to males and demonstrate an inverse correlation between sperm concentrations and particulate matter in the environment. This effect may be mediated by detrimental effects on the endocrine system or chromosomal abnormalities

There is sufficient evidence to show that maternal exposure to air pollutants during pregnancy either in the first trimester leads to low birth weight babies. Vehicular emissions, diesel exhaust emissions and construction activity are the primary source of air pollutants. Measures need to be taken to control pollution and increase awareness amongst the masses on the ill effects of air pollutants on reproductive health. Such measures are essential for the health of the generations to come.

* E-mail: mehtat@vsnl.com

Introduction

The anti-fertility effects of environmental pollutants have been known since the Roman times when the lead content of drinking water was suspected to be responsible for the declining population in the upper classes[1]. However, a serious resurgence of interest on the impact of environmental pollutants on fertility was brought about by the publication of Carlsen *et al.*[2]. On the basis of a meta analysis of over 12,000 semen samples, the authors concluded that there had been a genuine decline in semen quality in the past 50 years and consequently, male fertility. This paper was extensively criticized for the statistical methodology and the conclusions made were therefore questionable. This report generated extensive media attention and triggered many laboratories, the world over to perform retrospective analysis of their data to determine whether there was a decline in semen quality over the past few decades.

Several groups evaluated the semen quality in men over different periods of time. The findings of these studies were variable. Some groups observed a decline in semen quality while some did not observe any change in semen. Lifestyle changes and environmental pollutants are considered to be the two major factors responsible for a decline in semen quality[3].

Impact of Air Pollution on Male Fertility

Air Pollution and Semen Quality

One of the earliest studies which associated the impact of air pollution on reproductive health came from Teplice in the Czech Republic. The Telpice district is reported to have high level of air pollution with a large seasonal variation. The levels of particulate matter are highest in the winter months, which may be due to the high amount of coal burning for heating and power. While studying the overall impact of these pollutants on human health, they observed transient decrement in semen quality is associated with exposure to higher levels of air pollution[4]. Subsequently, a study by the US Environmental Protection Agency in the same district as compared with the neghbouring district, Prachatice in the Czech Republic, observed that periods of elevated air pollution were significantly associated with decrements in other semen measures including proportionately fewer motile sperm, proportionately fewer sperm with normal morphology or normal head shape, and proportionately more sperm with abnormal chromatin[5].

Sokol *et al.*[6] studied the air pollution indices *viz.*, ozone, particulate matter, nitrogen dioxide and carbon monoxide and its relation to semen quality in semen donors during a retrospective study. They found no relationship between the other pollutants and semen quality but exposure to ozone did adversely affect semen quality.

In a retrospective study, we too evaluated the mean sperm concentration in male partners of infertile couples undergoing a preliminary condition of their infertility condition during the period 1992 to 1996. The sperm concentration was correlated with the ambient air pollutant indices such as suspended particulate matter (SPM), nitrous oxide and sulphur dioxide. A significant negative correlation was observed between the ambient SPM levels and the sperm concentration[7]. Combustion emissions account for over half of the fine particles ($PM_{2.5}$) air pollution and most of the primary particulate organic matter in the environment. Contamination of the environment with particulate matter results from construction activity, vehicular emissions especially diesel emissions and coal burning. Extensive use of diesel generators to compensate for the poor supply of electricity also makes them a major source of SPM in the Indian environment.

Our findings corroborated the observations of Adamapolous *et al*[8] who reported a decline in sperm concentration and seminal volume during the period 1977 to 1993. Over the same period, they observed a marked deterioration in the air pollution indices in that area.

Endocrine Disrupting Activity of Diesel Exhaust

Low levels of diesel exhaust reduce the expression of several genes known to play key roles in gonadal development, including an enzyme necessary for testosterone synthesis. Mature male rats exposed to diesel exhaust during the fetal period showed an irreversible decrease in daily sperm production due to an insufficient number of Sertoli cells. Diesel exhaust particles (DEP) also contain substances with estrogenic, antiestrogenic and antiandrogenic activities. The neutral substance fraction of DEP has the causal substance that reduces estrogen receptor mRNA expression[9].

Chromosomal Abnormalities in Spermatozoa Associated with Air Pollution

Rubes *et al*[10] observed a significantly higher incidence of disomy in chromosome X and Y in men residing in Telpice as compared with the less polluted Prachatice in the Czech Republic. Further studies by the same group, reported that using repeated measures analysis, a significant association was found between exposure to periods of high air pollution (at or above the upper limit of US air quality standards) and the percentage of sperm with DNA fragmentation according to sperm chromatin structure assay (SCSA). They concluded that exposure to intermittent air pollution may result in sperm DNA damage and thereby increase the rates of male-mediated infertility, miscarriage, and other adverse reproductive outcomes[11].

The SCSA which has been developed to assay sperm DNA fragmentation was carried out to determine whether it correlated with increased exposure to air pollutants. A 2-year longitudinal study of men living a valley town with a reported abnormal level of infertility and spontaneous miscarriages and also a seasonal atmospheric smog pollution, showed, for the first time, that SCSA measurements of human sperm DNA fragmentation were detectable and correlated with dosage of air pollution while the classical semen measures were not correlated. Extensive DNA fragmentation probably cannot be repaired by the egg and the spontaneous abortion rate is approximately 2x higher if a man has more than 30 per cent of sperm showing DNA fragmentation[12].

Analysis of aneuploidy in human sperm by FISH showed that aneuploidy YY8 was associated with the season of heaviest air pollution. These findings are suggestive of an influence of air pollution on YY8 disomy. All these results indicate that air pollution may increase sperm DNA damage in human population, which may be even higher for susceptible groups[13].

Impact of Air Pollution on Female Fertility

Most studies on air pollution and fertility have focused on the male and there has been only one report on its impact on female fertility. Mohallem *et al*[14] carried out an experimental study exposing male and female mice to filtered air or to polluted air for 4 months. They observed that female mice exposed to air pollutants had a higher incidence of implantation failures and lower pregnancy rates as compared to those who had grown up with filtered air.

Impact of Air Pollution on Maternal Health and the Health of Newborn Babies

Altered Sex Ratio

Lichtenfels *et al*[15] found an altered secondary sex ratio in humans consistently exposed to air pollutants as indicated by a significant inverse correlation between particulate matter and secondary sex ratio. Subsequent animal studies in mice also corroborated these findings.

Low Birth Weights

Several reports clearly indicate that exposure of pregnant women to air pollutants lead to the birth of low birth weight babies. Women exposed to SPM greater than 2.5 microns in the first trimester of pregnancy lead to increased incidence of pre-term birth. Exposure to carbon monoxide >1.25 ppm increased the odds of pre term birth by 20-25 per cent [16].

Slama *et al.*[17] also reported that increase in maternal exposure to PM < 2.5 microns mainly from traffic emissions led to an increase in the birth of low birth weight babies.

Another epidemiological study comprised all singleton newborns (N = 3,988), born to women in 1998, who resided in the City of Kaunas. They found that the risk of pre term birth increased by 25 per cent (adjusted OR = 1.25, 95 per cent CI 1.07-1.46) per 10-microg/m^3 increase in NO_2 concentrations[18].

Seo *et al*[19] studied the relationship between maternal exposure to air pollution and birth weights. They observed that there was a significant increase in the risk of having low birth weight babies by an increase in exposure to all the air pollutants. Environmental health surveillance is a systemic, ongoing collection effort including the analysis of data correlated with environmentally-associated diseases and exposures.

Maternal exposure to air pollutants, NO_2, CO and particulate matter led to a decrease in birth weight[20]. The decrease was about 8.9 gms per interquartile increase in gestational exposure to gasses; while the impact of exposure to particulate matter led to a decrease in birth weight by early 14-16 gms per inter quartile increase in PM -10 or PM 2.5. On the other hand, Jalaluddin *et al*[21] did not find any correlation between the birth weights and air pollution indices in a study of 123840 singleton births in Sydney during the 1998 to 2000. However, they studied the air pollution indices in the 3 months preceding the birth. While the earlier studies report on exposure to air pollutants in the first trimester.

Increased Twinning

An increased rate of twinning has been observed in cattle that were bred in areas close to incinerators. To test whether the pollutants emitting from incinerators could be responsible for twinning in cattle as well as human, they studied the twinning rate in human in the area and found that the incidence of twinning was significantly higher in women who lived in the areas around the incinerators, which exhibit high levels of pollutions[22]. However, this has not been substantiated by any more reports.

References

1. Schragg SD and Dixon RL (1985). Occupational exposure associated with male reproductive dysfunction. Anat Rev Pharmacol Toxicol 25:567-592.
2. Carlsen E, Giwercman A, Keiding N, Skakkebaek NE (1992) Evidence for decreasing quality of semen during past 50 years. BMJ 12:305-306.
3. Mehta RH (2006) Factors impinging human fertility. Embryo Talk 1 (Suppl. 1): 14-20.
4. Srám RJ, Benes I, Binková B, Dejmek J, Horstman D, Kotsovec F, Otto D, Perreault SD, Rubes J, Selevan SG, Skalík I, Stevens RK, Lewtas J. (1996) Teplice program–the impact of air pollution on human health. Environ Health Perspect 104 Suppl 4:699-714.
5. Selevan SG, Borkovec L, Slott VL, Zudová Z, Rubes J, Evenson DP, Perreault SD. (2000) Semen quality and reproductive health of young Czech men exposed to seasonal air pollution. Environ Health Perspect 108:887-894.
6. Sokol RZ, Kraft P, Fowler IM, Mamet R, Kim E, Berhane KT (2006) Exposure to environmental ozone alters semen quality. Environ Health Perspect 114:360-365.

7. Mehta RH, Anand Kumar TC (1997) Declining semen quality in Bangloreans: A Preliminary report. Curr Sci 72:621-622.

8. Adampoulos DA, Pappa A, Nicopoulou S, Andreou E, Karametzanis M, Michopoulos J, Deligianni V, Simou M (1996) Seminal volume and total sperm number trends in men attending subfertility clinics in Athens area during the period 1977-1993. Hum Reprod 11:1936-1941.

9. Takeda K, Tsukue N, Yoshida S. (2004) Endocrine-disrupting activity of chemicals in diesel exhaust and diesel exhaust particles. Environ Sci 11:33-45.

10. Rubes J, Zudová Z, Vozdová M, Hajnová R, Urbanová J, Borkovec L, Nováková A. (2000) Air pollution and sperm quality. Cas Lek Cesk 139: 174-176.

11. Rubes J, Selevan SG, Evenson DP, Zudova D, Vozdova M, Zudova Z, Robbins WA, Perreault SD. (2005) Episodic air pollution is associated with increased DNA fragmentation in human sperm without other changes in semen quality. Hum Reprod 20:2776-2783

12. Evenson DP, Wixon R. (2005) Environmental toxicants cause sperm DNA fragmentation as detected by the Sperm Chromatin Structure Assay (SCSA (R)). Toxicol Appl Pharmacol 207 (Suppl. 2): 532-537.

13. Srám RJ, Binková B, Rössner P, Rubes J, Topinka J, Dejmek J. (1999) Adverse reproductive outcomes from exposure to environmental mutagens. Mutat Res 428: 203-215.

14. Mohallem SV, de Araújo Lobo DJ, Pesquero CR, Assunção JV, de Andre PA, Saldiva PH, Dolhnikoff M. (2005) Decreased fertility in mice exposed to environmental air pollution in the city of Sao Paulo. Environ Res 98:196-202.

15. Lichtenfels AJ, Gomes JB, Pieri PC, El Khouri Miraglia SG, Hallak J, Saldiva PH. (2007) Increased levels of air pollution and a decrease in the human and mouse male-to-female ratio in São Paulo, Brazil. Fertil Steril 87:230-232.

16. Ritz B, Wilhelm M, Hoggatt KJ, Ghosh JK. (2007) Ambient air pollution and preterm birth in the environment and pregnancy outcomes study at the University of California, Los Angeles. Am J Epidemiol 166:1045-1052.

17. Slama R, Morgenstern V, Cyrys J, Zutavern A, Herbarth O, Wichmann HE, Heinrich J; LISA Study Group. (2007) Traffic-related atmospheric pollutants levels during pregnancy and offspring's term birth weight: a study relying on a land-use regression exposure model. Environ Health Perspect 115: 1283-1292.

18. Maroziene L, Grazuleviciene R. (2002) Maternal exposure to low-level air pollution and pregnancy outcomes: a population-based study. Environ Health 1:6.

19. Seo JH, Ha EH, Kim OJ, Kim BM, Park HS, Leem JH, Hong YC, Kim YJ.(2007) Environmental health surveillance of low birth weight in Seoul using air monitoring and birth data. J Prev Med Pub Health 40:363-370.

20. Bell ML, Ebisu K, Belanger K.(2007) Ambient air pollution and low birth weight in Connecticut and Massachusetts. Environ Health Perspect 115:1118-1124.

21. Jalaludin B, Mannes T, Morgan G, Lincoln D, Sheppeard V, Corbett S. (2007) Impact of ambient air pollution on gestational age is modified by season in Sydney, Australia. Environ Health 6:16.

22. Lloyd OL, Lloyd MM, Williams FL, Lawson A. (1988) Twinning in human populations and in cattle exposed to air pollution from incinerators. Br J Ind Med 45:556-560.

Environmental & Occupational Exposures (2010) ***Pages 160–178***
Editors: **Sunil Kumar & R.R. Tiwari**
Published by: **DAYA PUBLISHING HOUSE, NEW DELHI**

Chapter 8

Pesticide Exposure and Male Reproduction with Reference to Oxidative Stress

Oli Sarkar and P.P. Mathur*

Department of Biochemistry and Molecular Biology, Pondicherry University, School of Life Sciences, Pondicherry – 605 014

ABSTRACT

Pesticides are widely used to protect crops, household plants and livestock from insects and fungi. However, some of these man-made chemicals possess structures similar to estrogen and are toxic to the male reproductive system. These estrogen-like compounds increase the production of reactive oxygen species (ROS) like hydrogen peroxide (H_2O_2), superoxide anion ($O_2^{\bullet -}$) and peroxyl radical ($ROO^{\bullet}$) and hamper the activities of antioxidant enzymes. The testis, epididymis and spermatozoa contain several antioxidant enzymes like superoxide dismutase (SOD), catalase (CAT), glutathione peroxidase (GPX), glutathione reductase (GR) and glutathione S-transferase (GST) that degrade cyto-toxic ROS into harmless metabolites. This ROS/ antioxidant system needs to be finely

* E-mail: ppmathur@gmail.com

balanced since developing spermatozoa require and produce ROS for their maturation process but once they attain maturity, ROS becomes toxic to sperm. Thus ROS are constantly produced and degraded in the testis, epididymis and by mature sperm. Pesticides that tamper with the oxidant/ antioxidant balance induce oxidative stress in male reproductive system. Estrogen-like pesticides (lindane, methoxychlor, TCDD [2, 3, 7, 8-tetrachlorodibenzo-*p*-dioxin], DDT [dichloro- diphenyl-trichloroethane] and vinclozolin) bring about decrease in the weights of reproductive organs and accessory glands, abnormal sperm with decreased viability, inhibition of testicular steroidogenesis, alteration in circulating testosterone, LH, and FSH levels and many other harmful effects. Studies have reported that maternal, fetal, neonatal or adult exposure to permitted or sub-NOAEL (No Observed Adverse Effect Level) amounts of estrogen-like pesticides causes immediate and trans-generational damage to male reproductive health and impair male fertility. In this article, we highlight the oxidative effects of pesticides on male reproductive system.

Introduction

Male Reproductive System

The male reproductive system consists of a pair of testes composed of a convoluted seminiferous tubule wherein spermatogenesis takes place. Each testis gives out in a rete testis that collects the testicular fluid, concentrates and pools in into the epididymis. Spermatids pass through the caput, corpus and cauda regions of epididymis, gain progressive motility and fertilizing ability and are stored there. Epididymal fluid passes via a pair of efferent ducts (vas deferens) into the bladder. The male rat has five pairs of accessory sex glands whose secretions contribute to the consistency of semen. A pair of seminal vesicles secretes vesicular fluid that aids and protects sperm from immune reactions during their transit through the female reproductive tract. Attached to each vesicle is a coagulating gland that joins the vas deferens to form an ejaculatory duct from the bladder to the urethra. A lobular mass of Cowper's glands secretes Cowper's fluid that serves to cleanse the bladder of urine prior to the passage of semen. A prostate gland, found at the base of bladder secretes fructose that provides the energy needed for sperm motility. A pair of preputial glands secretes smegma that has antibacterial and antiviral functions and lubricates the glans penis prior to ejaculation. A muscular penis serves to flush out semen from the bladder during ejaculation.

ROS and Oxidative Stress

Any chemical possessing one or more unpaired electrons is termed as a free radical. Free radicals that have high oxidizing ability are called reactive oxygen species (ROS). The most common ROS are superoxide anion ($O_2^{\bullet-}$), hydroxyl radical ($OH^{\bullet}$), peroxyl radical ($ROO^{\bullet}$), peroxynitrite anion ($NOO^{\bullet}$), nitric oxide ($NO^{\bullet}$) and hydrogen peroxide (H_2O_2). Increased ROS alter the redox state of cells causing cellular damage and such a state is called "oxidative stress". Cells have a set of enzymes that combat ROS and metabolize them into harmless byproducts. Detoxification process occurs as per the following steps: $O_2^{\bullet-}$- is converted to H_2O_2, then $OH^{\bullet}$ and finally H_2O. The first step (conversion of $O_2^{\bullet-}$ into H_2O_2 and O_2) is catalyzed by superoxide dismutase (SOD). SOD is a metalloprotein found as three isoforms differing in the metal cofactor (copper in SOD1, manganese in SOD2 and copper and zinc in SOD3)[1] The H_2O_2 produced after dismutation of $O_2^{\bullet-}$ is acted upon by catalase (CAT) or glutathione peroxidase (GPX)/ glutathione reductase (GR) system. CAT or GPX/ GR reduce H_2O_2 to H_2O and O_2. CAT is a hemeprotein that detoxifies $O_2^{\bullet-}$ produced by NADPH-oxidase and H_2O_2 into H_2O and O_2. In the presence of the electron donor reduced glutathione (GSH), the selenoprotein GPX removes $ROO^{\bullet}$ from H_2O_2 resulting in H_2O and oxidized glutathione (GSSG). GR reduces GSSG to regenerate GSH and completes the detoxification process[1–5]. However, if free radicals are not suitably metabolized, they are potentially harmful because they destabilize electrolytic balance within cells. Increased H_2O_2 has been shown to cause the peroxidation of poly unsaturated fatty acids (PUFA) found in membrane lipids thus compromising the function of plasma membrane in various cellular locales[6]. Thus, maintenance of suitable free radical levels is essential for proper cellular functions.

Male Reproductive System is Vulnerable to ROS

The role of ROS in male genital tract is a biphasic one. On one hand, free radicals have been shown to be important signal transducers in the testis and are implicated in germ cell-Sertoli cell junctions[7,8]. Small amounts of ROS aid sperm capacitation, whereby sperm head is freed of cholesterol and epididymal glycoproteins and ensure that sperm is competent to fertilize ovum. ROS has been shown to enhance hyperactivation and binding of sperm to zona pellucida to facilitate oocyte fusion. Acrosome reaction that allows the sperm contents to fuse with ovum is facilitated by the presence of small amounts of ROS[9-11]. On the other hand, high levels of ROS cause reduction in sperm number, motility, viability and alter sperm functions[12,13]. Oxidative stress has been shown to cause peroxidation of sperm membrane lipids and to bring about sperm DNA fragmentation[10,14]. Increased ROS has been shown to hinder the activities of 3β-hydroxysteroid dehydrogenase (3βHSD) and 17β-hydroxysteroid dehydrogenase (17βHSD), which catalyze the rate-limiting steps of steroidogenesis. The levels of steroid acute regulatory (StAR) protein are also affected by elevated ROS. Elevated ROS alters the function of Sertoli cells thus decreasing the level of androgen binding protein (ABP), hampering steroid transport and resulting in decreased circulating testosterone levels[15]. Semen of infertile men shows the presence of leucocytes and leucocytospermia has been linked with high ROS levels[16]. Thus, elevated ROS has been correlated with oxidative stress, leucocytospermia, androgen deprivation and infertility. Sperm are poorly equipped with ROS scavengers; however, testis and epididymis are rich with anti-oxidant enzymes. These continuously metabolize free radicals to maintain a homogenous environment suitable for germ cell development. During conditions of oxidative stress, the activity of these enzymes is down-regulated and results in the production of damaged sperm. Recent studies have suggested that exposure to certain chemicals could have an adverse effect on the oxidative status of the male reproductive system. A few of these toxicants will be discussed in the next section.

Pesticides Affecting the Male Reproductive System

Introduction

The cumulative effect of the green revolution has resulted in an abundance of man-made chemicals in the environment in the form of pesticides (methoxychlor, DDT), fungicides (vinclozolin), insecticides (lindane) and herbicides (TCDD). Among these, polychlorobenzenes (PCBs) and organochlorines (OCs) are considered especially toxic because they share structural similarity with the hormone estrogen, bind to estrogen receptor and disrupt endocrine metabolism in estrogen-dependent organs. Thus, PCBs and OCs are considered xeno-estrogens or endocrine disruptors. Although utilization of these compounds is monitored stringently, minute traces of PCBs and OCs are found in the environment. In their seminar paper, Colborn *et al.*, suggested that numerous endocrine defects seen in wildlife and human populations were due to prenatal and postnatal exposure to these endocrine disruptors[17].

Endocrine disruptors are known to affect testicular (spermatogenesis and steroidogenesis) and epididymal (capacitation and maturation) functions. Germline stem cells undergo a series of differentiation and proliferation steps to become elongate spermatids. This process of spermatogenesis is regulated by androgens that are synthesized in the interstitial cells and diffuse into seminiferous tubules to exert their actions. Elongate spermatids then continue their development in the epididymis where they gain progressive motility and fertilizing ability following changes in the plasma membrane. Testis and epididymis are host to high concentrations of ROS and any imbalance in the pro-oxidant/ anti- oxidant status hampers the production of viable spermatozoa. Therefore, male reproductive organs and male fertility are vulnerable targets of endocrine disruptors. Studies from our laboratory have shown the reproductive toxicity of PCBs and OCs. The following section describes briefly the molecular effects of some of these endocrine disrupting pesticides.

Lindane

Lindane [1, 2, 3, 4, 5, 6-hexachlorocyclohexane] is deemed "moderately toxic" by the WHO and its use as pesticide/insecticide is banned in more than fifty countries. However, it is still prevalently used in India as a pesticide and poses a major threat to both wildlife and human populations. Lindane is absorbed via digestive, cutaneous and respiratory routes and accumulates in adipose tissue[18]. It has a deleterious effect on liver, brain and blood by altering the oxidative status of those organs[19]. The reproductive No Observed Adverse Effect for Lindane (NOAEL) is 1.7 mg/kg body weight/ day. Recent studies have shown that sub-NOAEL doses of lindane can harm male reproductive organs by inducing oxidative stress[20].

In the testis, lindane damages seminiferous tubule morphology resulting in decreased spermatogenesis[18]. Following exposure to lindane, the testis was under oxidative stress characterized by decrease in activities of anti-oxidant enzymes and increase in the levels of H_2O_2 and peroxidation of membrane lipids[18,21]. The increased ROS present had an adverse effect on the activity of steroidogenic enzymes (3βHSD and 17βHSD), steroid regulatory (StAR) and transport (ABP) proteins resulting in decreased in circulatory testosterone levels[15,18]. Lindane exposure affects the functions of Sertoli cells concomitant with loss in steroidogenesis[15]. Prolonged exposure to lindane results in irreversible damage to testis and epididymis.

Lindane has been shown to affect the weight and differentiation of epididymis[22,23]. Lindane has been implicated in the increased generation of ROS and due to the high concentration of PUFA in epididymis, the organ is a target of ROS-induced oxidative damage[24]. Long-term exposure to lindane resulted in oxidative stress in the epididymis at doses well below the NOAEL dose. The activities of antioxidant enzymes showed irreversible losses in a dose-dependent manner, suggesting the bioaccumulation hazards of lindane[23]. Sperm count, motility and viability were decreased in adult rats following exposure to lindane. Thus the ROS-induced oxidative damage to the male reproductive system following exposure to lindane has numerous direct and indirect harmful effects.

Methoxychlor

Methoxychlor [1, 1, 1–trichloro- 2, 2- bis (*p*-methoxy phenyl) ethane] is widely sprayed as insecticide to protect crops, livestock and pets and was developed as a synthetic alternative to DDT. Due to its insolubility in water, it sediments on the ground and is transported into streams and other water bodies. Methoxychlor is thus ingested through oral and cutaneous routes and accumulates in adipose tissue. The reproductive NOAEL for methoxychlor is 18 mg/kg body weight/day. Methoxychlor is considered to be toxic to liver, kidney, heart and central nervous system[25].

Studies have shown that methoxychlor has estrogenic and anti-androgenic activity[26]. It is interesting to note that methoxychlor is metabolized rapidly within the body, but its mono- and bis-hydroxy metabolites are more toxic than methoxychlor itself[26]. Due to its estrogenic and anti-androgenic activity it is harmful to the male reproductive system[27,28]. Gestational or lactational exposure to methoxychlor caused rats to have smaller testis and epididymis, bigger prostate and low sperm counts[29,30]. Neonatal rats exposed to methoxychlor, even at high doses, showed normal testis and epididymis weights and morphology along with low sperm counts[31]. However, when rats were exposed from weaning till adulthood, they showed retarded sexual maturity, decreased epididymal size and lower seminal sperm count[29]. But adult rats injected with methoxychlor did not show alteration in testicular germ cell numbers despite having increased follicle-stimulating hormone (FSH) levels[32]. Studies have shown that methoxychlor is activated by monooxygenase to give rise to a free radical metabolite that binds to the microsomal component. However, antioxidant scavenging enzymes prevent the binding of this metabolite to microsomal component thereby allowing retention of the toxic metabolite[33,34]. Methoxychlor is also converted into mono-*o*-demethylated derivatives by cytochrome P450 1A2 (CYP1A2). The CYP system gives rise to ROS as byproducts, and thus the degradation of methoxychlor gives rise to ROS through direct and indirect methods both causing oxidative stress[35,36]. Oxidative stress in testis is known to hamper testicular steroidogenesis and may account for the decrease in testosterone production observed in methoxychlor-exposed rats[15,32]. Methoxychlor caused a reduction in the activities of antioxidant enzymes and concomitant increase in H_2O_2 levels[37].

Methoxychlor has been shown to decrease adult rat epididymis, seminal vesicle and prostate weight. Sperm count and progressive motility were affected after short term exposure to methoxychlor. Activities of antioxidant enzymes were significantly decreased following oral administration of methoxychlor. Vitamin E is an antioxidant present in cell membranes and maintains cell membrane integrity by limiting ROS-induced lipid peroxidation. Vitamin E had a protective action on methoxychlor-induced oxidative stress in epididymis[13]. Thus methoxychlor causes oxidative damage to male reproductive system reiterating the role of this pesticide as a stressor.

TCDD

TCDD [2, 3, 7, 8-tetrachlorodibenzo-*p*-dioxin] is a polychlorinated dibenzodioxin herbicide that garnered attention due to its use as the biological weapon "Agent Orange" in the

Vietnam War. TCDD is found in herbicides, residues from incineration of municipal waste, vehicular and metal industry emissions and bleaching of textile and paper. The reproductive NOAEL for TCDD is 63 mg/kg body weight/day. TCDD has also been detected in chlorine-bleached cigarette paper and is speculated to be a harmful hazard of smoking. TCDD is ingested by oral intake, inhalation or from mother to child during pregnancy and breastfeeding[38]. Due to its hydrophobic and lipophilic nature, TCDD accumulates in adipose tissue. TCDD is not easily metabolized or excreted and has long bioaccumulation time[39].

TCDD is known to mediate its cellular effects by translocating to the nucleus by interacting with cytosolic aryl hydrocarbon receptor (AhR), binding to AhR nuclear translocator (Arnt) and finally to the *cis*-acting dioxin responsive element (DRE)[40]. TCDD has been shown to cause oxidative stress by promoting interactions between AhR and xanthine oxidase system, inducing cytochrome P450 system, decreasing activities of antioxidant enzymes[37,41,42]. TCDD has been shown to affect the morphology of testis, affect Sertoli and Leydig cell function, decrease cholesterol uptake into Cytochrome P450 system resulting in androgen deprivation in adult rats[43–47]. During fetal life, a single high dose of TCDD did not alter testis weight but seminiferous tubules were dilated. Androgen production and sperm count were decreased in the offspring. StAR protein levels were increased but circulating testosterone, LH and FSH levels were diminished[48,49]. However, daily low-dose exposure caused retarded development.

Epididymis is highly sensitive to TCDD; exposure to sub-NOAEL doses of TCDD caused a significant decrease in activities of antioxidant enzymes and a state of oxidative stress therein[50]. A concomitant decrease in sperm count and increase in ratio of abnormal: normal sperm were observed[38,51]. Exposure to TCDD caused a decrease in weight of epididymis and accessory sex glands and demasculinized behavior[52–54]. It is interesting to note that oxidative stress following exposure to TCDD could be reversed by treatment with the ROS scavenger, vitamin E. Vitamin E is reported to impart a protective action against TCDD on testis, epididymis, accessory organs and daily sperm production[55]. Thus TCDD induces oxidative stress in the male reproductive system.

DDT

DDT [4, 4'- (2, 2, 2-trichloroethane-1, 1-diyl) bis (chlorobenzene) or dichloro- diphenyl- trichloroethane] is a synthetic pesticide used to combat the spread of insect-borne diseases (like malaria and filariasis) and agricultural pests. It is termed "moderately hazardous" by the WHO and its usage was banned in nearly hundred countries from 2004; however the agricultural use of DDT was banned in 1989 in India. It is hydrophobic and readily dissolves in organic solvents and lipids. DDT accumulates in adipose tissue and its presence is amplified through the food chain. The reproductive NOAEL for DDT is 50.4-mg/kg body weight/day. DDT occurs in the environment in contaminated water and soil. DDT is metabolized into dichloro diphenyldichloro ethylene (DDE) and dichloro diphenyl dichloroethane (DDD). DDE has been shown to bind to androgen receptor and competitively inhibit androgen binding. This is considered as a causative factor in the anti-androgenic action of DDT[56]. DDT and DDE have been implicated in demasculinization of males by suppression of testosterone synthesis, increased testosterone clearance, estrogenic activity and anti-androgenic activity[57,58]. At low doses, DDT reduces the anogenital distance and induces areolas in male rats. At middle doses, male rats show hypospadias, lack of accessory sex glands and female-like nipples. At high doses, adult rats show undescended testis and a lack of epididymis[59].

Vinclozolin

Vinclozolin [3-(3, 5-dichlorophenyl)-5-methyl-5-vinyloxazolidine-2, 4- dione] is a fungicide used to protect fruit (like grapes) and vegetable crops from infections by fungi (*Botrytis cinerea, Sclerotinia sclerotiorum* and *Rhizoctonia solani*)[60]. It is widely used in European, American and Asian countries including India to improve fruits and vegetables crop yield[60]. The reproductive NOAEL for vinclozolin is 4.9-mg/kg body weight/day. Vinclozolin inhibits the synthesis of ergosterol and this is implicated in its anti-fungal actions[60]. Although vinclozolin is weakly anti-androgenic, its metabolites butenoic acid (M1) and enanilide (M2) competitively bind androgen receptor and inhibit androgen action[61–63]. Vinclozolin causes oxygen activation leading to peroxidation of fungal membrane lipids[64].

Maternal exposure to vinclozolin resulted in male offspring with female-like shortened anogenital distance and nipple remnants. After puberty, these offspring showed improperly descended testis, epididymal granulomas, small or absent accessory glands and vaginal pouches. Although these offspring could mount receptive females they were unable to ejaculate properly. One in four offspring die prior to maturity due to bladder lesions or stones. However female offspring did not exhibit any debilitating deformities[61]. In rats exposed to vinclozolin at the time of sex differentiation (fetal days 8-14) there was a reduction in spermatogenic capacity for four generations (F1-F4)[65]. Rats exposed to vinclozolin at puberty showed widespread Leydig cell hypertrophy, impaired steroidogenesis and decreased circulating testosterone levels at puberty[66]. The same animals showed decreased testis weights and sperm count in adulthood[66]. When adult rats were exposed to sub-NOAEL doses of vinclozolin, there was a decrease in testis and epididymis weight, increase in circulating LH, FSH, testosterone and dehydrotestosterone levels in parental and F1 offspring. However the fertility index remained largely unaffected in parental generation, but was significantly decreased in F1 offspring[67]. Rats exposed to vinclozolin at puberty showed reduction in weights of epididymis, prostate and seminal vesicles, sloughing of epididymal tubules and decreased sperm count at puberty[66].

Role of Oxidative Stress in Infertility

Mature sperm are vulnerable targets of oxidative stress, since their structure enables them to be responsive to ROS that are needed for their capacitation and motility. For instance, sperm plasma membrane is rich in PUFA (a target of ROS) while sperm cytosol is underprovided with antioxidant enzymes and thus membrane lipids undergo peroxidation at mild pro-oxidant conditions. Oxidative stress has been showed to compromise the integrity of sperm DNA and hasten germ cell apoptosis[68]. Semen of infertile men showed high levels of ROS as opposed to decrease in antioxidant enzyme activity. Excess of ROS caused the improper shedding of germ cell residual body resulting in sperm with large residual cytoplasm. Such sperm are not viable, and lead to infertility in the subject. Interestingly, immature sperm produce ROS, and when this ROS attacks matured sperm during their co-transit through seminiferous tubule and epididymis, it leads to lower sperm counts, abnormal sperm and decreased fertility. Recent studies have proposed ROS as a marker of male factor infertility (MFI). Seminal ROS levels have been correlated with sperm concentration, motility and morphology and suggested as an index to assess male reproductive capacity[69]. However oxidative damage to sperm has been reported as a side effect of assisted reproductive technologies (ART)[70].

Assessment of Oxidative Stress

Oxidative stress in the male reproductive system is assessed in two ways: a non-invasive method that involves studying fertility by observing frequency, size and health of rat litter, and a molecular method that involves measuring free radical levels and scavenger enzyme activities in isolated organs, sperm and semen[71]. Short term testing (1-5 days) in rats is the preferred method to assess the oxidative potential of chemicals[72]. However, extrapolation of such results to humans often does not give an accurate indication of oxidative threat of potential toxicants. Trans-generational testing involving more parameters could offer a comprehensive method of assessing ROS-induced toxicity[67]. Assisted fertility methods require semen free of ROS-generating sperm and contaminating leukocytes and existing methods (like density gradient centrifugation, swim-up separation, magnetic cell separation (MACS) and one-step washing technique) need to be improved to increase the efficacy of ART[70].

Conclusions and Future Prospects

Although much has been studied about the estrogenic and anti-androgenic properties of pesticides as inducers of oxidative stress, the extent of toxicity has not been completely understood. For instance, there is inter-species variation in oxidative stress responses to same pesticide exposure[73]. But the mechanism(s) of this vulnerability/tolerance have not been elucidated. Characterization of genetic polymorphism of antioxidant enzymes and compilation of a weighted risk factor index would enable better detection and protection against oxidative stress[74]. Future studies may be directed at understanding and engineering tolerance to oxidative stress in mammals.

Acknowledgements

P. P. Mathur acknowledges the receipt of financial support from the Department of Science and Technology, Government of India under the projects SP/SO/B-65/99 and DST-FIST to the Department. The authors wish to acknowledge the staff of the Centre for Bioinformatics, Pondicherry University for computational facilities.

References

1. Mruk DD, Silvestrini B, Mo MY and Cheng CY (2002). Antioxidant superoxide dismutase–a review: its function, regulation in the testis, and role in male fertility. Contraception, 65: 305-11.
2. Sikka SC (1996). Oxidative stress and role of antioxidants in normal and abnormal sperm function. Front Biosci, 1: e78-86.
3. Sikka SC, Rajasekaran M and Hellstrom WJ (1995). Role of oxidative stress and antioxidants in male infertility. J Androl, 16: 464-8.
4. Fujii J, Iuchi Y, Matsuki S and Ishii T (2003). Cooperative function of antioxidant and redox systems against oxidative stress in male reproductive tissues. Asian J Androl, 5: 231-42.
5. Ochsendorf FR (1999). Infections in the male genital tract and reactive oxygen species. Hum Reprod Update, 5: 399-420.
6. Kim JG and Parthasarathy S (1998). Oxidation and the spermatozoa. Semin Reprod Endocrinol, 16: 235-9.
7. Sarkar O, Mathur PP and Mruk DD (2008). Nitric oxide-cGMP signaling: its role in cell junction dynamics during spermatogenesis. Immun Endoc Metab Agents Med Chem, In press.
8. Sarkar O, Xia WL and Mruk DD (2006). Adjudin-mediated junction restructuring in the seminiferous epithelium leads to displacement of soluble guanylate cyclase from adherens junctions. J Cell Phys, 208: 175-187.
9. Zini A, De Lamirande E and Gagnon C (1995). Low levels of nitric oxide promote human sperm capacitation *in vitro*. J Androl, 16: 424-31.
10. Aitken RJ; Clarkson JS and Fishel S (1989). Generation of reactive oxygen species, lipid peroxidation, and human sperm function. Biol Reprod, 41: 183-97.

11. de Lamirande E and Gagnon C (1993). A positive role for the superoxide anion in triggering hyperactivation and capacitation of human spermatozoa. Int J Androl, 16: 21-5.

12. Chitra KC, Latchoumycandane C and Mathur PP (2003). Induction of oxidative stress by bisphenol A in the epididymal sperm of rats. Toxicology, 185: 119-127.

13. Latchoumycandane C, Chitra KC and Mathur PP (2002). The effect of methoxychlor on the epididymal antioxidant system of adult rats. Reprod Toxicol, 16: 161-72.

14. Aitken RJ (1994). Pathophysiology of human spermatozoa. Curr Opin Obstet Gynecol, 6: 128-35.

15. Saradha B, Vaithinathan S and Mathur PP (2008). Single exposure to low dose of lindane causes transient decrease in testicular steroidogenesis in adult male Wistar rats. Toxicology, doi:10.1016/j.tox.2007.11.011.

16. Rajasekaran M, Hellstrom WJ, Naz RK and Sikka SC (1995). Oxidative stress and interleukins in seminal plasma during leukocytospermia. Fertil Steril, 64: 166-71.

17. Colborn T, vom Saal FS and Soto AM (1993). Developmental effects of endocrine-disrupting chemicals in wildlife and humans. Environ Health Perspect, 101: 378-84.

18. Pages N, Sauviat MP, Bouvet S and Goudey-Perriere F (2002). Reproductive toxicity of lindane. J Soc Biol, 196: 325-38.

19. Abdollahi M, Ranjbar A, Shadnia S, Nikfar S and Rezaie A (2004). Pesticides and oxidative stress: a review. Med Sci Monit, 10: RA141-7.

20. Chitra KC, Sujatha R, Latchoumycandane C and Mathur PP (2001). Effect of lindane on antioxidant enzymes in epididymis and epididymal sperm of adult rats. Asian J Androl, 3: 205-8.

21. Saradha B, Vaithinathan S and Mathur PP (2008). Lindane alters the levels of HSP70 and clusterin in adult rat testis. Toxicology, 243: 116-123.

22. Dalsenter PR, Faqi AS, Webb J, Merker HJ and Chahoud I (1996). Reproductive toxicity and tissue concentrations of lindane in adult male rats. Hum Exp Toxicol, 15: 406-10.

23. Saradha B and Mathur PP (2006). Induction of oxidative stress by lindane in epididymis of adult male rats. Environ Toxicol Pharmacol, 22: 90-96.

24. Lenzi A, Gandini L, Picardo M, Tramer F, Sandri G and Panfili E (2000). Lipoperoxidation damage of spermatozoa polyunsaturated fatty acids (PUFA): scavenger mechanisms and possible scavenger therapies. Front Biosci, 5: E1-E15.

25. Reuber MD (1980). Carcinogenicity and toxicity of methoxychlor. Environ Health Perspect, 36: 205-19.

26. Bulger WH, Muccitelli RM and Kupfer D (1978). Interactions of methoxychlor, methoxychlor base-soluble contaminant, and 2,2-bis(p-hydroxyphenyl)-1,1,1-trichloroethane with rat uterine estrogen receptor. J Toxicol Environ Health, 4: 881-93.

27. Maness SC, McDonnell DP and Gaido KW (1998). Inhibition of androgen receptor-dependent transcriptional activity by DDT isomers and methoxychlor in HepG2 human hepatoma cells. Toxicol Appl Pharmacol, 151: 135-42.

28. Lafuente A, Marquez N, Pousada Y, Pazo D and Esquifino AI (2000). Possible estrogenic and/or antiandrogenic effects of methoxychlor on prolactin release in male rats. Arch Toxicol, 74: 270-5.

29. Gray LE, Jr., Ostby J, Ferrell J, Rehnberg G, Linder R, Cooper R, Goldman J, Slott V and Laskey J (1989). A dose-response analysis of methoxychlor-induced alterations of reproductive development and function in the rat. Fundam Appl Toxicol, 12: 92-108.

30. Welshons WV, Nagel SC, Thayer KA, Judy BM and Vom Saal FS (1999). Low-dose bioactivity of xenoestrogens in animals: fetal exposure to low doses of methoxychlor and other xenoestrogens increases adult prostate size in mice. Toxicol Ind Health, 15: 12-25.

31. Chapin RE, Harris MW, Davis BJ, Ward SM, Wilson RE, Mauney MA, Lockhart AC, Smialowicz RJ, Moser VC, Burka LT and Collins BJ (1997). The effects of perinatal/juvenile methoxychlor exposure on adult rat nervous, immune, and reproductive system function. Fundam Appl Toxicol, 40: 138-57.

32. Okazaki K, Okazaki S, Nishimura S, Nakamura H, Kitamura Y, Hatayama K, Nakamura A, Tsuda T, Katsumata T, Nishikawa A and Hirose M (2001). A repeated 28-day oral dose toxicity study of methoxychlor in rats, based on the 'enhanced OECD test guideline 407' for screening endocrine-disrupting chemicals. Arch Toxicol, 75: 513-21.

33. Bulger WH, Temple JE and Kupfer D (1983). Covalent binding of [14C]methoxychlor metabolite(s) to rat liver microsomal components. Toxicol Appl Pharmacol, 68: 367-74.

34. Bulger WH and Kupfer D (1989). Characteristics of monooxygenase-mediated covalent binding of methoxychlor in human and rat liver microsomes. Drug Metab Dispos, 17: 487-94.

35. Stresser DM and Kupfer D (1998). Human cytochrome P450-catalyzed conversion of the proestrogenic pesticide methoxychlor into an estrogen. Role of CYP2C19 and CYP1A2 in O-demethylation. Drug Metab Dispos, 26: 868-74.

36. Bondy SC and Naderi S (1994). Contribution of hepatic cytochrome P450 systems to the generation of reactive oxygen species. Biochem Pharmacol, 48: 155-9.

37. Latchoumycandane C and Mathur PP (2002). Effect of methoxychlor on the antioxidant system in mitochondrial and microsome-rich fractions of rat testis. Toxicology, 176: 67-75.

38. Faqi AS, Dalsenter PR, Merker HJ and Chahoud I (1998). Reproductive toxicity and tissue concentrations of low doses of 2,3,7,8-tetrachlorodibenzo-*p*-dioxin in male offspring rats exposed throughout pregnancy and lactation. Toxicol Appl Pharmacol, 150: 383-92.

39. Enan E, El-Sabeawy F, Moran F, Overstreet J and Lasley B (1998). Interruption of estradiol signal transduction by 2,3,7,8-tetrachlorodibenzo-*p*-dioxin (TCDD) through disruption of the protein phosphorylation pathway in adipose tissues from immature and mature female rats. Biochem Pharmacol, 55: 1077-90.

40. Schmidt JV, Su GH, Reddy JK, Simon MC and Bradfield CA (1996). Characterization of a murine Ahr null allele: involvement of the Ah receptor in hepatic growth and development. Proc Natl Acad Sci U S A, 93: 6731-6.

41. Sugihara K, Kitamura S, Yamada T, Ohta S, Yamashita K, Yasuda M and Fujii-Kuriyama Y (2001). Aryl hydrocarbon receptor (AhR)-mediated induction of xanthine oxidase/ xanthine dehydrogenase activity by 2,3,7,8-tetrachlorodibenzo-*p*-dioxin. Biochem Biophys Res Commun, 281: 1093-9.

42. Poland A and Kimbrough RD (1984). Biological Mechanisms of Dioxin Action. Bambury Report 18. Cold Spring Harbor Laboratory, Cold Spring Harbor, NY.

43. Moore RW, Jefcoate CR and Peterson RE (1991). 2,3,7,8-Tetrachlorodibenzo-*p*-dioxin inhibits steroidogenesis in the rat testis by inhibiting the mobilization of cholesterol to cytochrome P450scc. Toxicol Appl Pharmacol, 109: 85-97.

44. Moore RW, Potter CL, Theobald HM, Robinson JA and Peterson RE (1985). Androgenic deficiency in male rats treated with 2,3,7,8-tetrachlorodibenzo-*p*-dioxin. Toxicol Appl Pharmacol, 79: 99-111.

45. Johnson L, Dickerson R, Safe SH, Nyberg CL, Lewis RP and Welsh TH, Jr. (1992). Reduced Leydig cell volume and function in adult rats exposed to 2,3,7,8-tetrachlorodibenzo-*p*-dioxin without a significant effect on spermatogenesis. Toxicology, 76: 103-18.

46. Rune GM, de Souza P, Krowke R, Merker HJ and Neubert D (1991). Morphological and histochemical pattern of response in rat testes after administration of 2,3,7,8-tetrachlorodibenzo-*p*-dioxin (TCDD). Histol Histopathol, 6: 459-67.

47. Lai KP, Wong MH and Wong CK (2005). Effects of TCDD in modulating the expression of Sertoli cell secretory products and markers for cell-cell interaction. Toxicology, 206: 111-23.

48. Haavisto TE, Myllymaki SA, Adamsson NA, Brokken LJ, Viluksela M, Toppari J and Paranko J (2006). The effects of maternal exposure to 2,3,7,8-tetrachlorodibenzo-*p*-dioxin on testicular steroidogenesis in infantile male rats. Int J Androl, 29: 313-22.

49. Bell DR, Clode S, Fan MQ, Fernandes A, Foster PM, Jiang T, Loizou G, MacNicoll A, Miller BG, Rose M, Tran L and White S (2007). Toxicity of 2,3,7,8-tetrachlorodibenzo-*p*-dioxin in the

developing male Wistar(Han) rat. II: Chronic dosing causes developmental delay. Toxicol Sci, 99: 224-33.

50. Latchoumycandane C, Chitra KC and Mathur PP (2003). 2,3,7,8-tetrachlorodibenzo- *p*-dioxin (TCDD) induces oxidative stress in the epididymis and epididymal sperm of adult rats. Arch Toxicol, 77: 280-4.

51. Gray LE, Wolf C, Mann P and Ostby JS (1997). In utero exposure to low doses of 2,3,7,8-tetrachlorodibenzo-*p*-dioxin alters reproductive development of female Long Evans hooded rat offspring. Toxicol Appl Pharmacol, 146: 237-44.

52. Mably TA, Moore RW, Goy RW and Peterson RE (1992). In utero and lactational exposure of male rats to 2,3,7,8-tetrachlorodibenzo-*p*-dioxin. 2. Effects on sexual behavior and the regulation of luteinizing hormone secretion in adulthood. Toxicol Appl Pharmacol, 114: 108-17.

53. Mably TA, Moore RW and Peterson RE (1992). In utero and lactational exposure of male rats to 2,3,7,8-tetrachlorodibenzo-*p*-dioxin. 1. Effects on androgenic status. Toxicol Appl Pharmacol, 114: 97-107.

54. Gray LE, Jr., Kelce WR, Monosson E, Ostby JS and Birnbaum LS (1995). Exposure to TCDD during development permanently alters reproductive function in male Long Evans rats and hamsters: reduced ejaculated and epididymal sperm numbers and sex accessory gland weights in offspring with normal androgenic status. Toxicol Appl Pharmacol, 131: 108-18.

55. Latchoumycandane C and Mathur PP (2002). Effects of vitamin E on reactive oxygen species-mediated 2,3,7,8-tetrachlorodibenzo-*p*-dioxin toxicity in rat testis. J Appl Toxicol, 22: 345-51.

56. Kelce WR, Stone CR, Laws SC, Gray LE, Kemppainen JA and Wilson EM (1995). Persistent DDT metabolite p,p′-DDE is a potent androgen receptor antagonist. Nature, 375: 581-5.

57. Guillette LJ, Jr., Gross TS, Masson GR, Matter JM, Percival HF and Woodward AR (1994). Developmental abnormalities of the gonad and abnormal sex hormone concentrations in juvenile alligators from contaminated and control lakes in Florida. Environ Health Perspect, 102: 680-8.

58. LeBlanc GA, Bain LJ and Wilson VS (1997). Pesticides: multiple mechanisms of demasculinization. Mol Cell Endocrinol, 126: 1-5.

59. Gray LE, Ostby J, Furr J, Wolf CJ, Lambright C, Parks L, Veeramachaneni DN, Wilson V, Price M, Hotchkiss A, Orlando E and Guillette L (2001). Effects of environmental antiandrogens on reproductive development in experimental animals. Hum Reprod Update, 7: 248-64.

60. Rankin GO, Teets VJ, Nicoll DW and Brown PI (1989). Comparative acute renal effects of three N-(3,5-dichlorophenyl) carboximide fungicides: N-(3,5-dichlorophenyl)succinimide, vinclozolin and iprodione. Toxicology, 56: 263-72.

61. Gray LE, Jr., Ostby JS and Kelce WR (1994). Developmental effects of an environmental antiandrogen: the fungicide vinclozolin alters sex differentiation of the male rat. Toxicol Appl Pharmacol, 129: 46-52.

62. Kelce WR, Monosson E, Gamcsik MP, Laws SC and Gray LE, Jr. (1994). Environmental hormone disruptors: evidence that vinclozolin developmental toxicity is mediated by antiandrogenic metabolites. Toxicol Appl Pharmacol, 126: 276-85.

63. Wong C, Kelce WR, Sar M and Wilson EM (1995). Androgen receptor antagonist versus agonist activities of the fungicide vinclozolin relative to hydroxyflutamide. J Biol Chem, 270: 19998-20003.

64. Choi GJ, Lee HJ and Cho KY (1996). Lipid Peroxidation and Membrane Disruption by Vinclozolin in Dicarboximide-Susceptible and Resistant Isolates of *Botrytis cinerea*. 55: 29-39.

65. Anway MD, Cupp AS, Uzumcu M and Skinner MK (2005). Epigenetic transgenerational actions of endocrine disruptors and male fertility. Science, 308: 1466-9.

66. Yu WJ, Lee BJ, Nam SY, Ahn B, Hong JT, Do JC, Kim YC, Lee YS and Yun YW (2004). Reproductive disorders in pubertal and adult phase of the male rats exposed to vinclozolin during puberty. J Vet Med Sci, 66: 847-53.

67. Matsuura I, Saitoh T, Ashina M, Wako Y, Iwata H, Toyota N, Ishizuka Y, Namiki M, Hoshino N and Tsuchitani M (2005). Evaluation of a two-generation reproduction toxicity study adding endpoints to detect endocrine disrupting activity using vinclozolin. J Toxicol Sci, 30 Spec No.: 163-188.

68. Agarwal A, Saleh RA and Bedaiwy MA (2003). Role of reactive oxygen species in the pathophysiology of human reproduction. Fertil Steril, 79: 829-43.

69. Agarwal A, Said TM, Bedaiwy MA, Banerjee J and Alvarez JG (2006). Oxidative stress in an assisted reproductive techniques setting. Fertil Steril, 86: 503-12.

70. Agarwal A, Sharma RK, Nallella KP, Thomas AJ, Jr., Alvarez JG and Sikka SC (2006). Reactive oxygen species as an independent marker of male factor infertility. Fertil Steril, 86: 878-85.

71. Gray LE, Jr., Ostby J, Sigmon R, Ferrell J, Rehnberg G, Linder R, Cooper R, Goldman J and Laskey J (1988). The development of a protocol to assess reproductive effects of toxicants in the rat. Reprod Toxicol, 2: 281-7.

72. Linder RE, Strader LF, Slott VL and Suarez JD (1992). Endpoints of spermatotoxicity in the rat after short duration exposures to fourteen reproductive toxicants. Reprod Toxicol, 6: 491-505.

73. Samanta L and Chainy GB (2002). Response of testicular antioxidant enzymes to hexachlorocyclohexane is species specific. Asian J Androl, 4: 191-4.

74. Saradha B, Vaithinathan S, Sarkar O and Mathur PP (2006). Reproductive Toxicants: Perspectives and Research Prospects. Embryo Talk, Suppl 1: 62-67.

Environmental & Occupational Exposures (2010) *Pages 179–235*
Editors: **Sunil Kumar & R.R. Tiwari**
Published by: **DAYA PUBLISHING HOUSE, NEW DELHI**

Chapter 9

Oxidative Stress and Reproductive Function with Special Reference to Environmental and Occupational Exposure

S.S. du Plessis[1], F. Lampiao[2]**, N. Desai[3]*** and A. Agarwal[4]*****

[1]Senior Lecturer and Head; [2]Researcher
Division of Medical Physiology, Faculty of Health Sciences, Stellenbosch University, PO Box 19063, Tygerberg, 7505, South Africa
[3]Research Fellow; [4]Director,
Center for Reproductive Medicine, Cleveland Clinic, 9500 Euclid Avenue, Desk A19.1, Cleveland, Ohio, 44195, USA

Introduction

The maintenance of intracellular homeostasis is a result of a complex interaction between pro-oxidants and antioxidants. Whenever there is an imbalance between the pro-oxidants and antioxidants (the body's scavenging ability) a state of oxidative stress (OS) develops. Normal aerobic metabolism is associated with the

E-mail: *ssdp@sun.ac.za; **fannuel@sun.ac.za; ***desain2@ccf.org;
****agarwaa@ccf.org

generation of pro-oxidant molecules named free radicals or reactive oxygen species (ROS) and reactive nitrogen species (RNS). These free radicals have a dual role and act as a double-edged sword in the reproductive function of both males and females. They can serve as key signaling molecules during normal physiological reproductive processes, but also have a role in pathologies involving human reproduction. Recent scientific evidence has revealed that OS may in fact be a common factor in some of the causes of male and female infertility. Infertility affects approximately 10-15 per cent of all couples trying to conceive and there is good substantiation that lifestyle and both environmental and occupational factors can impact on a man or woman's fertility *via* the generation of OS. Free radicals can negatively influence production and quality of gametes, sperm-oocyte interaction and fertilization, early embryo development and successful pregnancy.

This chapter addresses the role of OS in the physiological regulation of both male and female reproductive function as well as the pathological consequences thereof and mechanisms by which OS can lead to infertility. It furthermore aims to highlight the effect of environmental and occupational exposure contributing to increased OS and the consequent pathological implications on the respective reproductive systems and procreation.

Oxidative Stress

In a healthy body oxidants and antioxidants remain in balance. Whenever there is an imbalance between the pro-oxidants (free radical species) and the body's scavenging ability (antioxidants) to readily detoxify the reactive intermediates, a state of OS is initiated (Figure 9.1). OS therefore develops as a result of either an increase in oxidant generation; a decrease in antioxidant protection or a failure to repair oxidative damage.

OS can lead to pathological effects when oxidative damage is caused in a cell, tissue, or organ, due to free radicals such as ROS[25,127]. The level of OS is determined by the balance between the rate at which oxidative damage is induced (input) and the rate at which it is efficiently removed and repaired (output). The rate at which damage is caused is determined by how fast the ROS are generated and then inactivated by endogenous defense agents called antioxidants. The rate at which damage is removed is dependent on

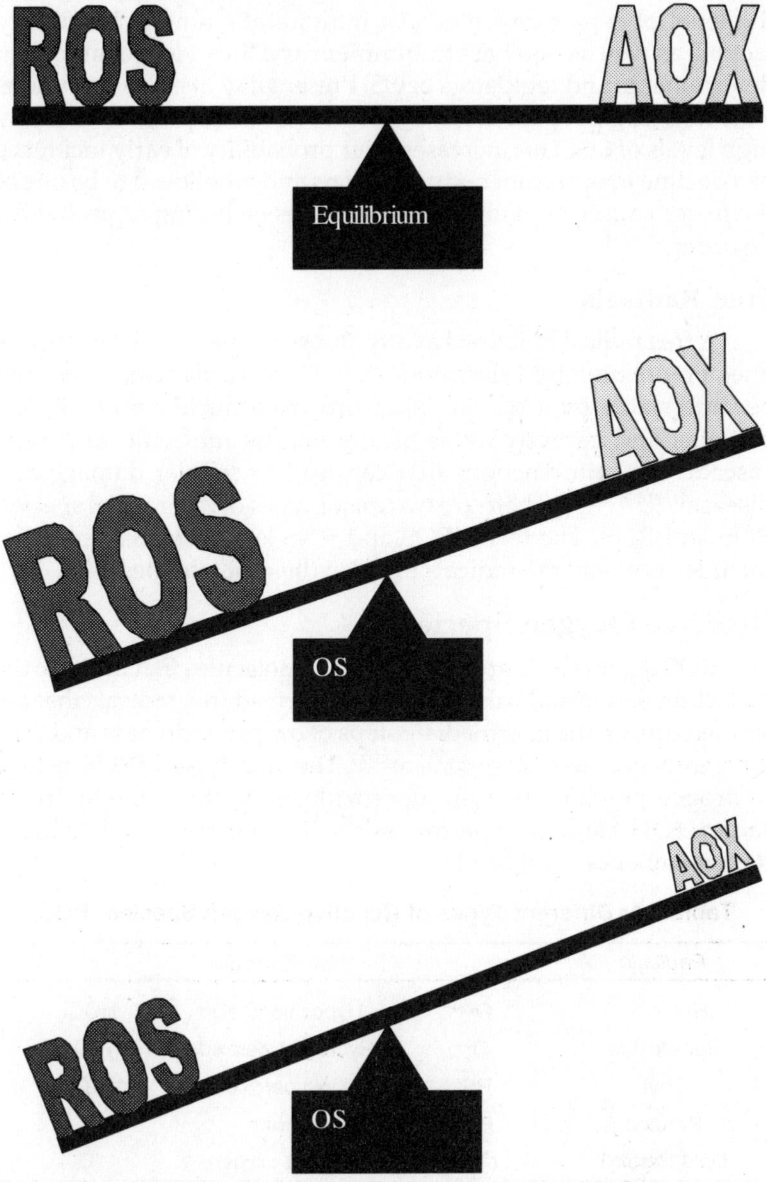

Figure 9.1: Mechanism of Oxidative Stress Development (ROS: Reactive oxygen species; AOX: Antioxidants; OS = Oxidative stress)

the level of repair enzymes. An individual's unique hereditary factors, as well as his/her environment and lifestyle are important determinants and regulators of OS. Present day lifestyle conditions lead to many people running the risk of developing abnormally high levels of OS. This increases their probability of early incidence of a decline in optimum body functions and is believed to be one of the major causes of many human diseases including reproductive disorders[13,87,113].

Free Radicals

A free radical is defined as any atom or molecule that possesses one or more unpaired electron(s)[199,231]. They are highly reactive and become stable by acquiring electrons from nucleic acids, lipids, proteins and carbohydrates of any nearby molecule causing a cascade of chain reactions that can lead to cellular damage and disease[11,40,196,237,253]. There are two major types of free radical species: ROS and RNS. The terms ROS and RNS is a collective term that includes not only the radicals but also their metabolites [39,41].

Reactive Oxygen Species

ROS represents a broad category of molecules that indicate the collection of non-radicals and oxygen-derived free radicals that are formed during the intermediate steps of oxygen reduction and exist inherently in all aerobic organisms[7,13]. The main types of ROS include hydrogen peroxide (H_2O_2), superoxide anion (O_2^{-}), the hydroxyl radical (OH^-) and lipid peroxides[7,106]. (For a more complete list of ROS members see Table 9.1)

Table 9.1: Different Types of Reactive Oxygen Species (ROS)

Radicals		*Non-Radicals*	
Hydroxyl	OH^-	Hypochloric acid	HOCl
Superoxide	O_2^{-}	Hydrogen peroxide	H_2O_2
Thyl	RS^-	Lipid peroxide	LOOH
Peroxyl	$RO_2^{\cdot}$	Ozone	O_3
Lipid Peroxyl	$LOO^{\cdot}$	Singlet oxygen	$^{-1}O_2$

Even under basal conditions, aerobic metabolism gives rise to the production of ROS, with the most important source probably being the leakage of activated oxygen from mitochondria during normal oxidative respiration[108]. Superoxide is formed when electrons leak from the electron transport chain, while when dismutated, it results in formation of H_2O_2. There are many different sources by which ROS are generated. *In vivo* most ROS come from endogenous sources as by-products of normal and essential metabolic reactions, such as energy generation from mitochondria during aerobic respiration and peroxisomal β-oxidation of fatty acids or when cells are exposed to various stress conditions from exogenous sources *e.g.* radiation from the sun/UV light, exposure to ionizing radiation (gamma radiation), consumption of alcohol in excess, cigarette smoke, environmental pollutants such as emission from automobiles and industries, metals, asbestos, metabolism of xenobiotics (detoxification reactions involving the liver cytochrome P-450 enzyme system), bacterial, fungal or viral infections (cytokines and inflammatory stimulation of phagocytosis by pathogens) and enzymatic disorders (Figure 9.2).

Due to their highly reactive nature ROS can combine readily with other molecules, directly causing oxidation that can lead to structural and functional changes and conversely result in cellular damage[11,71,106]. Under normal physiological conditions ROS must be neutralized continuously. This inactivation is done by a defense system consisting of enzymes and antioxidants[224,241].However, a small amount of ROS needs to be preserved as it is necessary to maintain normal cell function. In the event of excessive ROS production that exceeds the antioxidant defense mechanism of the cells, the result is OS and all of its accompanying effects.

Reactive Nitrogen Species

Nitrogen-derived free radicals are called RNS. Two common examples of RNS include nitric oxide ($NO^{\cdot}$) and peroxynitrite ($OONO^{-}$)[196,253] (For a more complete list of RNS members see Table 9.2). NO acts in a variety of tissues to regulate a diverse range of physiological processes (*e.g.* vasodilating properties), but with an unpaired electron NO is also a highly active free radical that can damage proteins, carbohydrates, nucleotides and lipids. NO is formed during the enzymatic conversion of L-arginine to L-citrulline by nitric oxide synthase (NOS)[74,182,207,255]. There are 3 types of NOS enzymes in humans namely: inducible NOS (iNOS), neuronal NOS (nNOS) and endothelial NOS (e-NOS).

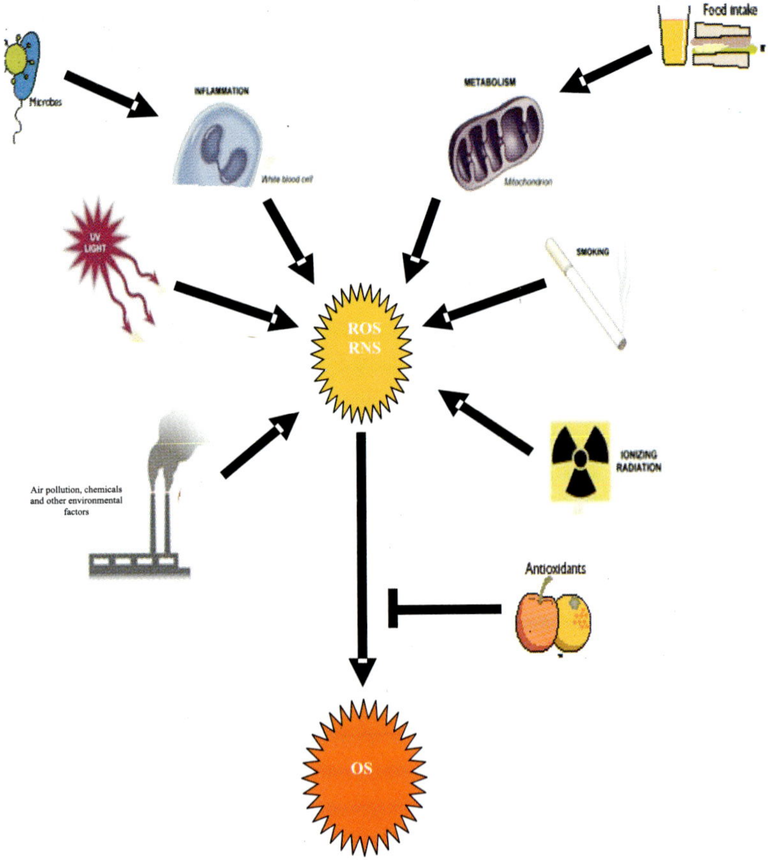

Figure 9.2: Endogenous and Exogenous Sources of Reactive Oxygen Species (ROS) and Reactive Nitrogen Species (RNS) Leading to Oxidative Stress (OS)

Table 9.2: Different Types of Reactive Nitrogen Species (RNS)

Nitric oxide	$NO^{\cdot}$	Nitryl chloride	NO_2Cl
Peroxynitrite	$OONO^-$	Nitrogen dioxide	$NO_2^{\cdot}$
Peroxynitrous acid	ONOOH	Dinitrogen trioxide	N_2O_3
Nitroxyl anion	NO^-	Nitrous acid	HNO_2
Nitrosyl cation	NO^+		

Antioxidants

Organisms have developed efficient protective mechanisms against excessive accumulation of oxidants. There are both enzymatic and non-enzymatic antioxidants in the body[196,253] that neutralize ROS by elaborate antioxidant defense systems[6]. Under normal conditions ROS are neutralized and cleared from the cell by these scavenging molecules in order to prevent overproduction, while under pathological conditions these molecules will help minimize oxidative damage, repair it or even prevent it. Catalase, superoxide dismutase (SOD), glutathione (GSH) peroxidase and GSH reductase are enzymatic or natural antioxidants that can neutralize excessive ROS. Non-enzymatic antioxidants, also known as synthetic antioxidants or dietary supplements, include Vitamin C, Vitamin E, Vitamin A, pyruvate, GSH, taurine and hypotaurine, zinc, selenium, beta carotene and carotene[6,16,196,237,253]. Both male and female genital tracts are rich in antioxidants[98,131,227,272].

Mechanism of Cell Injury Due to Oxidative Stress

Pathological levels of OS can lead to cell injury and dysfunction *via* various mechanisms, including lipid peroxidation, deoxyribonucleic acid (DNA) damage, redox-dependant signaling pathways and apoptosis.

Polyunsaturated fatty acids in cell membranes are targets for attack from ROS, thereby causing lipid peroxidation. Break down or peroxidation of fatty acids can result in the loss of membrane fluidity as well as the formation of various oxidatively modified products which are toxic to cells[130,217]. Phosphodiester backbones and DNA bases are sites that are highly susceptible to OS and ROS mediated peroxidative damage resulting in DNA fragmentation.

Redox-dependant signaling due to increases in ROS has been implicated in modifying the activity of various intracellular signaling molecules and pathways. It has been shown to activate tyrosine kinases, while inhibiting tyrosine phosphatase activity. Modifying the activity of the mitogen activated protein kinases (MAPK), particularly p38MAPK, JNK and ERK[41] may also initiate a chain of reactions ultimately leading to apoptosis[6]. Apoptosis is a process of programmed cell death that occurs under several physiological and pathological situations. It represents a common mechanism whereby the body naturally removes old, damaged and senescent cells.

Apoptosis may occur spontaneously or in response to specific stimuli including OS[54]. The process of apoptosis may also be accelerated by ROS-induced DNA damage[224].

Oxidative Stress and Normal Female Reproductive Function

Several oxidative and antioxidant systems have been reported to be present in various female reproductive tissues[40,46,106,132,191]. In the female reproductive tract, the functions of ROS can also be conflicting. As mentioned earlier, free radical generation under controlled conditions is advocated to play an important role in normal physiological functioning of the female reproductive system[7,11,233,241]. ROS has been reported to act as physiological mediator in hormone signaling, ovarian steroidogenesis, germ cell function, corpus luteum formation, luteolysis and modulation of cyclical changes in the human endometrium[11.230,232,233,241]. OS also plays a role during pregnancy and parturition[85,171,176].

Oxidative Stress and Ovarian Function

OS plays a role in the physiology of ovarian function. ROS most likely exert a regulatory role in folliculogenesis, oocyte maturation, ovulation, corpus luteum function and ovarian steroidogenesis[132,208,234,239]. Various biomarkers of OS have been demonstrated to be present in normally cycling human ovaries[221,236]. Cu-Zn-SOD and Mn-SOD have been detected by immuno-histochemical staining in ovarian tissue[239] and El Mouatassim[79] argued that the expression of these enzymes combined with GSH peroxidase indicates that they are markers for oocyte maturation. It furthermore indicates that the oocytes are exposed to OS and that the enzymatic antioxidants act as catalysts in neutralizing ROS.

RNS and specifically NO are also involved in the modulation of folliculogenesis and steroidogenesis[109,207]. It was shown that follicular NO increase during the secretory phase and peak at mid-cycle of the menstrual cycle[157]. NO concentrations in follicular fluid have also been negatively correlated with mature oocytes, fertilization, embryo quality and rate of cleavage[44,45]. Duleba[88] demonstrated that OS influenced theca-interstitial cells in a dose-dependant manner *in vitro* with the highest doses of OS inhibiting proliferation.

Mn-SOD and Cu-Zn-SOD expression were also observed in luteinized granulosa and theca cells. As these SOD's and other antioxidant enzymes are cyclically expressed in the steroid producing cells of the ovaries, it therefore implies that ROS play a role in corpus luteum (CL) formation and steroidogenesis[234]. eNOS was also expressed in the CL, with the highest expression during the luteal phase[91,202], thereby suggesting a role for NO in luteolysis.

Oxidative Stress and the Endometrium

Both eNOS and iNOS have been found to be expressed in the endometrium, endometrial vessels and glandular surface epithelial cells[238,248]. NO is important for menstruation as it regulates the microvasculature of the endometrium. ROS on the other hand helps bring about changes in the endometrium during the secretory phase in order to prepare it for implantation.

ROS has been implicated to play a putative role in the modulation of recurring changes in the human endometrium. Sugino described a cyclical variation in SOD expression in the endometrium, whereby SOD activity decreases in the late secretory phase with simultaneous increases in ROS levels[232]. It was furthermore shown that withdrawal of ovarian steroids (progesterone and estrogen) stimulates prostaglandin F2α production through nuclear factor kappaβ activation *via* oxygen radicals in human endometrial stromal cells cultured *in vitro*, thereby linking these effects to endometrial shedding[231]. All of these influences are potentially very relevant to the regulation of menstruation.

Oxidative Stress and Female Infertility

The inability to conceive, following 12 or more months of unprotected intercourse, affects about 10 per cent of the population of reproductive years and is classified by the ASRM as infertility[1]. Almost 50 per cent of cases are due to female causes, more than 30 per cent due to male causes and the rest of the cases are unexplained[77,80].

Various reviews have revealed a connection between reproductive toxicity and involvement of electron transfer-ROS-OS[144]. When there is an excess of free radicals in the female reproductive system, they precipitate pathologies in the reproductive tract[11]. It is well known that OS contributes widely to female infertility as it has been demonstrated to be involved in many of the causes of infertility such as endometriosis, tubal factor infertility, polycystic ovarian disease, unexplained infertility, embryonic development, preterm labor and recurrent pregnancy loss[10,11,15,46,201,259] (Figure 9.3). Increased levels of ROS in the female reproductive tract environment can have detrimental effects on the gametes and embryos. All of these aforementioned pathological effects are exerted by various mechanisms including lipid damage, DNA damage, inhibition of protein synthesis, mitochondrial alterations and depletion of ATP[59, 107, 119, 146, 164, 195, 204].

Oxidative Stress and Endometriosis

Women of reproductive age often suffer from a common gynecological disorder, endometriosis, which is characterized by the growth of endometrial glands and stroma outside the uterus. It is suggested that OS is present in the peritoneal cavity of endometriosis sufferers as markers of increased lipid peroxidation (lysophosphatidyl choline) have been accounted for by both Murphy [173] and Shanti [216]. Elevated levels of lipid peroxidation combined with significantly lower concentrations of SOD were also reported in peritoneal fluid of woman with endometriosis [163, 237]. A possible source of ROS and contributor to the OS may be the increased number and activation of macrophages detected in the peritoneal cavity of patients with this disease [237].

Despite the fact that various other studies failed to report higher ROS levels in peritoneal fluid of patients with endometriosis[46, 260], antioxidant treatment experiments were able to show an inhibitory effect on OS induced proliferation of endometrial stromal cells *in vitro*. RU486, an antiprogestational agent with antioxidant activity, showed a marked reduction in propagation of both stromal and epithelial cells[88, 174]. This furthermore implicates OS to be involved as one of the many causative factors in the etiopathogenesis of endometriosis.

NOS activity was reported to be higher in peritoneal macrophages isolated *in vitro*[186, 265], while iNOS was more expressed in endometrial tissue from endometriosis sufferers. Both eNOS expression and SOD were also found to be increased in patients with endometriosis[187].

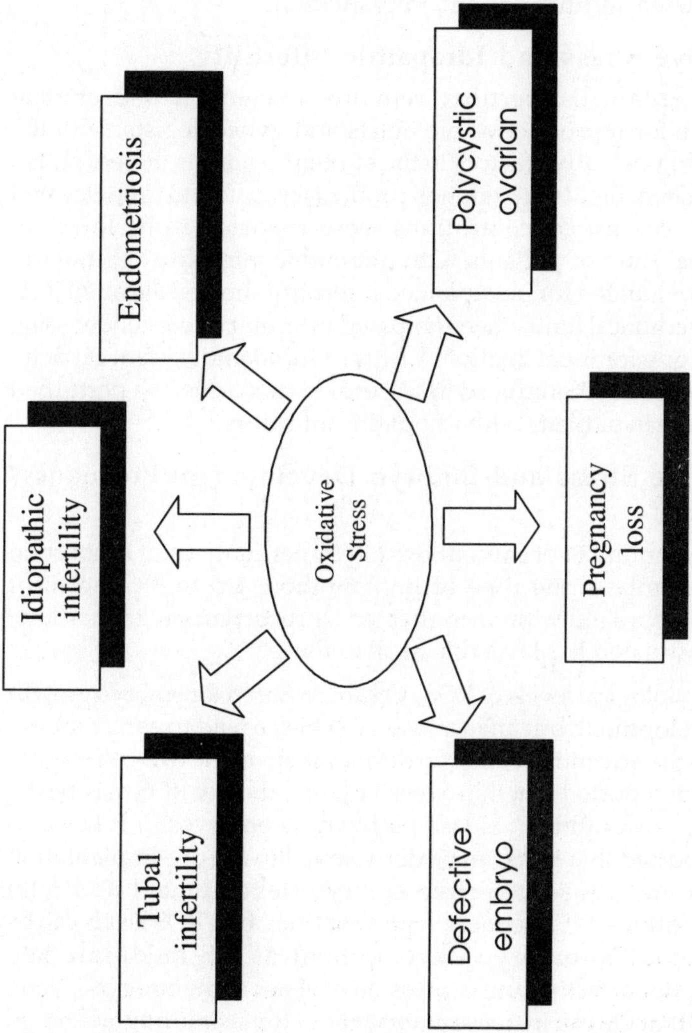

Figure 9.3: The Role of Oxidative Stress (OS) in Female Infertility

The infertility linked with endometriosis can possibly be explained by the deleterious effects of the associated OS on oocytes, spermatozoa, fertilization and implantation.

Oxidative Stress and Idiopathic Infertility

Unexplained infertility remains a scientific and clinical challenge for reproductive biologists and gynecologists, with the underlying causative factors in the etiopathogenesis thereof still to be elucidated. Lipid peroxidation products were found to be elevated and antioxidant concentrations were reported to be lower in peritoneal fluid of patients with idiopathic infertility[198]. Similarly females evaluated for unexplained infertility showed elevated ROS in their peritoneal fluid when compared to fertile patients undergoing laparoscopy for tubal ligation[260]. This reduced antioxidant capacity and increased ROS-induced lipid peroxidation reflects a perturbed redox state in patients with idiopathic infertility.

Oxidative Stress and Embryo Development/Pregnancy/ Abortion

A vast number of conceptions (30-50 per cent) result in abortion predominanly at the time of implantation. Up to 3 per cent of reproductive aged woman is affected by recurrent pregnancy loss. OS is postulated to play a role in all of these[10, 60].

Physiological levels of ROS/OS are required for embryo growth and development, but an increase in ROS can lead to early embryo block by the arresting of embryo development in the two-cell stage[106, 180]. Burton reported that the excessive generation of ROS may be the result of the xanthine oxidase pathway in embryos [52]. It has also been reported that ROS can be detrimental to the pre-implantation embryo and cause defective embryo development and fetal embryopathies[106, 110]. Dennery report that elevated ROS levels can be detrimental to embryo development as OS modulate key transcriptional factors and expression of genes in the embryo[73]. Yang showed that OS can increase embryonic cytoplasmic fragmentation and apoptosis, leading to either embryonic death/abortion or congenital abnormalities[269]

Pregnancy is associated with an inflammatory response characterized by leukocyte activation[116, 209]. In pregnancies complicated by preeclampsia this leukocyte activation response was further exacerbated [209].

The pathophysiology of miscarriage might be partially explained by placental OS and preeclampsia[73]. Recently it has been proposed that OS modulates the expression of cytokine receptors in the placenta, cytotrophoblasts, vascular endothelial cells and smooth muscle cells[42]. Agarwal *et al.*, suggests that the redox state has a critical role in modulating implantation and affecting preimplantation embryonic growth[10].

Oxidative Stress and Male Reproductive Function

Until recently ROS were exclusively considered to be toxic to human spermatozoa however, a strong body of evidence advocates that physiological levels of ROS has a positive role in the control of human sperm function[18, 19, 21, 70, 93].

Aitken[27] was the first to report that limited amounts of ROS was necessary for normal sperm physiology by showing that low levels of ROS enhance sperm-*zona pellucida* binding, which could be reversed by Vitamin E supplementation. The generation of physiological levels of ROS appears to be an important part of the capacitation process whereby spermatozoa gain the ability to respond to signals presented by the oocyte-cumulus complex. This subsequently initiates a cascade of cellular interactions that ultimately can lead to fertilization[21]. ROS, and in particular both superoxide anion and H_2O_2, is specifically necessary for stimulating the tyrosine phosphorylation events associated with capacitation[32, 153]. De Lamirande and Gagnon[69] furthermore found that incubating spermatozoa with low concentrations of H_2O_2 not only stimulates capacitation, but also leads to hyperactivation, acrosome reaction and oocyte fusion. Low concentrations of NO have also been shown to promote sperm capacitation, acrosome reaction, hyperactivation and *zona pellucida* binding[215, 270, 271]. NO regulates cAMP and exert its effect on capacitation of spermatozoa *via* the action of adenyl cyclase.

Just as in the female reproductive system it is important to note that ROS, within physiological ranges, is a necessary for successful male reproductive function ROS must therefore be continuously inactivated *in vivo* to maintain physiological levels and normal sperm function. As the sperm head is very condensed and the cytoplasm highly reduced during the final stages of maturation, it is deficient in cytoplasmic enzymes. Seminal plasma allows compensating for this deficiency as it contains an array of antioxidant defense mechanisms in order to protect spermatozoa against oxidants[35, 38, 75, 222, 223].

Oxidative Stress and Male Infertility

The most common defined cause of human infertility is defective sperm function[118]. Male factor infertility contributes between 30–50 per cent towards all cases of couple infertility. It is distinguished from female infertility in being a disease that is largely focused on the germ cells [21]. Female infertility is mostly of somatic cell origin and has an endocrine basis often amenable to pharmacological treatment. Most infertile men are endocrinologically normal and produce sufficient spermatozoa, but these gametes are mostly not normal as judged by functional and morphological characteristics[21]. Commonly recorded deficiencies of spermatozoa include their capacity to move and penetrate cervical mucus as well as ability to acrosome react, bind to the *zona pellucida* and fuse with the oocyte's vitelline membrane[17, 63, 162, 273]. Spermatozoa seem to suffer from a pathological condition that simultaneously affects many different aspects of sperm function. It is hypothesized that oxidative stress could account for such a multiplicity of defects in individual semen samples (Figure 9.4) and is therefore most likely the fundamental mediator of defective sperm function[62]. As early as 1943, the presence of free radicals was reported by MacLeod[21, 165]. He noted that the loss of motility by human spermatozoa in an oxygenated medium could be abrogated by the addition of catalase and thereby concluding that human spermatozoa generated H_2O_2 [21].

Spermatozoa are often unable to prevent oxidative damage by free radicals as they lack cytoplasmic enzymes. They are also particularly susceptible to ROS-induced damage because their plasma membranes contain large quantities of polyunsaturated fatty acids[211].

Origin of Oxidants in the Male Reproductive System

Semen is made up of various cell types including mature and immature spermatozoa, round cells from different stages of spermatogenesis, leukocytes and epithelial cells[13]. Of these, leukocytes and immature spermatozoa are the two main sources of ROS[95] (Figure 9.5).

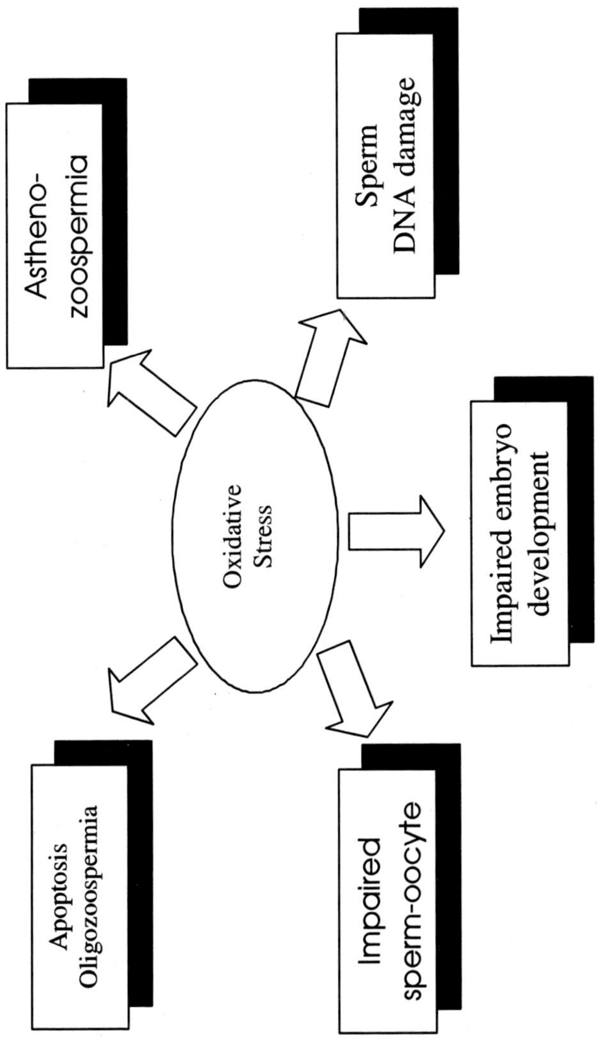

Figure 9.4: Role of Oxidative Stress (OS) in Male Infertility

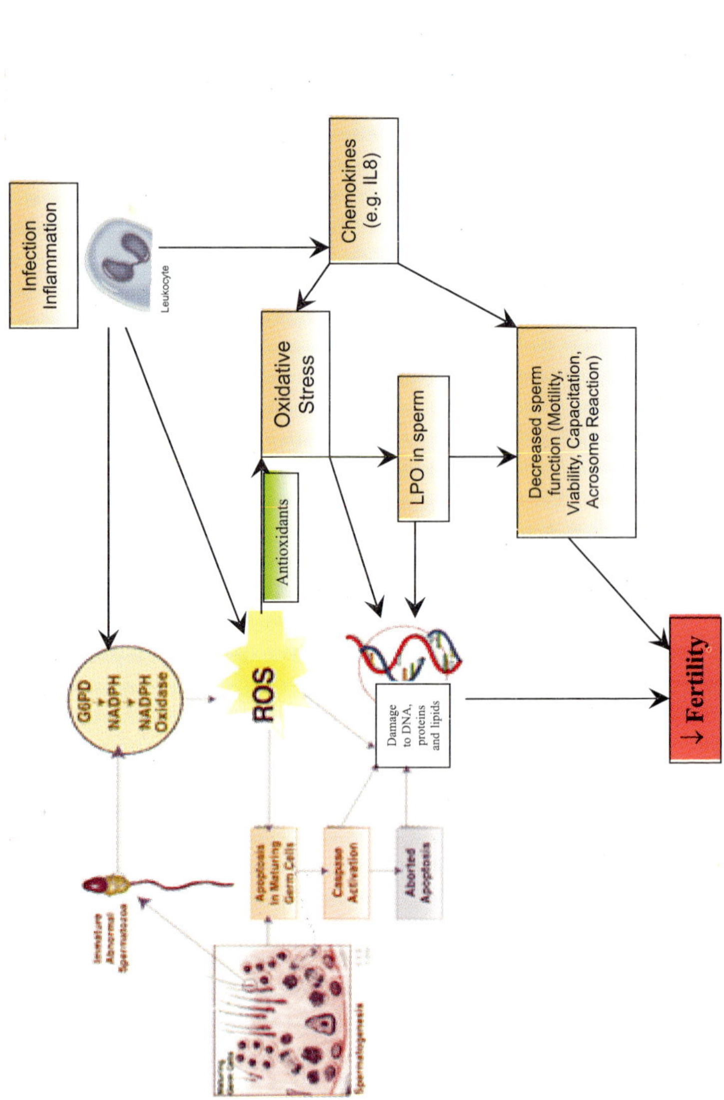

Figure 9.5: Possible Mechanisms of ROS/OS Induced Decrease in Sperm Function, DNA Damage and Fertility (OS: Oxidative stress; ROS: Reactive oxygen species; LPO: Lipid peroxidation)

Generation of ROS by Spermatozoa

As mentioned previously it is well established that all actively respiring cells generate ROS as a consequence of electron leakage from intracellular redox activities. It is understandable that spermatozoa do generate ROS. Spermatozoa may generate ROS either *via* the nicotinamide adenine dinucleotide phosphate (NADPH) oxidase system at the level of the sperm plasma membrane[25] or the NADH-dependent oxido-reductase system at the level of the mitochondria[97]. The latter (mitochondrial system) seems to be the main source of ROS in the spermatozoa from infertile males[197].

An important pathological source of ROS is immature spermatozoa. The presence of excess residual cytoplasm (specifically in the midpiece/cytoplasmic droplet) appears to be associated with excessive redox activity observed in spermatozoa of infertile patients[103]. The etiology of impaired sperm function due to the presence of excess residual cytoplasm involves the induction of excessive redox activity and OS[102]. This is due to surplus glucose-6-phosphate dehydrogenase and creatine phosphokinase enhancing cytoplasmic generation of NADPH, thereby fueling the production of free radicals by a proposed sperm NADPH oxidase[21]. Human spermatozoa generate superoxide which can dismutate spontaneously or enzymatically to H_2O_2 and also lead to the formation of the potent oxidant OH^-[36].

Gil-Guzman *et al.*[101] demonstrated that ROS production is negatively correlated with semen quality including normal morphology according to the World Health Organization (WHO) classification[261] and Tygerberg strict criteria[148]. The same group also found that ROS production was higher in immature sperm fractions than in mature subsets obtained after isolate gradient fractionation. Furthermore nuclear DNA damage of mature spermatozoa was also directly correlated to the number of immature (ROS-producing) sperm. These findings allowed for speculation that oxidative damage of mature sperm by ROS-producing immature sperm during their co-migration from seminiferous tubules to the epididymis may be an important cause of male infertility[15].

Leukocytes as Sources of ROS

ROS produced by leukocytes forms the first line of defense in any infectious process. During inflammation and infection, activated leukocytes can produce significantly higher amounts of ROS than non-activated leukocytes[197]. ROS is positively correlated with interleukin-8, a potent stimulator of pro-inflammatory cytokines, thereby also suppressing the scavenging effect of oxidants[114, 179, 200]. Leukocytes are present throughout the male reproductive tract and are found in almost every human ejaculate[245]. Despite ROS being released as part of the defense system in the reproductive tract, it can still damage the spermatozoa present[6]. Leukocytes, particularly neutrophils and macrophages, are associated with excessive ROS production in the male reproductive tract and this ultimately cause sperm dysfunction[20, 114, 184, 190, 212, 218]. Leukocytes act either directly by ROS synthesis or indirectly by stimulating other neighboring white cells or spermatozoa *via* soluble factors (cytokines) to ROS production[95, 97, 184]. ROS production by leukocytes is also via the NADPH oxidase enzyme system.

Leukocytospermia is defined by the WHO as the presence of $>1x10^6$ peroxidase-positive leukocytes per milliliter of semen. Sharma *et al.*, reported that seminal leukocytes might cause OS even at concentrations below the WHO cutoff value[218].

Consequences of OS

Excessive ROS production and the consequent development of OS may affect the quality and number of spermatozoa reaching the oocyte in the female reproductive tract. OS can also impair fertilization by precluding initiation of sperm-oocyte fusion[22], while ROS can also impair embryo development and the health of the offspring[14] (Figure 9.4).

Impaired Motility

Motility is a unique and indispensible attribute of human spermatozoa. Impaired sperm motility has been associated with OS[24, 185] and increased generation of ROS has been correlated with a reduction in motility[12, 37, 125, 158]. This can be the result of the induction of lipid peroxidation[23, 28, 36] or the rapid depletion of ATP, due to excessive ROS, resulting in decreased phosphorylation of axonemal proteins[68] and sperm immobilization[136]

Apoptosis and Decreased Sperm Concentration

Oligozoospermic patients (decreased sperm concentration) have a reduced chance of fertilizing the oocyte and initiating pregnancy[224].

The severity of oligozoospermia has been correlated to increased ROS levels[189]. Apoptosis that occurs during adult life helps discard cells that have an altered function or no function at all[254]. With regard to normal physiological male reproductive conditions, abnormal spermatozoa are removed from the semen due to apoptosis *via* caspase activation, while it may also be responsible for controlling the overproduction of male gametes[210, 226]. Apoptosis is strictly regulated by intrinsic genetic control[226], as well as by extrinsic factors such as irradiation[111], chemotherapy[138] and toxins[156]. Spontaneous germ cell apoptosis have been found in spermatogonia, spermatocytes and spermatids in the testis of normal men[115, 134] Pathological levels of ROS can cause increased stimulation of apoptosis of spermatozoa which can result in their death and lead to a reduced sperm count. Gandini *et al.*, reported that oligoasthenozoospermic subjects showed a significantly higher percentage of apoptosis than normozoospermic men[94]. Agarwal *et al.*, furthermore reported that mature spermatozoa from infertility patients showed significantly higher levels of apoptosis compared to mature spermatozoa from normal donors[15]. These levels of apoptosis were also significantly correlated with levels of seminal ROS.

Aitken postulate that, in view of reports of declining sperm counts during the last few decades and increased environmental exposure to ROS and changing lifestyle factors, a possible association between oxidative damage to spermatozoa and declining sperm count in the general population exist[19].

Impaired Sperm-Oocyte Fusion

The release of SOD might be the inherent mechanism to help prevent unnecessary production of ROS at the time of gamete fusion [166]. Irregularities in SOD production can lead to both spermatozoa and oocyte damage due to increased ROS generation. The effects of ROS on the sperm membrane are predominantly responsible for the inability of the sperm to fuse with the oocyte. This lipid peroxidation process leads to a loss of membrane fluidity and reduced membrane enzyme and ion channel activity. As a result spermatozoa are unable to initiate the required biochemical reactions associated with acrosome reaction, *zona pellucida* binding and oocyte penetration[29, 105]. Various other studies have also reported that acrosomal exocytosis and sperm-oocyte fusion is inhibited by OS and correlated with high levels of redox activity in spermatozoa[26,27,120].

Sperm DNA Damage

The plasma membrane of human spermatozoa is not the only sub-cellular structure susceptible to OS. The chromatin of the sperm nucleus is also vulnerable to DNA damage[19,21,22]. The characteristic tight packaging of the sperm DNA helps to protect it from oxidative insult[251]. Poor compaction and incomplete protamination of sperm chromatin increase their vulnerability[22,48]. It has been shown that men with poor semen quality exhibit sperm nuclear genome fragmentation that is often accompanied by oxidative DNA damage[121,211]. OS has also been correlated with high frequencies of single and double DNA strand breaks[31,251]. Spermatozoa from leukocytospermic patients have been shown to have excessive DNA and structural damage. Various authors suggest that DNA damage commonly observed in spermatozoa from infertile men is mediated by high ROS levels[89,90,140,235].

As the sperm contributes half of the genomic material to the offspring, normal sperm genetic material is required for fertilization, embryo and fetus development and postnatal child wellbeing[6,14,105]. Aitken explains that at low levels of OS, sperm DNA is damaged but the spermatozoa still exhibit a normal ability to fertilize. This elucidates the importance of sperm DNA damage in mediating the paternal impact of occupational or environmental toxicants on morbidity in children and young adults[21]. As an example a male smoker's body is exposed to OS and his spermatozoa will show elevated levels of DNA fragmentation and oxidative base changes[33,90]. This DNA damage does not necessarily impact on the fertility of the male smoker[21], but may make a significant contribution to the increased levels of childhood cancer seen in the offspring of such subjects[129].

Aitken propose that non-specific oxidative damage to DNA in male germ cells create a predisposition to mutational change in the embryo[21]. There is furthermore a substantial risk that spermatozoa carrying damaged DNA are being selected during assisted reproductive techniques (ART) specifically such as intracytoplasmic sperm injection (ICSI) as the natural selection barriers (*e.g.* peroxidative damage to the sperm plasma membrane) is bypassed[19,

[250]. This subsequent injection of a spermatozoon with DNA damage into an oocyte can lead to congenital abnormalities[19, 219].

Environmental and Occupational Exposure and Lifestyle Factors Contributing to OS

Fertility is dependent on normal male and female reproductive function. While there are distinct structural, mechanical and hormonal deficits that can affect fertility, environmental and occupational exposure as well as lifestyle factors can also contribute to OS and lead to reproductive pathologies. ROS can also damage your body *via* external sources as our surroundings increasingly bombard us with ROS. These environmental attacks overwhelm the body's natural ability to prevent damage with our own supply of endogenous antioxidants.

Many chemicals contribute to increasing the toxic load and have the potential to disrupt fertility. These include: organic solvents, pesticides, alcohol, cigarette smoke, some chemicals used in the plastics industry, cleaning products, chemicals used in personal care products and some preservatives. Due to the industrial revolution and specifically during the past century the rapid expansion of particularly the chemicals industry has resulted in the release of a superfluity of xenobiotics into the environment[30, 206]. These alien molecules have worked their way into our lives in a variety of forms including pesticides, herbicides, cosmetics, cleaning materials, waste, pharmaceuticals and industrial by-products[30]. It is becoming increasingly apparent that a major target of this chemical barrage is the reproductive system, as numerous studies have associated occupational exposure to pesticides, herbicides, industrial agents and heavy metals with impaired fertility. These xenobiotics can possibly be metabolized to molecules (quinones) that can cause cellular damage by either binding to DNA or generating ROS species, ultimately creating a state of OS. Westernization and prosperity are some aspects that can influence lifestyle choices. There is good evidence that diet and lifestyle can impact on man's fertility. These lifestyle factors *e.g.* diet (nutrient-poor diet, high insulin levels and obesity) smoking, vigorous exercise and emotional stress can also contribute to development of OS and exert a role on reproductive function. The remainder of this section will highlight and deal with only a few occupational and environmental exposures as well as lifestyle factors that contribute to generation of OS and affecting human reproduction.

Psychological Stress

It has been demonstrated that mental stress creates OS. Mental stress is associated with lower antioxidant levels (GSH and SOD) and higher levels of pro-oxidants [82]. Various studies have shown a correlation between stress and semen quality. One such study in particular reported that students have lower sperm counts and sperm quality during the highly stressful periods of examinations[84]. Eskiocak and co-workers were also able to link periods of psychological stress with a reduction in sperm quality mediated by an increase in seminal plasma ROS generation and a reduction in antioxidant protection[83, 247].

Diet and Obesity

OS is also a nutritional issue. It occurs when reactive oxygen molecules are produced at a higher rate in the body than they are neutralized by anti-oxidants and this result in structural and genetic damage to cells.

Nutritional deficient diets lacking antioxidant vitamins and synergistic minerals do not enable the quenching of reactive oxygen molecules. For example Vitamin C and Vitamin E are essential antioxidants that protect the body's cells from damage from OS and free radicals. Vitamin C is the most abundant antioxidant in the semen of fertile men, and it contributes to the maintenance of healthy sperm by protecting the sperm's DNA from free radical damage[228].

Vitamin E is a fat-soluble vitamin that helps protect the sperm's cell membrane from damage. Studies have shown that Vitamin E improves sperm motility and morphology. Vitamin C functions to regenerate Vitamin E, thus these vitamins may work together to improve sperm function[81, 89, 228, 243]. Selenium on the other hand is a mineral that also functions as an antioxidant. Selenium supplements have been shown to increase sperm motility, and a combination of selenium and Vitamin E has been shown to decrease damage from free radicals and improve sperm motility in infertile men [112].

High body mass index (BMI), overweight and obese subjects are also at danger of infertility. Men with BMI's greater than 25 are at increased risk of infertility due to reduction in sperm concentration and increased DNA fragmentation. Obesity decreases the levels of circulating testosterone and increases levels of estradiol[141, 143, 181].

Obesity furthermore leads to a condition known as the metabolic syndrome (MS). MS is characterized by a group of abnormalities including overweight, dyslipidemia, hypertension, and impaired glucose metabolism. It has been known for sometime now that obesity and the MS are associated with infertility. In males, the MS cause infertility through several mechanisms. Firstly, the excess adipose tissue leads to the conversion of testosterone to estrogen which subsequently results in the development of secondary hypogonadism through hypothalamic-pituitary-gonadal axis inhibition[86]. Secondly, it leads to infertility *via* increased scrotal temperatures due to the accumulation of suprapubic and inner thigh fat in severely obese men. Lastly, MS and several of its components, namely, obesity, insulin resistance, and dyslipidemia, are associated with systemic proinflammatory states and increased OS[65, 66]. OS cause sperm membrane lipid peroxidation which results in the impairment of sperm motility, DNA damage and impaired sperm-oocyte interaction[140, 249]. Conversely, obesity produces OS as adipose tissue releases pro-inflammatory cytokines that increase leukocyte production of ROS[225].

Alcohol Consumption

There is a growing body of evidence suggesting that alcohol is one of the lifestyle factors that are suspected to have a detrimental effect on reproductive health in men and women. Impotence, testicular atrophy, and loss of sexual interest are often associated with alcoholism in men[50]. Muthusami and Chinnaswami showed that there was a significant reduction of follicle stimulating hormone (FSH), luteinizing hormone (LH) levels as well as testosterone levels in alcoholics when compared to non-alcoholics[175]. Furthermore, they reported that semen volume, sperm count, motility, and number of morphologically normal sperm were significantly decreased in alcoholics when compared to non-alcoholics[104]. Excessive alcohol consumption has also been linked to a decrease in the percentage of normal sperm in asthenozoospermic patients[104], while Maneesh *et al.*, suggested the presence of OS within the testicle by reporting a significant reduction in testosterone, increase in lipid peroxidation byproducts and a drop in antioxidants[167]. In females, it has also been reported that alcohol consumption is a predictor for infertility problems[244]. The association between alcohol and infertility is of great concern because the use of alcohol is widespread. In many countries, it is common to start drinking alcohol during the teenage years as it is considered as a common form of social entertainment.

Many processes and factors are involved in causing alcohol induced OS. One way alcohol cause detrimental effects on the reproductive function of both males and females is *via* its ability to induce OS through generating ROS molecules in response to the metabolism of ethanol by the microsomal ethanol-oxidizing system (MEOS)[64, 160]. Alcohol metabolism results in NADH formation which enhances activity of the respiratory chain, including heightened oxygen use and excessive ROS formation[13]. ROS are cellular renegades and wreak havoc in biological system by tissue damage, altering biochemical compounds, corroding cell membranes and killing out rightly[263]. Alcohol also induces hypoxia that results in tissue damage. Many alcohol abusers also have diets deficient in protective antioxidants[139, 264].

Smoking

Tobacco smoke contains nearly 4000 harmful substances (*e.g.* alkaloids, nitrosamines, nicotine, hydroxycotine etc.). Many of these substances generate ROS and RNS[61, 246]. It is well established that smoking has detrimental effects on the male reproductive system as it has been significantly correlated with lower sperm count, motility and morphology[149, 213, 256]. This is most likely due to higher levels of OS induced by smoking. Semen of smokers shows a 100-fold increase in OS and up to 5x higher cadmium levels[213].

Saleh *et al.*, demonstrated that cigarette smoking leads to an increase in ROS levels and decreases in ROS-TAC scores. It was furthermore reported that smokers have high levels of leukocytospermia and suggested that OS develops due to ROS generation by activated leukocytes[213]. It was also reported that smokers have decreased levels of seminal plasma antioxidants such as Vitamin C[172] and Vitamin E[90].

Various compounds of cigarette smoke (*i.e.* polycyclic aromatic hydrocarbons) and smoking metabolites may act as chemotactic stimuli and thereby induce an inflammatory response, leading to the recruitment of leukocytes with subsequent generation of ROS [205, 213]. Sperm motility correlates negatively with the amount of cotinine and hydroxycotinine in seminal plasma[68, 256]. A recent study showed that motility is one of the first sperm parameters affected and asthenozoospermia may be an early indicator of reduced semen quality in light smokers. The incidence of teratozoospermia was also significantly higher in heavy smokers when compared to non-smokers[96].

Smoking significantly reduced GSH peroxidase concentrations in the liquor folliculi. The follicular fluid microenvironment is important for follicular maturation and granulose cell function. Reduced concentrations of GSH peroxidase, a protective enzyme, may affect the fertilizing ability of the oocytes and down regulation of GSH peroxidase in the follicular fluid is significantly associated with low fertilization rates[191, 239].

Studies have shown that heavy paternal or maternal smoking can even affect reproductive parameters of their offspring during especially adolescence[128, 205].

Cell Phone Radiation

Stopczyk *et al.*, demonstrated that microwaves produced by mobiles significantly depleted SOD-1 activity while a significant increase in the concentration of malonyldialdehyde (MDA) after 1, 5, and 7 min of exposure was observed in a suspension of human blood platelets[229]. On the grounds of these results the authors conclude that OS after exposure to microwaves may be the reason for many adverse changes in cells and may cause a number of systemic disturbances in the human body. Many animal studies also demonstrated that cell phone radiation can increase levels of MDA and decrease the levels of antioxidant enzymes, while other studies consistently reported that cell phone radiation leads to a decrease in male fertility. Epidemiological studies also without fail found positive correlations with decreases in sperm parameters[8, 72]. Recently, Friedman *et al.*, showed that radiofrequency electromagnetic waves (RF-EMW) stimulate plasma membrane NADH oxidase in mammalian cells and cause production of ROS[92]. A recent study provided evidence that cell phone radiation can lead to generation of ROS[9]. Results showed a significant increase in ROS production in exposed samples and a decrease in sperm motility, viability, and ROS-TAC score in exposed samples[9]. A plausible explanation for the ROS production is that it is due to stimulation of the spermatozoa's plasma membrane redox system (increase in the activity of spermatozoal NADH oxidase) by RF-EMW or the effect of EMW on leukocytes present in the neat semen. This may be attributed to an after RF-EMW exposure. Electromagnetic wave–dependent decrease in melatonin, an antioxidant, can also predispose sperm to oxidative stress[51].

Although many animal, as well as *in vitro* studies have provided evidence that cell phone radiation may lead to decrease in sperm parameters due to OS, considerable research is still required to confirm this evidence.

Heat Stress and Exercise

It is well known that the testicles should be cooler than the rest of the body for optimal spermatogenesis. Just as the harmful effects of a varicocele on sperm production is believed to result from the excessive warming of the testicular area (caused by dilated veins), similarly various recreational (*e.g.* cycling, hot tubs or prolonged baths) and occupational (*e.g.* long distance driving, furnace operators) activities can lead to increasing testicular temperature. It is generally assumed that these raised temperatures lead to amplified rates of oxidative DNA damage and hence more mutations in the resulting spermatozoa[124]. Furthermore, obesity and the accompanying accumulation of adipose tissue within the groin region also results in raising testicular temperature. This has been linked to the development of OS in the testis and reduced sperm quality[43, 123, 194].

The creation of ROS is also an unwanted side effect of aerobic exercise and respiration. Because consumption of oxygen increases up to 20 times greater than the level at rest during high activity, ROS can leak from an elevated oxygen flow through mitochondrial electron-transport pathways. High impact exercise is thus linked with OS since muscle aerobic metabolism creates a large amount of ROS[193]. Manna *et al.*, showed that increasing levels of exercise led to a reduction in sperm count and motility and a corresponding increase in biochemical signs of testicular OS in a rodent model[168].

Heavy Metal Toxicity

Even moderate exposures to toxic metals such as lead and cadmium has been conclusively linked to sperm oxidative damage and can significantly reduce semen quality by directly affecting sperm[4,117] and increasing DNA oxidation [177,268]. Other metals such as aluminum, vanadium, and mercury are believed to also have effects on male fertility, though there is less research in these areas. The increase in infertility and miscarriage observed in the partners of welders and battery/paint factory workers could possibly be due to oxidative damage to sperm DNA initiated by the inhalation of metal fumes[49,99]. An assessment of heavy metal status may be necessary during infertility treatment depending on the lifestyle and occupational exposures of the couples affected[56,133,242].

Lead is reported to cause OS by disturbing the pro-oxidant and antioxidant balance[117]. Various animal models as well as *in vitro* studies have been performed to study and elucidate the mechanisms through which lead exert its effects on reproduction. Lead has inhibitory effects on the delta amino levulanic acid (ALA) synthase enzyme. Inhibition of this enzyme leads to the accumulation of ALA resulting in the generation of ROS. Lead can also cause peroxidation of polyunsaturated fatty acids (PUFA) in plasma membranes. Spermatozoa are more susceptible to lead induced OS due to the high content of PUFA in their plasma membrane. Another target of lead is the enzymatic antioxidant systems of the cell[117]. Lead has been shown to inhibit the activity of SOD, catalase and glutathione peroxidase by inhibiting the functional sulphydril group of these enzymes. It has been shown that elevated blood levels of lead (BLL;± 33.6µg/dL) increased ROS generation in rat spermatozoa, while relatively lower BLL (±18.6µg/dL) resulted in a significant decrease in SOD activity in rat testicular tissue [117]. Epidemiological studies reported that BLL of about 23.4µg/dL (humans) might be a risk factor for prostate cancer through generation of free radicals[16], while another study showed that occupational lead exposure leading to raised BLL affects fecundity of male workers[220]. The 3rd NHNES reported an inverse correlation between BLL (2.8 µg/dL) with levels of serum Vitamin C, carotenoids and Vitamin E in 10,098 adult participants[154].

The toxicity of cadmium to the reproductive system is well established. Many animal studies suggest a role for cadmium as a pro-oxidant. Cadmium exposure causes alterations in transcription of genes and expression of L type voltage-dependent calcium channels [47]. These channels regulate calcium as well as cadmium entry into the cell. Altered expression of these channels on the sperm tail is correlated with abnormal sperm motility. Chronic low dose exposure to cadmium is associated with a decrease in motility. The negative effects of cadmium may be mediated by indirect generation of hydroxyl radical, superoxide anion, H_2O_2 or NO, and reducing the zinc concentration. Chronic zinc deficiency is associated with increased sensitivity to OS mainly because zinc serves as an antioxidant and has a protective effect on spermatogenesis[47]. In support of this theory it was shown that chronic low dose cadmium exposure produced a time- and dose-dependent reduction in sperm motility. A recent study also reported that there is an association between blood cadmium levels and endometriosis[126].

Plastics Industry Chemicals

Many chemicals can exert an effect on reproductive function, especially those used in the plastics industry. Bisphenol A (BPA) is mainly used in the coverings of food containers (*e.g.* milk, water, and infant bottles) and dental materials. Potential human exposure occurs due to migration of BPA from the food container into food. Infants are more susceptible because of the use of BPA in infant bottles and packaging of canned infant formula. BPA can also migrate from dental sealants and composites (fillings), ultimately ending up in the systemic circulation[142, 152]. Its capability to mimic estradiol receptors is well reported in the literature. In a study on rat brain, Obata demonstrated the generation of hydroxyl radicals in the striatum after BPA exposure [183]. Chitra reported that BPA generates ROS in various rat tissues including the reproductive organs [57]. BPA was shown to increase the levels of H_2O_2 and TBARS (thiobarbituric acid reactive substance) in rat testis. This subsequently leads to the depletion of the antioxidant defense system. Kabuto *et al.*, also reported that BPA administration induces overproduction of H_2O_2 in the kidneys, liver and testes of rats. It has also been described that exposure to BPA during fetal life and infancy may lead to underdevelopment of the brain and testis due to oxidative injury[135].

Phthalate esters are used mainly in the plastics industry to provide flexibility and resilience to various plastic products. They are widely used in many consumer products such as plastic bags, inflatable recreational toys, blood storage bags, plastic clothing, soaps and shampoo. Di (2-ethyhexyl) phthalate (DEHP) is one of the most commonly used and best-studied phthalate esters in the plastics industry[2,100,122,192]. Animal studies provided clear evidence of developmental and reproductive toxicity due to DEHP; however human studies have not provided sufficient evidence of reproductive toxicity. DEHP and its most toxic metabolite mono (2-ethylhexyl) phthalate (MEHP) induced testicular atrophy in laboratory animals. Oral administration of phthalate esters to rats is reported to increase the generation of ROS within the testis with a concomitant decrease in antioxidant levels, culminating in impaired spermatogenesis[155]. In the last decade many studies have reported the capability of phthalates to induce OS in various tissues including the testis. Manojkumar *et al.*, demonstrated a decrease in the concentration of Vitamin E in blood stored in DEHP-plasticized bags[169], while Kasahara *et al.*, reported that DEHP causes germ cell apoptosis *via* the induction of OS[137]. MEHP enhances the generation of ROS in mitochondria and low concentrations of MEHP induce the release of cytochrome C from the mitochondria. It was also suggested that MEHP causes redox-mediated activation of nuclear factor-kB and upregulation of Fas ligand on Sertoli cells and subsequent apoptosis of germ cells[137]. Comparable to the pro-oxidant effect of cadmium, DEHP leads to the depletion of zinc in the testis and this might be one of the possible mechanisms how DEHP can exert its negative effect on reproductive function *via* the induction of OS[188].

Agriculture Fertilizers and Pesticides

Chemical fertilizers are being used worldwide by farmers resulting in an excess of nitrate and ammonium in agricultural areas. Lots of evidence has been documented regarding nitrogen saturation of soil and the effect thereof on crops, grasslands and surrounding areas or the impact of nitrogen loading on aquatic ecosystems [3,257,258]. Un-ionized ammonia can be neurotoxic and rapidly lethal, while nitrate can be reduced to nitrite causing methemoglobinemia, a condition where the blood can no longer bind oxygen[159]. Newborn humans are particularly susceptible to nitrate poisoning because fetal hemoglobin is more readily oxidized to methemoglobin[147]. Embryos and larvae of some aquatic species such as fishes and amphibians have been reported to be very sensitive to high levels of chemical fertilizers in water due to increased OS[170,262]. These fertilizers can also stimulate NO production. It has been reported in humans that excess NO negatively affects sperm motility, viability, acrosome reaction as well as ability to penetrate the oocytes[266].

Various pesticides and herbicides such as lindane, methoxychlor and dioxin-TCDD[58, 150, 151] have all been linked with testicular OS in rodent models. Carbendazim (Methyl-2-benzimidazole carbamate) is a systemic broad-spectrum fungicide controlling various fungal pathogens. It also functions as a preservative in the paint, textile and leather industry, as well as a preservative of fruits[214]. Carbendazim has been reported to have harmful effects on various aspects of male reproduction in hamsters, mice, rats and humans. Its detrimental effects on male reproduction include decreased mean testes weight, low sperm count, reduced seminiferous tubule diameters[53], decreased sperm motility and increased abnormal sperm morphology[34]. A study done in rats revealed that carbendazim's deleterious effects on male reproduction are mediated *via* its ability to increase OS, by impairing steroidogenic enzymes and antioxidant cellular defenses. It also enhanced H_2O_2, hydroxyl radicals and lipid peroxidation in the Leydig cells[203]. Chlorpyrifos, an organophosphate pesticide, is another agricultural chemical that can lead to ROS-induced DNA strand breaks, as well as lipid peroxidation[145].

Solvents

Toluene is widely used as an organic solvent in various industries and commercial products. It is found in paint, rubber and is also used as a component of gasoline. Household products such as adhesives and various cleaning fluids also contain toluene[78]. Humans are mainly exposed to toluene *via* vapor inhalation. Recent investigations have shown that toluene may induce reproductive dysfunctions. It has been reported that occupational exposure to high concentrations of toluene vapor increases the risk for miscarriage in pregnant women[161, 240]. In a study done in male rats, toluene administration led to a decrease in epididymal sperm count and the serum concentrations of testosterone[178]. In both these studies, toluene was reported to mediate its reproductive toxicity via oxidative damage by either decreasing the antioxidant status [78] or inducing excessive ROS generation[178].

In the female reproductive system, another solvent namely xylene has been implicated in increasing the number of fetal resorbtions, delaying fetal development, reducing birth weight, reducing serum progesterone and estrogen levels as well as preventing ovulation in rodents[252]. Abnormally high xylene concentration have also been reported to be in the blood and semen of workers exposed to a working environment where the air concentration of xylene exceeded the maximum allowable concentration. These men were reported to have decreased sperm vitality, motility and acrosin activity[267]. Studies have shown that xylene is capable of inducing complete inhibition of mitochondrial respiration and is known to usually enhance mitochondrial ROS generation[5, 55] This ability propensity of xylene to generate ROS is more than likely the basis of its harmful effects on both male and female reproduction.

Conclusion

There is an escalating body of literature on the evidence of OS influencing the entire reproductive span of men and women[67]. OS plays a role from gametogenesis to fertilization and embryo development. ROS and RNS are responsible for OS and acts as necessary evils or double-edged swords in human reproduction. These products are required at physiological levels for normal reproductive function, while increased production or decreased scavenging result in fertility impairments such as decreased sperm function, endometriosis and abortions or congenital abnormalities in the offspring due to DNA damage. The main damage results from the ROS-induced alteration of macromolecules such as polyunsaturated fatty acids in membrane lipids, essential proteins, and DNA.

This chapter emphasizes the powerful function of OS in reproduction as well as in the induction of impaired reproductive function. An expanding body of evidence now supports a role for OS as a significant cause of infertility. This role encompasses not just the etiology of impaired fertility but also the origins of genetic disease in the offspring. It is possible that multiple pathways for creating OS are involved and it is therefore important that the biochemical mechanisms responsible for creating OS are understood. A variety of environmental and/or genetic factors can induce OS in the reproductive systems of both males and females. Internally ROS are byproducts of normal enzyme or chemical reactions while our surroundings also bombard us with ROS from external sources.

Resolving the various factors contributing to the creation of OS is strategically important because such data will help design methods for both the treatment and prevention of pathologies involving OS in the reproductive systems. Treatment with appropriate antioxidants in order to reduce the severity of OS is theoretically plausible. These treatments should not only improve fertilizing potential, but also reduce the risk of adverse genetic outcomes in the offspring[21]. This suggests the need for a healthy environment. Despite the common association between compromised gamete quality and OS, couples are rarely screened for OS nor treated for this condition. Instead they are offered mechanical treatment such as ICSI. Direct treatment of OS may allow for natural conception, thereby conserving scarce and costly medical resources[76, 247]. It is therefore of utmost importance to establish the minimum well tolerated concentration and define the physiological levels of ROS in the reproductive tracts.

OS generating and contributing lifestyle factors to be avoided include smoking, alcohol abuse, cell phone radiation, excessive exercise and psychological stress. If your work, hobby or lifestyle brings you into contact with environmental dangers such as pesticides, solvents, organic fumes, heavy metals, excessive heat or radiation exposure, you may be unknowingly affecting your reproductive function due to OS damage.

References

1. (2004) Definition of "infertility". Fertil Steril 82 Suppl 1:S206.
2. (2005) Third National Report on Human Exposure to Environmental Chemicals. Center for Disease Control.
3. Aber JD (1992) Nitrogen cycling and nitrogen saturation in temperate forest ecosystems. Trends in Ecology and Evolution 7:220-223.
4. Acharya UR, Acharya S, Mishra M (2003) Lead acetate induced cytotoxicity in male germinal cells of Swiss mice. Ind Health 41:291-294.
5. Adam-Vizi V (2005) Production of reactive oxygen species in brain mitochondria: contribution by electron transport chain and non-electron transport chain sources. Antioxid Redox Signal 7:1140-1149.
6. Agarwal A, Allamaneni SS (2004) Oxidants and antioxidants in human fertility. Middle East Fertility Society Journal 9:187-197.

7. Agarwal A, Allamaneni SS (2004) Role of free radicals in female reproductive diseases and assisted reproduction. Reprod Biomed Online 9:338-347.

8. Agarwal A, Deepinder F, Sharma RK, Ranga G, Li J (2008) Effect of cell phone usage on semen analysis in men attending infertility clinic: an observational study. Fertil Steril 89:124-128.

9. Agarwal A, Desai NR, Makker K, Varghese A, Mouradi R, Sabanegh E, Sharma R (2008) Effects of radiofrequency electromagnetic waves (RF-EMW) from cellular phones on human ejaculated semen: an *in vitro* pilot study. Fertil Steril.

10. Agarwal A, Gupta S, Sharma R (2005) Oxidative stress and its implications in female infertility–a clinician's perspective. Reprod Biomed Online 11:641-650.

11. Agarwal A, Gupta S, Sharma RK (2005) Role of oxidative stress in female reproduction. Reprod Biol Endocrinol 3:28.

12. Agarwal A, Ikemoto I, Loughlin KR (1994) Relationship of sperm parameters with levels of reactive oxygen species in semen specimens. J Urol 152:107-110.

13. Agarwal A, Prabakaran SA (2005) Mechanism, measurement, and prevention of oxidative stress in male reproductive physiology. Indian J Exp Biol 43:963-974.

14. Agarwal A, Said TM (2003) Role of sperm chromatin abnormalities and DNA damage in male infertility. Hum Reprod Update 9:331-345.

15. Agarwal A, Saleh RA, Bedaiwy MA (2003) Role of reactive oxygen species in the pathophysiology of human reproduction. Fertil Steril 79:829-843.

16. Ahamed M, Siddiqui MK (2007) Low-level lead exposure and oxidative stress: current opinions. Clin Chim Acta 383:57-64.

17. Aiken J, Buckingham D, Harkiss D (1994) Analysis of the extent to which sperm movement can predict the results of ionophore-enhanced functional assays of the acrosome reaction and sperm-oocyte fusion. Hum Reprod 9:1867-1874.

18. Aitken RJ (1997) Molecular mechanisms regulating human sperm function. Mol Hum Reprod 3:169-173.

19. Aitken RJ (1999) The Amoroso Lecture. The human spermatozoon–a cell in crisis? J Reprod Fertil 115:1-7.
20. Aitken RJ, Baker HW (1995) Seminal leukocytes: passengers, terrorists or good samaritans? Hum Reprod 10:1736-1739.
21. Aitken RJ, Baker MA (2004) Oxidative stress and male reproductive biology. Reprod Fertil Dev 16:581-588.
22. Aitken RJ, Baker MA, Sawyer D (2003) Oxidative stress in the male germ line and its role in the aetiology of male infertility and genetic disease. Reprod Biomed Online 7:65-70.
23. Aitken RJ, Buckingham D, Harkiss D (1993) Use of a xanthine oxidase free radical generating system to investigate the cytotoxic effects of reactive oxygen species on human spermatozoa. J Reprod Fertil 97:441-450.
24. Aitken RJ, Buckingham DW, Brindle J, Gomez E, Baker HW, Irvine DS (1995) Analysis of sperm movement in relation to the oxidative stress created by leukocytes in washed sperm preparations and seminal plasma. Hum Reprod 10:2061-2071.
25. Aitken RJ, Buckingham DW, West KM (1992) Reactive oxygen species and human spermatozoa: analysis of the cellular mechanisms involved in luminol- and lucigenin-dependent chemiluminescence. J Cell Physiol 151:466-477.
26. Aitken RJ, Clarkson JS (1987) Cellular basis of defective sperm function and its association with the genesis of reactive oxygen species by human spermatozoa. J Reprod Fertil 81:459-469.
27. Aitken RJ, Clarkson JS, Fishel S (1989) Generation of reactive oxygen species, lipid peroxidation, and human sperm function. Biol Reprod 41:183-197.
28. Aitken RJ, Harkiss D, Buckingham D (1993) Relationship between iron-catalysed lipid peroxidation potential and human sperm function. J Reprod Fertil 98:257-265.
29. Aitken RJ, Irvine DS, Wu FC (1991) Prospective analysis of sperm-oocyte fusion and reactive oxygen species generation as criteria for the diagnosis of infertility. Am J Obstet Gynecol 164:542-551.
30. Aitken RJ, Koopman P, Lewis SE (2004) Seeds of concern. Nature 432:48-52.

31. Aitken RJ, Krausz C (2001) Oxidative stress, DNA damage and the Y chromosome. Reproduction 122:497-506.

32. Aitken RJ, Paterson M, Fisher H, Buckingham DW, van Duin M (1995) Redox regulation of tyrosine phosphorylation in human spermatozoa and its role in the control of human sperm function. J Cell Sci 108 (Pt 5):2017-2025.

33. Aitken RJ, Sawyer D (2003) The human spermatozoon–not waving but drowning. Adv Exp Med Biol 518:85-98.

34. Akbarsha MA, Kadalmani B, Girija R, Faridha A, Hamid KS (2001) Spermatotoxic effect of carbendazim. Indian J Exp Biol 39:921-924.

35. Alvarez JG, Storey BT (1983) Taurine, hypotaurine, epinephrine and albumin inhibit lipid peroxidation in rabbit spermatozoa and protect against loss of motility. Biol Reprod 29:548-555.

36. Alvarez JG, Touchstone JC, Blasco L, Storey BT (1987) Spontaneous lipid peroxidation and production of hydrogen peroxide and superoxide in human spermatozoa. Superoxide dismutase as major enzyme protectant against oxygen toxicity. J Androl 8:338-348.

37. Armstrong JS, Rajasekaran M, Chamulitrat W, Gatti P, Hellstrom WJ, Sikka SC (1999) Characterization of reactive oxygen species induced effects on human spermatozoa movement and energy metabolism. Free Radic Biol Med 26:869-880.

38. Armstrong JS, Rajasekaran M, Hellstrom WJ, Sikka SC (1998) Antioxidant potential of human serum albumin: role in the recovery of high quality human spermatozoa for assisted reproductive technology. J Androl 19:412-419.

39. Aruoma OI, Grootveld M, Bahorun T (2006) Free radicals in biology and medicine: from inflammation to biotechnology. Biofactors 27:1-3.

40. Attaran M, Pasqualotto E, Falcone T, Goldberg JM, Miller KF, Agarwal A, Sharma RK (2000) The effect of follicular fluid reactive oxygen species on the outcome of *in vitro* fertilization. Int J Fertil Womens Med 45:314-320.

41. Bahorun T, Soobratte MA, Luximon-Ramma V, Aruoma OI (2006) Free Radicals and Antioxidants in Cardiovascular Health and Disease. Internet Journal of Medical Update.

42. Banerjee S, Smallwood A, Moorhead J, Chambers AE, Papageorghiou A, Campbell S, Nicolaides K (2005) Placental expression of interferon-gamma (IFN-gamma) and its receptor IFN-gamma R2 fail to switch from early hypoxic to late normotensive development in preeclampsia. J Clin Endocrinol Metab 90:944-952.

43. Banks S, King SA, Irvine DS, Saunders PT (2005) Impact of a mild scrotal heat stress on DNA integrity in murine spermatozoa. Reproduction 129:505-514.

44. Barrionuevo MJ, Schwandt RA, Rao PS, Graham LB, Maisel LP, Yeko TR (2000) Nitric oxide (NO) and interleukin-1beta (IL-1beta) in follicular fluid and their correlation with fertilization and embryo cleavage. Am J Reprod Immunol 44:359-364.

45. Bedaiwy MA, Falcone T, Mohamed MS, Aleem AA, Sharma RK, Worley SE, Thornton J, Agarwal A (2004) Differential growth of human embryos *in vitro*: role of reactive oxygen species. Fertil Steril 82:593-600.

46. Bedaiwy MA, Falcone T, Sharma RK, Goldberg JM, Attaran M, Nelson DR, Agarwal A (2002) Prediction of endometriosis with serum and peritoneal fluid markers: a prospective controlled trial. Hum Reprod 17:426-431.

47. Benoff S, Auborn K, Marmar JL, Hurley IR (2008) Link between low-dose environmentally relevant cadmium exposures and asthenozoospermia in a rat model. Fertil Steril 89:e73-79.

48. Bianchi PG, Manicardi GC, Bizzaro D, Bianchi U, Sakkas D (1993) Effect of deoxyribonucleic acid protamination on fluorochrome staining and in situ nick-translation of murine and human mature spermatozoa. Biol Reprod 49:1083-1088.

49. Bonde JP (1993) The risk of male subfecundity attributable to welding of metals. Studies of semen quality, infertility, fertility, adverse pregnancy outcome and childhood malignancy. Int J Androl 16 Suppl 1:1-29.

50. Boyden TW, Pamenter RW (1983) Effects of ethanol on the male hypothalamic-pituitary-gonadal axis. Endocr Rev 4:389-395.

51. Burch JB, Reif JS, Yost MG, Keefe TJ, Pitrat CA (1998) Nocturnal excretion of a urinary melatonin metabolite among electric utility workers. Scand J Work Environ Health 24:183-189.

52. Burton GJ, Hempstock J, Jauniaux E (2003) Oxygen, early embryonic metabolism and free radical-mediated embryopathies. Reprod Biomed Online 6:84-96.

53. Carter SD, Hess RA, Laskey JW (1987) The fungicide methyl 2-benzimidazole carbamate causes infertility in male Sprague-Dawley rats. Biol Reprod 37:709-717.

54. Chandra J, Samali A, Orrenius S (2000) Triggering and modulation of apoptosis by oxidative stress. Free Radic Biol Med 29:323-333.

55. Chen Q, Vazquez EJ, Moghaddas S, Hoppel CL, Lesnefsky EJ (2003) Production of reactive oxygen species by mitochondria: central role of complex III. J Biol Chem 278:36027-36031.

56. Chia SE, Xu B, Ong CN, Tsakok FM, Lee ST (1994) Effect of cadmium and cigarette smoking on human semen quality. Int J Fertil Menopausal Stud 39:292-298.

57. Chitra KC, Latchoumycandane C, Mathur PP (2003) Induction of oxidative stress by bisphenol A in the epididymal sperm of rats. Toxicology 185:119-127.

58. Chitra KC, Sujatha R, Latchoumycandane C, Mathur PP (2001) Effect of lindane on antioxidant enzymes in epididymis and epididymal sperm of adult rats. Asian J Androl 3:205-208.

59. Cooke MS, Evans MD, Dizdaroglu M, Lunec J (2003) Oxidative DNA damage: mechanisms, mutation, and disease. Faseb J 17:1195-1214.

60. Cramer DW, Wise LA (2000) The epidemiology of recurrent pregnancy loss. Semin Reprod Med 18:331-339.

61. Cross CE, Halliwell B, Borish ET, Pryor WA, Ames BN, Saul RL, McCord JM, Harman D (1987) Oxygen radicals and human disease. Ann Intern Med 107:526-545.

62. Cummins JM, Jequier AM, Kan R (1994) Molecular biology of human male infertility: links with aging, mitochondrial genetics, and oxidative stress? Mol Reprod Dev 37:345-362.

63. Cummins JM, Pember SM, Jequier AM, Yovich JL, Hartmann PE (1991) A test of the human sperm acrosome reaction following ionophore challenge. Relationship to fertility and other seminal parameters. J Androl 12:98-103.

64. Dahchour A, Lallemand F, Ward RJ, De Witte P (2005) Production of reactive oxygen species following acute ethanol or acetaldehyde and its reduction by acamprosate in chronically alcoholized rats. Eur J Pharmacol 520:51-58.

65. Dandona P, Aljada A, Chaudhuri A, Mohanty P, Garg R (2005) Metabolic syndrome: a comprehensive perspective based on interactions between obesity, diabetes, and inflammation. Circulation 111:1448-1454.

66. Davi G, Falco A (2005) Oxidant stress, inflammation and atherogenesis. Lupus 14:760-764.

67. de Bruin JP, Dorland M, Spek ER, Posthuma G, van Haaften M, Looman CW, te Velde ER (2002) Ultrastructure of the resting ovarian follicle pool in healthy young women. Biol Reprod 66:1151-1160.

68. de Lamirande E, Gagnon C (1992) Reactive oxygen species and human spermatozoa. II. Depletion of adenosine triphosphate plays an important role in the inhibition of sperm motility. J Androl 13:379-386.

69. de Lamirande E, Gagnon C (1993) Human sperm hyperactivation in whole semen and its association with low superoxide scavenging capacity in seminal plasma. Fertil Steril 59:1291-1295.

70. de Lamirande E, Gagnon C (1994) Reactive oxygen species (ROS) and reproduction. Adv Exp Med Biol 366:185-197.

71. de Lamirande E, Gagnon C (1995) Impact of reactive oxygen species on spermatozoa: a balancing act between beneficial and detrimental effects. Hum Reprod 10 Suppl 1:15-21.

72. Deepinder F, Makker K, Agarwal A (2007) Cell phones and male infertility: dissecting the relationship. Reprod Biomed Online 15:266-270.

73. Dennery PA (2004) Role of redox in fetal development and neonatal diseases. Antioxid Redox Signal 6:147-153.

74. Dong M, Shi Y, Cheng Q, Hao M (2001) Increased nitric oxide in peritoneal fluid from women with idiopathic infertility and endometriosis. J Reprod Med 46:887-891.

75. Donnelly ET, McClure N, Lewis SE (1999) Antioxidant supplementation *in vitro* does not improve human sperm motility. Fertil Steril 72:484-495.

76. Du Plessis SS, Makker K, Desai KM, Agarwal A (2008) Impact of oxidative stress on IVF. Expert Rev Obstet Gynecol 3:539-554.

77. Duckitt K (2003) Infertility and subfertility. Clin Evid:2044-2073.

78. Edelfors S, Hass U, Hougaard KS (2002) Changes in markers of oxidative stress and membrane properties in synaptosomes from rats exposed prenatally to toluene. Pharmacol Toxicol 90:26-31.

79. El Mouatassim S, Guerin P, Menezo Y (1999) Expression of genes encoding antioxidant enzymes in human and mouse oocytes during the final stages of maturation. Mol Hum Reprod 5:720-725..

80. Eskandari N (2003) Infertility. In: Cherney A NL (ed) Current Obstetrics and Gynecologi Diagnosis and Treatment. 9th edn. McGraw-Hill New York, pp 979-1000.

81. Eskenazi B, Kidd SA, Marks AR, Sloter E, Block G, Wyrobek AJ (2005) Antioxidant intake is associated with semen quality in healthy men. Hum Reprod 20:1006-1012.

82. Eskiocak S, Gozen AS, Kilic AS, Molla S (2005) Association between mental stress and some antioxidant enzymes of seminal plasma. Indian J Med Res 122:491-496.

83. Eskiocak S, Gozen AS, Taskiran A, Kilic AS, Eskiocak M, Gulen S (2006) Effect of psychological stress on the L-arginine-nitric oxide pathway and semen quality. Braz J Med Biol Res 39:581-588.

84. Eskiocak S, Gozen AS, Yapar SB, Tavas F, Kilic AS, Eskiocak M (2005) Glutathione and free sulphydryl content of seminal plasma in healthy medical students during and after exam stress. Hum Reprod 20:2595-2600.

85. Fainaru O, Almog B, Pinchuk I, Kupferminc MJ, Lichtenberg D, Many A (2002) Active labour is associated with increased oxidisibility of serum lipids ex vivo. Bjog 109:938-941.

86. Fejes I, Koloszar S, Zavaczki Z, Daru J, Szollosi J, Pal A (2006) Effect of body weight on testosterone/estradiol ratio in oligozoospermic patients. Arch Androl 52:97-102.

87. Fiers W, Beyaert R, Declercq W, Vandenabeele P (1999) More than one way to die: apoptosis, necrosis and reactive oxygen damage. Oncogene 18:7719-7730.

88. Foyouzi N, Berkkanoglu M, Arici A, Kwintkiewicz J, Izquierdo D, Duleba AJ (2004) Effects of oxidants and antioxidants on proliferation of endometrial stromal cells. Fertil Steril 82 Suppl 3:1019-1022.

89. Fraga CG, Motchnik PA, Shigenaga MK, Helbock HJ, Jacob RA, Ames BN (1991) Ascorbic acid protects against endogenous oxidative DNA damage in human sperm. Proc Natl Acad Sci U S A 88:11003-11006.

90. Fraga CG, Motchnik PA, Wyrobek AJ, Rempel DM, Ames BN (1996) Smoking and low antioxidant levels increase oxidative damage to sperm DNA. Mutat Res 351:199-203.

91. Friden BE, Runesson E, Hahlin M, Brannstrom M (2000) Evidence for nitric oxide acting as a luteolytic factor in the human corpus luteum. Mol Hum Reprod 6:397-403.

92. Friedman J, Kraus S, Hauptman Y, Schiff Y, Seger R (2007) Mechanism of short-term ERK activation by electromagnetic fields at mobile phone frequencies. Biochem J 405:559-568.

93. Gagnon C, Iwasaki A, De Lamirande E, Kovalski N (1991) Reactive oxygen species and human spermatozoa. Ann N Y Acad Sci 637:436-444.

94. Gandini L, Lombardo F, Paoli D, Caponecchia L, Familiari G, Verlengia C, Dondero F, Lenzi A (2000) Study of apoptotic DNA fragmentation in human spermatozoa. Hum Reprod 15:830-839.

95. Garrido N, Meseguer M, Simon C, Pellicer A, Remohi J (2004) Pro-oxidative and anti-oxidative imbalance in human semen and its relation with male fertility. Asian J Androl 6:59-65.

96. Gaur DS, Talekar M, Pathak VP (2007) Effect of cigarette smoking on semen quality of infertile men. Singapore Med J 48:119-123.

97. Gavella M, Lipovac V (1992) NADH-dependent oxidoreductase (diaphorase) activity and isozyme pattern of sperm in infertile men. Arch Androl 28:135-141.

98. Gavella M, Lipovac V, Vucic M, Rocic B (1996) Superoxide anion scavenging capacity of human seminal plasma. Int J Androl 19:82-90.

99. Gennart JP, Buchet JP, Roels H, Ghyselen P, Ceulemans E, Lauwerys R (1992) Fertility of male workers exposed to cadmium, lead, or manganese. Am J Epidemiol 135:1208-1219.

100. Gesler RM (1973) Toxicology of di-2-ethylhexyl phthalate and other phthalic acid ester plasticizers. Environ Health Perspect 3:73-79.

101. Gil-Guzman E, Ollero M, Lopez MC, Sharma RK, Alvarez JG, Thomas AJ, Jr., Agarwal A (2001) Differential production of reactive oxygen species by subsets of human spermatozoa at different stages of maturation. Hum Reprod 16:1922-1930.

102. Gomez E, Buckingham DW, Brindle J, Lanzafame F, Irvine DS, Aitken RJ (1996) Development of an image analysis system to monitor the retention of residual cytoplasm by human spermatozoa: correlation with biochemical markers of the cytoplasmic space, oxidative stress, and sperm function. J Androl 17:276-287.

103. Gomez E, Irvine DS, Aitken RJ (1998) Evaluation of a spectrophotometric assay for the measurement of malondialdehyde and 4-hydroxyalkenals in human spermatozoa: relationships with semen quality and sperm function. Int J Androl 21:81-94.

104. Goverde HJ, Dekker HS, Janssen HJ, Bastiaans BA, Rolland R, Zielhuis GA (1995) Semen quality and frequency of smoking and alcohol consumption–an explorative study. Int J Fertil Menopausal Stud 40:135-138.

105. Griveau JF, Le Lannou D (1997) Reactive oxygen species and human spermatozoa: physiology and pathology. Int J Androl 20:61-69.

106. Guerin P, El Mouatassim S, Menezo Y (2001) Oxidative stress and protection against reactive oxygen species in the pre-implantation embryo and its surroundings. Hum Reprod Update 7:175-189.

107. Halliwell B, Gutteridge JM (1988) Free radicals and antioxidant protection: mechanisms and significance in toxicology and disease. Hum Toxicol 7:7-13.

108. Halliwell B, Gutteridge JM, Cross CE (1992) Free radicals, antioxidants, and human disease: where are we now? J Lab Clin Med 119:598-620.

109. Hanafy KA, Krumenacker JS, Murad F (2001) NO, nitrotyrosine, and cyclic GMP in signal transduction. Med Sci Monit 7:801-819.

110. Harvey AJ, Kind KL, Thompson JG (2002) REDOX regulation of early embryo development. Reproduction 123:479-486.

111. Hasegawa M, Zhang Y, Niibe H, Terry NH, Meistrich ML (1998) Resistance of differentiating spermatogonia to radiation-induced apoptosis and loss in p53-deficient mice. Radiat Res 149:263-270.

112. Hawkes WC, Turek PJ (2001) Effects of dietary selenium on sperm motility in healthy men. J Androl 22:764-772.

113. Hayes JD, McLellan LI (1999) Glutathione and glutathione-dependent enzymes represent a co-ordinately regulated defence against oxidative stress. Free Radic Res 31:273-300.

114. Hendin BN, Kolettis PN, Sharma RK, Thomas AJ, Jr., Agarwal A (1999) Varicocele is associated with elevated spermatozoal reactive oxygen species production and diminished seminal plasma antioxidant capacity. J Urol 161:1831-1834.

115. Hikim AP, Wang C, Lue Y, Johnson L, Wang XH, Swerdloff RS (1998) Spontaneous germ cell apoptosis in humans: evidence for ethnic differences in the susceptibility of germ cells to programmed cell death. J Clin Endocrinol Metab 83:152-156.

116. Holthe MR, Staff AC, Berge LN, Lyberg T (2004) Leukocyte adhesion molecules and reactive oxygen species in preeclampsia. Obstet Gynecol 103:913-922.

117. Hsu PC, Guo YL (2002) Antioxidant nutrients and lead toxicity. Toxicology 180:33-44.

118. Hull MG, Glazener CM, Kelly NJ, Conway DI, Foster PA, Hinton RA, Coulson C, Lambert PA, Watt EM, Desai KM (1985) Population study of causes, treatment and outcome of infertility. Br Med J (Clin Res Ed) 291:1693-1697.

119. Hyslop PA, Hinshaw DB, Halsey WA, Jr., Schraufstatter IU, Sauerheber RD, Spragg RG, Jackson JH, Cochrane CG (1988) Mechanisms of oxidant-mediated cell injury. The glycolytic and mitochondrial pathways of ADP phosphorylation are major intracellular targets inactivated by hydrogen peroxide. J Biol Chem 263:1665-1675.

120. Ichikawa T, Oeda T, Ohmori H, Schill WB (1999) Reactive oxygen species influence the acrosome reaction but not acrosin activity in human spermatozoa. Int J Androl 22:37-42.

121. Irvine DS, Twigg JP, Gordon EL, Fulton N, Milne PA, Aitken RJ (2000) DNA integrity in human spermatozoa: relationships with semen quality. J Androl 21:33-44.

122. Ishihara M, Itoh M, Miyamoto K, Suna S, Takeuchi Y, Takenaka I, Jitsunari F (2000) Spermatogenic disturbance induced by di-(2-ethylhexyl) phthalate is significantly prevented by treatment with antioxidant vitamins in the rat. Int J Androl 23:85-94.

123. Ishii T, Matsuki S, Iuchi Y, Okada F, Toyosaki S, Tomita Y, Ikeda Y, Fujii J (2005) Accelerated impairment of spermatogenic cells in SOD1-knockout mice under heat stress. Free Radic Res 39:697-705.

124. Ivell R (2007) Lifestyle impact and the biology of the human scrotum. Reprod Biol Endocrinol 5:15.

125. Iwasaki A, Gagnon C (1992) Formation of reactive oxygen species in spermatozoa of infertile patients. Fertil Steril 57:409-416.

126. Jackson LW, Zullo MD, Goldberg JM (2008) The association between heavy metals, endometriosis and uterine myomas among premenopausal women: National Health and Nutrition Examination Survey 1999-2002. Hum Reprod 23:679-687.

127. Janssen YM, Van Houten B, Borm PJ, Mossman BT (1993) Cell and tissue responses to oxidative damage. Lab Invest 69:261-274.

128. Jensen MS, Mabeck LM, Toft G, Thulstrup AM, Bonde JP (2005) Lower sperm counts following prenatal tobacco exposure. Hum Reprod 20:2559-2566.

129. Ji BT, Shu XO, Linet MS, Zheng W, Wacholder S, Gao YT, Ying DM, Jin F (1997) Paternal cigarette smoking and the risk of childhood cancer among offspring of nonsmoking mothers. J Natl Cancer Inst 89:238-244.

130. Jones R, Mann T, Sherins R (1979) Peroxidative breakdown of phospholipids in human spermatozoa, spermicidal properties of fatty acid peroxides, and protective action of seminal plasma. Fertil Steril 31:531-537.

131. Jozwik M, Jozwik M, Kuczynski W, Szamatowicz M (1997) Nonenzymatic antioxidant activity of human seminal plasma. Fertil Steril 68:154-157.

132. Jozwik M, Wolczynski S, Jozwik M, Szamatowicz M (1999) Oxidative stress markers in preovulatory follicular fluid in humans. Mol Hum Reprod 5:409-413.

133. Jurasovic J, Cvitkovic P, Pizent A, Colak B, Telisman S (2004) Semen quality and reproductive endocrine function with regard to blood cadmium in Croatian male subjects. Biometals 17:735-743.

134. Jurisicova A, Lopes S, Meriano J, Oppedisano L, Casper RF, Varmuza S (1999) DNA damage in round spermatids of mice with a targeted disruption of the Pp1c gamma gene and in testicular biopsies of patients with non-obstructive azoospermia. Mol Hum Reprod 5:323-330.

135. Kabuto H, Amakawa M, Shishibori T (2004) Exposure to bisphenol A during embryonic/fetal life and infancy increases oxidative injury and causes underdevelopment of the brain and testis in mice. Life Sci 74:2931-2940.

136. Kao SH, Chao HT, Chen HW, Hwang TI, Liao TL, Wei YH (2008) Increase of oxidative stress in human sperm with lower motility. Fertil Steril 89:1183-1190.

137. Kasahara E, Sato EF, Miyoshi M, Konaka R, Hiramoto K, Sasaki J, Tokuda M, Nakano Y, Inoue M (2002) Role of oxidative stress in germ cell apoptosis induced by di(2-ethylhexyl)phthalate. Biochem J 365:849-856.

138. Kemp CJ, Sun S, Gurley KE (2001) p53 induction and apoptosis in response to radio- and chemotherapy *in vivo* is tumor-type-dependent. Cancer Res 61:327-332.

139. Koch OR, Pani G, Borrello S, Colavitti R, Cravero A, Farre S, Galeotti T (2004) Oxidative stress and antioxidant defenses in ethanol-induced cell injury. Mol Aspects Med 25:191-198.

140. Kodama H, Yamaguchi R, Fukuda J, Kasai H, Tanaka T (1997) Increased oxidative deoxyribonucleic acid damage in the spermatozoa of infertile male patients. Fertil Steril 68:519-524.

141. Koloszar S, Fejes I, Zavaczki Z, Daru J, Szollosi J, Pal A (2005) Effect of body weight on sperm concentration in normozoospermic males. Arch Androl 51:299-304.

142. Korasli D, Ziraman F, Ozyurt P, Cehreli SB (2007) Microleakage of self-etch primer/adhesives in endodontically treated teeth. J Am Dent Assoc 138:634-640.

143. Kort HI, Massey JB, Elsner CW, Mitchell-Leef D, Shapiro DB, Witt MA, Roudebush WE (2006) Impact of body mass index values on sperm quantity and quality. J Androl 27:450-452.

144. Kovacic P, Jacintho JD (2001) Reproductive toxins: pervasive theme of oxidative stress and electron transfer. Curr Med Chem 8:863-892.

145. Kovacic P, Pozos RS (2006) Cell signaling (mechanism and reproductive toxicity): redox chains, radicals, electrons, relays, conduit, electrochemistry, and other medical implications. Birth Defects Res C Embryo Today 78:333-344.

146. Kowaltowski AJ, Vercesi AE (1999) Mitochondrial damage induced by conditions of oxidative stress. Free Radic Biol Med 26:463-471.

147. Kross BC, Ayebo AD, Fuortes LJ (1992) Methemoglobinemia: nitrate toxicity in rural America. Am Fam Physician 46:183-188.

148. Kruger TF, Acosta AA, Simmons KF, Swanson RJ, Matta JF, Veeck LL, Morshedi M, Brugo S (1987) New method of

evaluating sperm morphology with predictive value for human *in vitro* fertilization. Urology 30:248-251.

149. Kunzle R, Mueller MD, Hanggi W, Birkhauser MH, Drescher H, Bersinger NA (2003) Semen quality of male smokers and nonsmokers in infertile couples. Fertil Steril 79:287-291.

150. Latchoumycandane C, Chitra KC, Mathur PP (2003) 2,3,7,8-tetrachlorodibenzo- p-dioxin (TCDD) induces oxidative stress in the epididymis and epididymal sperm of adult rats. Arch Toxicol 77:280-284.

151. Latchoumycandane C, Mathur PP (2002) Induction of oxidative stress in the rat testis after short-term exposure to the organochlorine pesticide methoxychlor. Arch Toxicol 76:692-698.

152. Le HH, Carlson EM, Chua JP, Belcher SM (2008) Bisphenol A is released from polycarbonate drinking bottles and mimics the neurotoxic actions of estrogen in developing cerebellar neurons. Toxicol Lett 176:149-156.

153. Leclerc P, de Lamirande E, Gagnon C (1997) Regulation of protein-tyrosine phosphorylation and human sperm capacitation by reactive oxygen derivatives. Free Radic Biol Med 22:643-656.

154. Lee DH, Lim JS, Song K, Boo Y, Jacobs DR, Jr. (2006) Graded associations of blood lead and urinary cadmium concentrations with oxidative-stress-related markers in the U.S. population: results from the third National Health and Nutrition Examination Survey. Environ Health Perspect 114:350-354.

155. Lee E, Ahn MY, Kim HJ, Kim IY, Han SY, Kang TS, Hong JH, Park KL, Lee BM, Kim HS (2007) Effect of di(n-butyl) phthalate on testicular oxidative damage and antioxidant enzymes in hyperthyroid rats. Environ Toxicol 22:245-255.

156. Lee J, Richburg JH, Younkin SC, Boekelheide K (1997) The Fas system is a key regulator of germ cell apoptosis in the testis. Endocrinology 138:2081-2088.

157. Lee KS, Joo BS, Na YJ, Yoon MS, Choi OH, Kim WW (2000) Relationships between concentrations of tumor necrosis factor-alpha and nitric oxide in follicular fluid and oocyte quality. J Assist Reprod Genet 17:222-228.

158. Lenzi A, Culasso F, Gandini L, Lombardo F, Dondero F (1993) Placebo-controlled, double-blind, cross-over trial of glutathione therapy in male infertility. Hum Reprod 8:1657-1662.

159. Lewis WMJ, Morris DP (1986) Toxicity of nitrite to fish: a review. Transaction of the American Fisheries Society 115:183-194.

160. Lieber CS (2004) The discovery of the microsomal ethanol oxidizing system and its physiologic and pathologic role. Drug Metab Rev 36:511-529.

161. Lindbohm ML (1995) Effects of parental exposure to solvents on pregnancy outcome. J Occup Environ Med 37:908-914.

162. Liu DY, Baker HW (1994) A new test for the assessment of sperm-zona pellucida penetration: relationship with results of other sperm tests and fertilization *in vitro*. Hum Reprod 9:489-496.

163. Liu Y, Luo L, Zhao H (2001) Levels of lipid peroxides and superoxide dismutase in peritoneal fluid of patients with endometriosis. J Tongji Med Univ 21:166-167.

164. Lopes S, Jurisicova A, Sun JG, Casper RF (1998) Reactive oxygen species: potential cause for DNA fragmentation in human spermatozoa. Hum Reprod 13:896-900.

165. MacLeod J (1943) The role of oxygen in the metabolism and motility of human spermatozoa. Am J Physiol 138:512-518.

166. Maiorino M, Ursini F (2002) Oxidative stress, spermatogenesis and fertility. Biol Chem 383:591-597.

167. Maneesh M, Dutta S, Chakrabarti A, Vasudevan DM (2006) Alcohol abuse-duration dependent decrease in plasma testosterone and antioxidants in males. Indian J Physiol Pharmacol 50:291-296.

168. Manna I, Jana K, Samanta PK (2004) Effect of different intensities of swimming exercise on testicular oxidative stress and reproductive dysfunction in mature male albino Wistar rats. Indian J Exp Biol 42:816-822.

169. Manojkumar V, Padmakumaran Nair KG, Santhosh A, Deepadevi KV, Arun P, Lakshmi LR, Kurup PA (1998) Decrease in the concentration of vitamin E in blood and tissues caused by di(2-ethylhexyl) phthalate, a commonly used plasticizer in blood storage bags and medical tubing. Vox Sang 75:139-144.

170. Marco A, Quilchano C, Blaustein AR (1999) Sensitivity to nitrate and nitrite in some pond-breeding amphibians from Pacific Northwest. Environmental Toxicology and Chemistry 18:2836-2839.

171. Mocatta TJ, Winterbourn CC, Inder TE, Darlow BA (2004) The effect of gestational age and labour on markers of lipid and protein oxidation in cord plasma. Free Radic Res 38:185-191.

172. Mostafa T, Anis TH, El-Nashar A, Imam H, Othman IA (2001) Varicocelectomy reduces reactive oxygen species levels and increases antioxidant activity of seminal plasma from infertile men with varicocele. Int J Androl 24:261-265.

173. Murphy AA, Palinski W, Rankin S, Morales AJ, Parthasarathy S (1998) Macrophage scavenger receptor(s) and oxidatively modified proteins in endometriosis. Fertil Steril 69:1085-1091.

174. Murphy AA, Zhou MH, Malkapuram S, Santanam N, Parthasarathy S, Sidell N (2000) RU486-induced growth inhibition of human endometrial cells. Fertil Steril 74:1014-1019.

175. Muthusami KR, Chinnaswamy P (2005) Effect of chronic alcoholism on male fertility hormones and semen quality. Fertil Steril 84:919-924.

176. Myatt L, Cui X (2004) Oxidative stress in the placenta. Histochem Cell Biol 122:369-382.

177. Naha N, Chowdhury AR (2006) Inorganic lead exposure in battery and paint factories: effect on human sperm structure and functional activity. J Uoeh 28:157-171.

178. Nakai N, Murata M, Nagahama M, Hirase T, Tanaka M, Fujikawa T, Nakao N, Nakashima K, Kawanishi S (2003) Oxidative DNA damage induced by toluene is involved in its male reproductive toxicity. Free Radic Res 37:69-76.

179. Nallella KP, Allamaneni SS, Pasqualotto FF, Sharma RK, Thomas AJ, Jr., Agarwal A (2004) Relationship of interleukin-6 with semen characteristics and oxidative stress in patients with varicocele. Urology 64:1010-1013.

180. Nasr-Esfahani MH, Aitken JR, Johnson MH (1990) Hydrogen peroxide levels in mouse oocytes and early cleavage stage embryos developed *in vitro* or *in vivo*. Development 109:501-507.

181. Nguyen RH, Wilcox AJ, Skjaerven R, Baird DD (2007) Men's body mass index and infertility. Hum Reprod 22:2488-2493.

182. O'Bryan MK, Zini A, Cheng CY, Schlegel PN (1998) Human sperm endothelial nitric oxide synthase expression: correlation with sperm motility. Fertil Steril 70:1143-1147.

183. Obata T, Kubota S (2000) Formation of hydroxy radicals by environmental estrogen-like chemicals in rat striatum. Neurosci Lett 296:41-44.

184. Ochsendorf FR (1999) Infections in the male genital tract and reactive oxygen species. Hum Reprod Update 5:399-420.

185. Oehninger S, Blackmore P, Mahony M, Hodgen G (1995) Effects of hydrogen peroxide on human spermatozoa. J Assist Reprod Genet 12:41-47.

186. Osborn BH, Haney AF, Misukonis MA, Weinberg JB (2002) Inducible nitric oxide synthase expression by peritoneal macrophages in endometriosis-associated infertility. Fertil Steril 77:46-51.

187. Ota H, Igarashi S, Hatazawa J, Tanaka T (1998) Endothelial nitric oxide synthase in the endometrium during the menstrual cycle in patients with endometriosis and adenomyosis. Fertil Steril 69:303-308.

188. Park JD, Habeebu SS, Klaassen CD (2002) Testicular toxicity of di-(2-ethylhexyl)phthalate in young Sprague-Dawley rats. Toxicology 171:105-115.

189. Pasqualotto FF, Sharma RK, Nelson DR, Thomas AJ, Agarwal A (2000) Relationship between oxidative stress, semen characteristics, and clinical diagnosis in men undergoing infertility investigation. Fertil Steril 73:459-464.

190. Pasqualotto FF, Sharma RK, Potts JM, Nelson DR, Thomas AJ, Agarwal A (2000) Seminal oxidative stress in patients with chronic prostatitis. Urology 55:881-885.

191. Paszkowski T, Clarke RN, Hornstein MD (2002) Smoking induces oxidative stress inside the Graafian follicle. Hum Reprod 17:921-925.

192. Peakall DB (1975) Phthalate esters: Occurrence and biological effects. Residue Rev 54:1-41.

193. Peake JM, Suzuki K, Coombes JS (2007) The influence of antioxidant supplementation on markers of inflammation and the relationship to oxidative stress after exercise. J Nutr Biochem 18:357-371.

194. Perez-Crespo M, Pintado B, Gutierrez-Adan A (2008) Scrotal heat stress effects on sperm viability, sperm DNA integrity and the offspring sex ratio in mice. Mol Reprod Dev 75:40-47.

195. Pierce GB, Parchment RE, Lewellyn AL (1991) Hydrogen peroxide as a mediator of programmed cell death in the blastocyst. Differentiation 46:181-186.

196. Pierce JD, Cackler AB, Arnett MG (2004) Why should you care about free radicals? Rn 67:38-42; quiz 43.

197. Plante M, de Lamirande E, Gagnon C (1994) Reactive oxygen species released by activated neutrophils, but not by deficient spermatozoa, are sufficient to affect normal sperm motility. Fertil Steril 62:387-393.

198. Polak G, Koziol-Montewka M, Gogacz M, Blaszkowska I, Kotarski J (2001) Total antioxidant status of peritoneal fluid in infertile women. Eur J Obstet Gynecol Reprod Biol 94:261-263.

199. Portz DM, Elkins TE, White R, Warren J, Adadevoh S, Randolph J (1991) Oxygen free radicals and pelvic adhesion formation: I. Blocking oxygen free radical toxicity to prevent adhesion formation in an endometriosis model. Int J Fertil 36:39-42.

200. Potts JM, Pasqualotto FF (2003) Seminal oxidative stress in patients with chronic prostatitis. Andrologia 35:304-308.

201. Pressman EK, Cavanaugh JL, Mingione M, Norkus EP, Woods JR (2003) Effects of maternal antioxidant supplementation on maternal and fetal antioxidant levels: a randomized, double-blind study. Am J Obstet Gynecol 189:1720-1725.

202. Preutthipan S, Chen SH, Tilly JL, Kugu K, Lareu RR, Dharmarajan AM (2004) Inhibition of nitric oxide synthesis potentiates apoptosis in the rabbit corpus luteum. Reprod Biomed Online 9:264-270.

203. Rajeswary S, Kumaran B, Ilangovan R, Yuvaraj S, Sridhar M, Venkataraman P, Srinivasan N, Aruldhas MM (2007) Modulation of antioxidant defense system by the environmental

fungicide carbendazim in Leydig cells of rats. Reprod Toxicol 24:371-380.

204. Ray SD, Lam TS, Rotollo JA, Phadke S, Patel C, Dontabhaktuni A, Mohammad S, Lee H, Strika S, Dobrogowska A, Bruculeri C, Chou A, Patel S, Patel R, Manolas T, Stohs S (2004) Oxidative stress is the master operator of drug and chemically-induced programmed and unprogrammed cell death: Implications of natural antioxidants *in vivo*. Biofactors 21:223-232.
205. Richthoff J, Elzanaty S, Rylander L, Hagmar L, Giwercman A (2008) Association between tobacco exposure and reproductive parameters in adolescent males. Int J Androl 31:31-39.
206. Robaire B, Hales BF (2003) Mechanisms of action of cyclophosphamide as a male-mediated developmental toxicant. Adv Exp Med Biol 518:169-180.
207. Rosselli M, Keller PJ, Dubey RK (1998) Role of nitric oxide in the biology, physiology and pathophysiology of reproduction. Hum Reprod Update 4:3-24.
208. Sabatini L, Wilson C, Lower A, Al-Shawaf T, Grudzinskas JG (1999) Superoxide dismutase activity in human follicular fluid after controlled ovarian hyperstimulation in women undergoing *in vitro* fertilization. Fertil Steril 72:1027-1034.
209. Sacks GP, Studena K, Sargent K, Redman CW (1998) Normal pregnancy and preeclampsia both produce inflammatory changes in peripheral blood leukocytes akin to those of sepsis. Am J Obstet Gynecol 179:80-86
210. Sakkas D, Mariethoz E, Manicardi G, Bizzaro D, Bianchi PG, Bianchi U (1999) Origin of DNA damage in ejaculated human spermatozoa. Rev Reprod 4:31-37.
211. Saleh RA, Agarwal A (2002) Oxidative stress and male infertility: from research bench to clinical practice. J Androl 23:737-752.
212. Saleh RA, Agarwal A, Kandirali E, Sharma RK, Thomas AJ, Nada EA, Evenson DP, Alvarez JG (2002) Leukocytospermia is associated with increased reactive oxygen species production by human spermatozoa. Fertil Steril 78:1215-1224.
213. Saleh RA, Agarwal A, Sharma RK, Nelson DR, Thomas AJ, Jr. (2002) Effect of cigarette smoking on levels of seminal oxidative

stress in infertile men: a prospective study. Fertil Steril 78:491-499.

214. Selmanoglu G, Barlas N, Songur S, Kockaya EA (2001) Carbendazim-induced haematological, biochemical and histopathological changes to the liver and kidney of male rats. Hum Exp Toxicol 20:625-630.

215. Sengoku K, Tamate K, Yoshida T, Takaoka Y, Miyamoto T, Ishikawa M (1998) Effects of low concentrations of nitric oxide on the zona pellucida binding ability of human spermatozoa. Fertil Steril 69:522-527.

216. Shanti A, Santanam N, Morales AJ, Parthasarathy S, Murphy AA (1999) Autoantibodies to markers of oxidative stress are elevated in women with endometriosis. Fertil Steril 71:1115-1118.

217. Sharma RK, Agarwal A (1996) Role of reactive oxygen species in male infertility. Urology 48:835-850.

218. Sharma RK, Pasqualotto AE, Nelson DR, Thomas AJ, Jr., Agarwal A (2001) Relationship between seminal white blood cell counts and oxidative stress in men treated at an infertility clinic. J Androl 22:575-583.

219. Shen HM, Chia SE, Ong CN (1999) Evaluation of oxidative DNA damage in human sperm and its association with male infertility. J Androl 20:718-723.

220. Shiau CY, Wang JD, Chen PC (2004) Decreased fecundity among male lead workers. Occup Environ Med 61:915-923.

221. Shiotani M, Noda Y, Narimoto K, Imai K, Mori T, Fujimoto K, Ogawa K (1991) Immunohistochemical localization of superoxide dismutase in the human ovary. Hum Reprod 6:1349-1353.

222. Sies H (1993) Strategies of antioxidant defense. Eur J Biochem 215:213-219.

223. Sikka SC (1996) Oxidative stress and role of antioxidants in normal and abnormal sperm function. Front Biosci 1:e78-86.

224. Sikka SC (2004) Role of oxidative stress and antioxidants in andrology and assisted reproductive technology. J Androl 25:5-18.

225. Singer G, Granger DN (2007) Inflammatory responses underlying the microvascular dysfunction associated with obesity and insulin resistance. Microcirculation 14:375-387.

226. Sinha Hikim AP, Swerdloff RS (1999) Hormonal and genetic control of germ cell apoptosis in the testis. Rev Reprod 4:38-47.

227. Smith R, Vantman D, Ponce J, Escobar J, Lissi E (1996) Total antioxidant capacity of human seminal plasma. Hum Reprod 11:1655-1660.

228. Song GJ, Norkus EP, Lewis V (2006) Relationship between seminal ascorbic acid and sperm DNA integrity in infertile men. Int J Androl 29:569-575.

229. Stopczyk D, Gnitecki W, Buczynski A, Kowalski W, Buczynska M, Kroc A (2005) [Effect of electromagnetic field produced by mobile phones on the activity of superoxide dismutase (SOD-1)–*in vitro* researches]. Ann Acad Med Stetin 51 Suppl 1:125-128.

230. Sugino N, Karube-Harada A, Sakata A, Takiguchi S, Kato H (2002) Nuclear factor-kappa B is required for tumor necrosis factor-alpha-induced manganese superoxide dismutase expression in human endometrial stromal cells. J Clin Endocrinol Metab 87:3845-3850.

231. Sugino N, Karube-Harada A, Taketani T, Sakata A, Nakamura Y (2004) Withdrawal of ovarian steroids stimulates prostaglandin F2alpha production through nuclear factor-kappaB activation via oxygen radicals in human endometrial stromal cells: potential relevance to menstruation. J Reprod Dev 50:215-225.

232. Sugino N, Shimamura K, Takiguchi S, Tamura H, Ono M, Nakata M, Nakamura Y, Ogino K, Uda T, Kato H (1996) Changes in activity of superoxide dismutase in the human endometrium throughout the menstrual cycle and in early pregnancy. Hum Reprod 11:1073-1078.

233. Sugino N, Takiguchi S, Kashida S, Karube A, Nakamura Y, Kato H (2000) Superoxide dismutase expression in the human corpus luteum during the menstrual cycle and in early pregnancy. Mol Hum Reprod 6:19-25.

234. Sugino N, Takiguchi S, Ono M, Tamura H, Shimamura K, Nakamura Y, Tsuruta R, Sadamitsu D, Ueda T, Maekawa T, Kato H (1996) Nitric oxide concentrations in the follicular fluid and apoptosis of granulosa cells in human follicles. Hum Reprod 11:2484-2487.

235. Sun JG, Jurisicova A, Casper RF (1997) Detection of deoxyribonucleic acid fragmentation in human sperm: correlation with fertilization *in vitro*. Biol Reprod 56:602-607.

236. Suzuki T, Sugino N, Fukaya T, Sugiyama S, Uda T, Takaya R, Yajima A, Sasano H (1999) Superoxide dismutase in normal cycling human ovaries: immunohistochemical localization and characterization. Fertil Steril 72:720-726.

237. Szczepanska M, Kozlik J, Skrzypczak J, Mikolajczyk M (2003) Oxidative stress may be a piece in the endometriosis puzzle. Fertil Steril 79:1288-1293.

238. Taguchi M, Alfer J, Chwalisz K, Beier HM, Classen-Linke I (2000) Endothelial nitric oxide synthase is differently expressed in human endometrial vessels during the menstrual cycle. Mol Hum Reprod 6:185-190.

239. Tamate K, Sengoku K, Ishikawa M (1995) The role of superoxide dismutase in the human ovary and fallopian tube. J Obstet Gynaecol 21:401-409.

240. Taskinen H, Kyyronen P, Hemminki K, Hoikkala M, Lajunen K, Lindbohm ML (1994) Laboratory work and pregnancy outcome. J Occup Med 36:311-319.

241. Taylor C (2001) Antioxidants and reactive oxygen species in human fertility. Environmental Toxicology and Pharmacoloy 10:189-198.

242. Telisman S, Cvitkovic P, Jurasovic J, Pizent A, Gavella M, Rocic B (2000) Semen quality and reproductive endocrine function in relation to biomarkers of lead, cadmium, zinc and copper in men. Environ Health Perspect 108:45-53.

243. Therond P, Auger J, Legrand A, Jouannet P (1996) alpha-Tocopherol in human spermatozoa and seminal plasma: relationships with motility, antioxidant enzymes and leukocytes. Mol Hum Reprod 2:739-744.

244. Tolstrup JS, Kjaer SK, Holst C, Sharif H, Munk C, Osler M, Schmidt L, Andersen AM, Gronbaek M (2003) Alcohol use as predictor for infertility in a representative population of Danish women. Acta Obstet Gynecol Scand 82:744-749.

245. Tomlinson MJ, White A, Barratt CL, Bolton AE, Cooke ID (1992) The removal of morphologically abnormal sperm forms by phagocytes: a positive role for seminal leukocytes? Hum Reprod 7:517-522.

246. Traber MG, van der Vliet A, Reznick AZ, Cross CE (2000) Tobacco-related diseases. Is there a role for antioxidant micronutrient supplementation? Clin Chest Med 21:173-187, x.

247. Tremellen K (2008) Oxidative stress and male infertility–a clinical perspective. Hum Reprod Update 14:243-258.

248. Tseng L, Zhang J, Peresleni T, Goligorsky MS (1996) Cyclic expression of endothelial nitric oxide synthase mRNA in the epithelial glands of human endometrium. J Soc Gynecol Investig 3:33-38.

249. Twigg J, Fulton N, Gomez E, Irvine DS, Aitken RJ (1998) Analysis of the impact of intracellular reactive oxygen species generation on the structural and functional integrity of human spermatozoa: lipid peroxidation, DNA fragmentation and effectiveness of antioxidants. Hum Reprod 13:1429-1436.

250. Twigg J, Irvine DS, Houston P, Fulton N, Michael L, Aitken RJ (1998) Iatrogenic DNA damage induced in human spermatozoa during sperm preparation: protective significance of seminal plasma. Mol Hum Reprod 4:439-445.

251. Twigg JP, Irvine DS, Aitken RJ (1998) Oxidative damage to DNA in human spermatozoa does not preclude pronucleus formation at intracytoplasmic sperm injection. Hum Reprod 13:1864-1871.

252. Ungvary G, Tatrai E, Hudak A, Barcza G, Lorincz M (1980) Studies on the embryotoxic effects of ortho-, meta- and para-xylene. Toxicology 18:61-74.

253. Van Langendonckt A, Casanas-Roux F, Donnez J (2002) Oxidative stress and peritoneal endometriosis. Fertil Steril 77:861-870.

254. Vaux DL, Korsmeyer SJ (1999) Cell death in development. Cell 96:245-254.

255. Vega M, Johnson MC, Diaz HA, Urrutia LR, Troncoso JL, Devoto L (1998) Regulation of human luteal steroidogenesis *in vitro* by nitric oxide. Endocrine 8:185-191.

256. Vine MF, Tse CK, Hu P, Truong KY (1996) Cigarette smoking and semen quality. Fertil Steril 65:835-842.

257. Vitousek PM, Aber J, Howarth RW, Likens GE, Matson PA, Schindler DW, Schlesinger WH, Tilman GD (1997) Human alteration of the global nitrogen cycle: sources and consequences. Ecological Application 7:737-750.

258. Vitousek PM, Hattenschwiler S, Olander L, Allison S (2002) Nitrogen and nature. Ambio 31:97-101.

259. Wall PD, Pressman EK, Woods JR, Jr. (2002) Preterm premature rupture of the membranes and antioxidants: the free radical connection. J Perinat Med 30:447-457.

260. Wang Y, Sharma RK, Falcone T, Goldberg J, Agarwal A (1997) Importance of reactive oxygen species in the peritoneal fluid of women with endometriosis or idiopathic infertility. Fertil Steril 68:826-830.

261. WHO (1999) Laboratory manual for the examination of human semen and sperm-cervical mucus interaction. 4th ed. Cambridge University Press New York.

262. Williams EM, Eddy FB (1989) Effect of nitrite on the embryonic development of Atlantic salmon (Salmo salar). Canadian Journal of Fisheries and Aquatic Science 46:1726-1729.

263. Wiseman H, Halliwell B (1996) Damage to DNA by reactive oxygen and nitrogen species: role in inflammatory disease and progression to cancer. Biochem J 313 (Pt 1): 17-29.

264. Wu D, Cederbaum AI (2003) Alcohol, oxidative stress, and free radical damage. Alcohol Res Health 27:277-284.

265. Wu MY, Chao KH, Yang JH, Lee TH, Yang YS, Ho HN (2003) Nitric oxide synthesis is increased in the endometrial tissue of women with endometriosis. Hum Reprod 18:2668-2671.

266. Wu TP, Huang BM, Tsai HC, Lui MC, Liu MY (2004) Effects of nitric oxide on human spermatozoa activity, fertilization and mouse embryonic development. Arch Androl 50:173-179.

267. Xiao G, Pan C, Cai Y, Lin H, Fu Z (1999) Effect of benzene, toluene, xylene on the semen quality of exposed workers. Chin Med J (Engl) 112:709-712.

268. Xu DX, Shen HM, Zhu QX, Chua L, Wang QN, Chia SE, Ong CN (2003) The associations among semen quality, oxidative DNA damage in human spermatozoa and concentrations of cadmium, lead and selenium in seminal plasma. Mutat Res 534:155-163.

269. Yang HW, Hwang KJ, Kwon HC, Kim HS, Choi KW, Oh KS (1998) Detection of reactive oxygen species (ROS) and apoptosis in human fragmented embryos. Hum Reprod 13:998-1002.

270. Yeoman RR, Jones WD, Rizk BM (1998) Evidence for nitric oxide regulation of hamster sperm hyperactivation. J Androl 19:58-64.

271. Zini A, De Lamirande E, Gagnon C (1995) Low levels of nitric oxide promote human sperm capacitation *in vitro*. J Androl 16:424-431.

272. Zini A, Garrels K, Phang D (2000) Antioxidant activity in the semen of fertile and infertile men. Urology 55:922-926.

273. Zouari R, De Almeida M, Rodrigues D, Jouannet P (1993) Localization of antibodies on spermatozoa and sperm movement characteristics are good predictors of *in vitro* fertilization success in cases of male autoimmune infertility. Fertil Steril 59:606-612.

Environmental & Occupational Exposures (2010) ***Pages* 236–257**
Editors: **Sunil Kumar & R.R. Tiwari**
Published by: **DAYA PUBLISHING HOUSE, NEW DELHI**

Chapter 10

Inevitable Contaminant of Water-Fluoride: A Non-Skeletal Study on Rats

*D. Agrawal[1], J.B.S. Kachhawa[2], T.I. Khan[1] and R.S. Gupta[2]**

[1]Centre for Advanced Studies, Department of Zoology, University of Rajasthan, Jaipur – 302 004
[2]Indira Gandhi Centre for Human Ecology, Environmental and Population Studies, University of Rajasthan, Jaipur – 302 004

ABSTRACT

Chronic fluoride intoxication (fluorosis) is a worldwide health problem and is endemic in areas where fluoride content is high in drinking water. Fluorosis, which was considered to be a problem related to teeth only, has now turned up to be a serious health hazard. It not only affects the body of a person but also renders them socially and culturally crippled. In India it is estimated that 62 million people (17 out of the 32 states) are affected with dental, skeletal and/or non-skeletal fluorosis. In the perception of Rajasthan, most of the districts have been

* E-mail: gupta_rs@hotmail.com

declared as fluorosis prone areas. Therefore, the impact of fluoride on non-skeletal system and male reproduction has been reviewed in this chapter.

Introduction

Fluorine is the 13th most abundant element available in the earth crust. The main source of fluoride intake by the human population is water, food, dental health products, medicines as well as pesticides, insecticides and fertilizers residues, and even inhaling it in the air we breathe[1].

To a certain extent (as per WHO; 0.6 ppm) fluoride ingestion is useful for bone and teeth development, but excessive ingestion causes a disease known as fluorosis. The WHO[2] standards permit only 1.5 mg/L as a safe limit of fluoride in drinking water for human consumption. In India, fluoride contamination of the top aquifer system is endemic in many locations including Andhra Pradesh, Tamil Nadu, Karnataka, Gujarat, Rajasthan, Punjab, Haryana, Bihar, Kerala and West Bengal[3,4].

A Survey conducted by PHED Rajasthan State[5] (1991-1993) revealed that the degree of fluoride problem is very serious in 7 districts (Ajmer, Bhilwara, Nagaur, Dausa, Jaipur, Tonk, Jalore) and serious in 10 districts (Alwar, Barmer, Bharatpur, Dungarpur, Jaisalmer, Sikar, Pali, Sawaimadhopur, Karoli, Sirohi), less serious in 9 districts (Banswara, Junjhunu, Udaipur, Churu, Dholpur, Ganganagar, Rajsamand, Jodhpur, Hanumangarh) and insignificant in 6 districts (Baran, Bundi, Bikaner, Chittorgarh, Jhalawar and Kota).

Fluorosis mainly manifests in three forms–dental, skeletal and non-skeletal. Fluoride intoxication is associated with depletion of energy production through inhibition of the Kreb's cycle[6], muscle atrophy[7,8], liver toxicity[9,10] and kidney toxicity[11].

The effect of fluoride on male and female fertility has become an area of growing concern. Various studies showed that fluoride causes adverse effects on both male and female fertility[12–14].

In order to evaluate the effect of sodium fluoride on male fertility, the present study was carried out with water samples of different levels of fluoride and alteration in their biochemical parameters were studied.

Material and Methods

Experiment had been carried out on mature male albino rats of Wistar strain. Healthy adult male rats were fed on a balanced diet of palates. They were kept in plastic cages under 12hrs light and 12hrs dark cycles and temperature at 25° C, water was provided *ad libitum.* 50 male rats were divided into 5 groups of 10 each and treated as under:

Group I–Served as control

Group II–Treated with fluoridated water of 8ppm concentration

Group III–Treated with fluoridated water of 10ppm concentration

Group IV–Treated with fluoridated water of 15ppm concentration

Group V–Treated with fluoridated water of 20ppm concentration

The period was 180 days for all treatment groups. On the day 181st final body weight were noted and whole groups were sacrificed by using light ether anaesthesia. The reproductive organs as well as vital organs including thyroid were dissected out, trimmed free of fat and each organ was weighed on a torsion balance. Blood was collected from heart and used for various hematological analyses and serum separated was stored at –20°C for biochemical analysis.

Sperm Dynamics

The testis and epididymis was removed immediately after anaesthesia. Sperm motility in cauda epididymis and sperm density in testis as well as in cauda epididymis was assessed by the method of Prasad *et al.*[15] (1972).

Haematological Studies

Blood was collected from heart and total erythrocyte count, total leucocyte count, Blood sugar, Blood urea was evaluated.

Serum Analysis

Blood collected from heart was kept to clot at room temperature and serum was separated. Parameters studied were alkaline phosphatase, SGOT, SGPT and Bilirubin.

Tissue Biochemistry

Fresh tissues of testis and accessory sex organs were processed for the estimation of glycogen[16], protein[17], cholesterol[18] and sialic acid[19]. Fructose[20] was determined in the seminal vesicle.

Hormone Analysis

Serum was analyzed for testosterone[21], T3, T4 and TSH[22].

Statistical Analysis

All the values of body and organ weights, biochemical estimation were averaged, standard error of mean were calculated and Student's 't' test was applied for general comparison.

Results

Body Weight

The treatment with fluoride for 180 days to rats did not cause any significant change in the body weight.

Organ Weight

Fluoride water treatment to rats caused a significant reduction ($p < 0.001$) in the weight of testes in comparison to control. The weight of testes was decreased by 40.25 per cent, 40.81 per cent, 42.69 per cent and 44.03 per cent in rats of group II, III, IV and V respectively in comparison to control. On the other hand the weight of epididymis, ventral prostate, seminal vesicle, kidney was also decreased in significant to highly significant manner. However a non-significant change was observed at all dose levels in weight of liver with respect to control level. The weight of thyroid gland decreased in all treated groups, conversely the reduction was significant ($p<0.01$) in group II and highly significant ($p<0.001$) in group III, IV and V when compared with group I. (Table 10.1)

Sperm Dynamics

The motility of spermatozoa in cauda epididymis was decreased by 52.41 per cent, 56.94 per cent, 64.30 per cent and 66.12 per cent in rats of group II, III, IV and V respectively in comparison to control. The fluoridated water exposed rats showed a significant ($p<0.001$) reduction in testicular sperm density as well as in cauda epididymal sperm density at all dose levels when compared with controls (Table 10.2).

Table 10.1: Effect of Fluoride on Body and Organ Weight in Male Albino Rats

Treatment	Organ Weight-mg\100gm Body Weight						
	Testes	Epididymis	Ventral-prostate	Seminal Vesicle	Kidney	Liver	Thyroid
Group-I Control or Vehicle treated	1402.19±6.21	429.31±7.45	378.54±13.4	710.05±14.45	747.43±12.98	4140.75±101.34	10.33±0.09
Group-II 8ppm Fluoride water	837.73 ±9.05**	325.23±9.54**	243.91 ±13.09**	639.56±20.79 ns	813.74±14.94*	4251.86±177.36 ns	9.38±0.21*
Group-III 10ppm Fluoride water	829.93±8.31**	311.64±10.78**	237.23±12.67**	631.98±19.87*	825.63±13.78*	4278.63±199.05 ns	9.31±0.19**
Group-IV 15ppm Fluoride water	803.56±8.42**	304.56±11.57**	236.76±11.89**	627.33±21.03*	839.04±14.23*	4329.11±176.83 ns	8.98±0.18**
Group-V 20ppm Fluoride water	784.81±8.63**	301.73±11.75**	235.89 ±9.02**	619.23±18.45*	850.74±14.87**	4375.91±107.45 ns	8.53±0.11**

Group II, III, IV and V compared with group I.

ns: Non significant; *: $P < 0.01$ significant; *: $P < 0.001$ Highly significant.

Table 10.2: Effect of Fluoride on Sperm Dynamics and Fertility in Male Albino Rats

Treatment	*Sperm Motility (per cent)*	*Sperm Density (million\ml)*	
		Testes	*Cauda Epididymis*
Group-I: Control or Vehicle treated	72.52±3.45	6.54±0.49	74.54±3.49
Group-II 8ppm Fluoride water	34.51±0.59**	3.12±0.12**	15.07±1.97**
Group-III 10ppm Fluoride water	31.23±1.54**	3.07±0.06**	13.83±2.01**
Group-IV 15ppm Fluoride water	25.89±1.39**	2.83±0.10**	11.03±1.66**
Group-V 20ppm Fluoride water	24.57±1.43**	2.59±0.13**	7.98±1.34**

Group II, III, IV and V compared with group I

ns: Non significant; *: P < 0.01 significant; *: P < 0.001 Highly significant.

Hematology

Results pertaining to effects of fluoride on blood parameters in male rats are given in (Table 10.3).

The treatment of fluoridated water for 180 days decreased R.B.C. count in highly significant ($p<0.001$) manner in all groups in comparison to control rats. A significant increase in W.B.C. counts ($p<0.01$) of 16.75, 18.92, 21.25 and 23.45 per cent was observed in groups II, III, IV and V respectively in comparison to control rats. Blood sugar and blood urea levels increased in all treated groups significantly in comparison to control.

Serum Analysis

Results pertaining to effects of fluoride on serum parameters in male rats are given in (Table 10.3).

The activity of serum alkaline phosphatase was significantly increased in all treated rats, when compared with control rats. SGOT and SGPT concentration increased significantly ($p<0.001$) in all groups after the administration of fluoridated water for 180 days.

Table 10.3: Effect of Fluoride on Blood Analysis in Male Albino Rats

Treatment	*R.B.C. Count (million/mm³)*	*W.B.C. Count (per mm³)*	*Blood Sugar (mg/dl)*	*Blood Urea (mg/dl)*	*Alkaline Phosphatase (µg ip/hr)*	*SGOT (units/L)*	*SGPT (units/L)*	*Bilirubin (µg/dl)*
Group-I Control or Vehicle treated	5.33±0.11	5250.05±50.08	89.12±6.39	35.43±1.97	3.09±0.04	34.81±1.17	22.82±1.89	0.99±0.04
Group-II 8ppm Fluoride water	3.89±0.27**	6129.19±194.67*	103.48±3.49^{ns}	77.97±5.78**	4.03±0.09**	73.29±2.98**	63.39±2.09**	1.32±0.05**
Group-III 10ppm Fluoride water	3.59±0.29**	6243.16±209.58*	113.37±4.23*	87.35±6.23**	4.27±0.07**	84.41±3.25**	75.86±2.85**	1.43±0.07**
Group-IV 15ppm Fluoride water	3.25±0.17**	6365.77±202.44**	115.03±3.19*	95.07±4.59**	4.69±0.07**	95.78±3.34**	87.76±2.44**	1.57±0.04**
Group-V 20ppm Fluoride water	2.97±0.14**	6481.32±193.41**	117.52±4.09*	102.39±4.93**	4.81±0.03**	101.23±2.89**	93.25±1.17**	1.75±0.01**

Group II, III, IV and V compared with group I.

ns: Non significant; *: P < 0.01 significant; *: P < 0.001 Highly significant.

Bilirubin concentration also increased significantly in all groups after the administration of fluoridated water for 180 days.

Tissue Biochemistry

Protein and sialic acid contents were decreased significantly in testes and cauda epididymis. Significant decline ($P<0.001$) was also noticed in glycogen content of testis and fructose content in seminal vesicle whereas significant elevation was observed in testicular cholesterol content in all treated groups (Table 10.4).

Hormone Analysis

Fluoridated water exposure caused significant reduction ($p<0.001$) in the serum testosterone level at all dose levels when compared with controls (Figure 10.1). A percentage reduction of 52.74, 59.66, 70.64 and 75.89 were observed in-group II, III, IV and V respectively in comparison to control rats. There was a significant declined level of T3 (Figure 10.2) and T4 (Figure 10.3) in all the treated groups however serum TSH level showed a significant ($p<0.01$) increase. A percentage increase of TSH 36.55, 41.24, 64.85 and 80.63 were observed in-group II, III, IV and V respectively in comparison to control rats (Figure 10.4).

Discussion

In the present study, significant loss in the weight of the testes and accessory sex organs *i.e.* epididymis, seminal vesicle and ventral prostate after the administration of fluoride at different dose levels was observed. Accessory sex organs are androgen dependent and thus reflect the availability of androgen. The availability of androgen is directly related to the weight of accessory sex organs[23]. After the exposure of fluoride, it was observed that the toxic effect of fluoride causes retardation in the growth of testes, cauda and caput epididymis and ventral prostate[24]. Significant decrease in thyroid weight suggests toxic effect of fluoride on thyroid gland. Decrease in thyroid weight might be due to follicular regression (epithelial cells). About 75 per cent of the weight of the entire thyroid gland consists of thyroglobulin protein[25]. Decrease in the content of thyroglobulin protein may also account for the decrease in thyroid weight. Earlier investigators[26] have also observed decrease in thyroid weight due to fluoride toxicity.

Table 10.4: Effect of Fluoride on Tissue Biochemistry in Male Albino Rats

Treatment	*Protein (mg/gm)*		*Sialic Acid (mg/gm)*		*Glycogen (mg/gm)*	*Cholesterol (mg/gm)*	*Fructose (mg/gm)*	*Ascorbic Acid (mg/gm)*
	Testes	*Cauda Epididymis*	*Testes*	*Testes*	*Seminal Vesicle*	*Adrenal Gland*	*Testes*	*Seminal Vesicle*
Group-I Control or Vehicle treated	229.14±3.41	248.18±4.04	5.54±0.08	5.21±0.04	2.87±0.16	8.99±0.53	5.57±0.21	4.28±0.39
Group-II 8ppm Fluoride water	171.97±3.71**	180.67±3.65**	3.74±0.05**	3.85±0.09**	3.88±0.15*	15.98±0.59**	7.98±0.29**	5.21±0.17 ns
Group-III 10ppm Fluoride water	169.04±3.99**	174.85±3.91**	3.69±0.04**	3.78±0.07**	4.02±0.12**	16.77±0.56**	8.51±0.37**	5.43±0.27 ns
Group-IV 15ppm Fluoride water	153.78±3.23**	162.81±3.59**	3.46±0.02**	3.50±0.05**	4.19±0.10**	18.03±.41**	9.37±0.18**	5.57±0.32 ns
Group-V 20ppm Fluoride water	140.52±2.95**	150.82±3.11**	3.31±0.03**	3.25±0.03**	4.29±0.09**	20.86±0.35**	10.03±0.21**	5.69±0.29*

Group II, III, IV and V compared with group I.

ns: Non significant; *: P < 0.01 significant; *: P < 0.001 Highly significant.

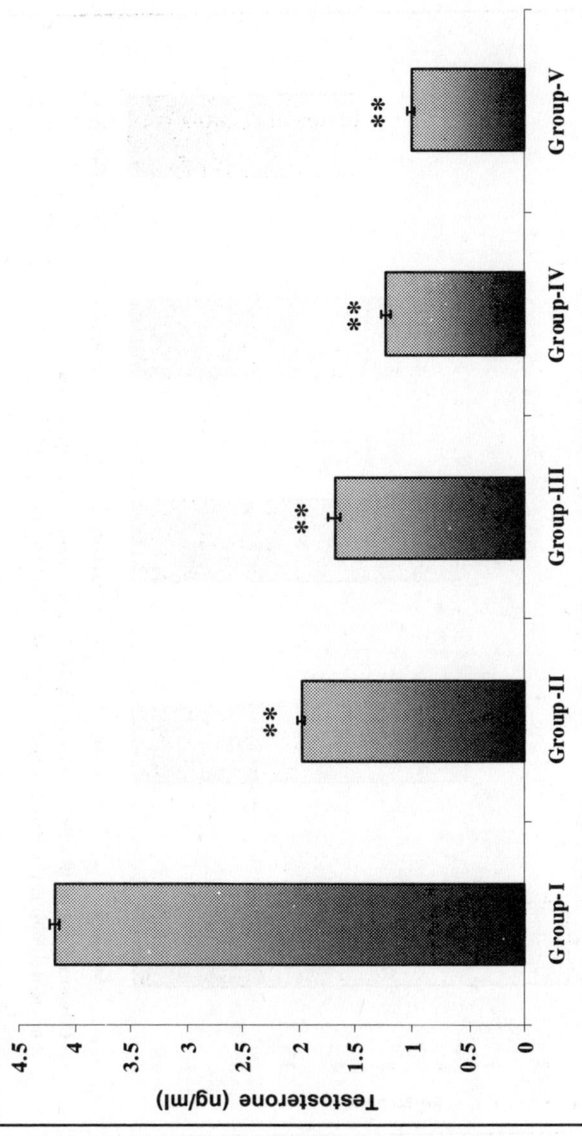

(Mean ± SEM of 10 animals) Group II, III, IV and V compared with group I
**=P<0.001 Highly significant

Figure 10.1: Effect of Fluoride on Testosterone in Male Albino Rats

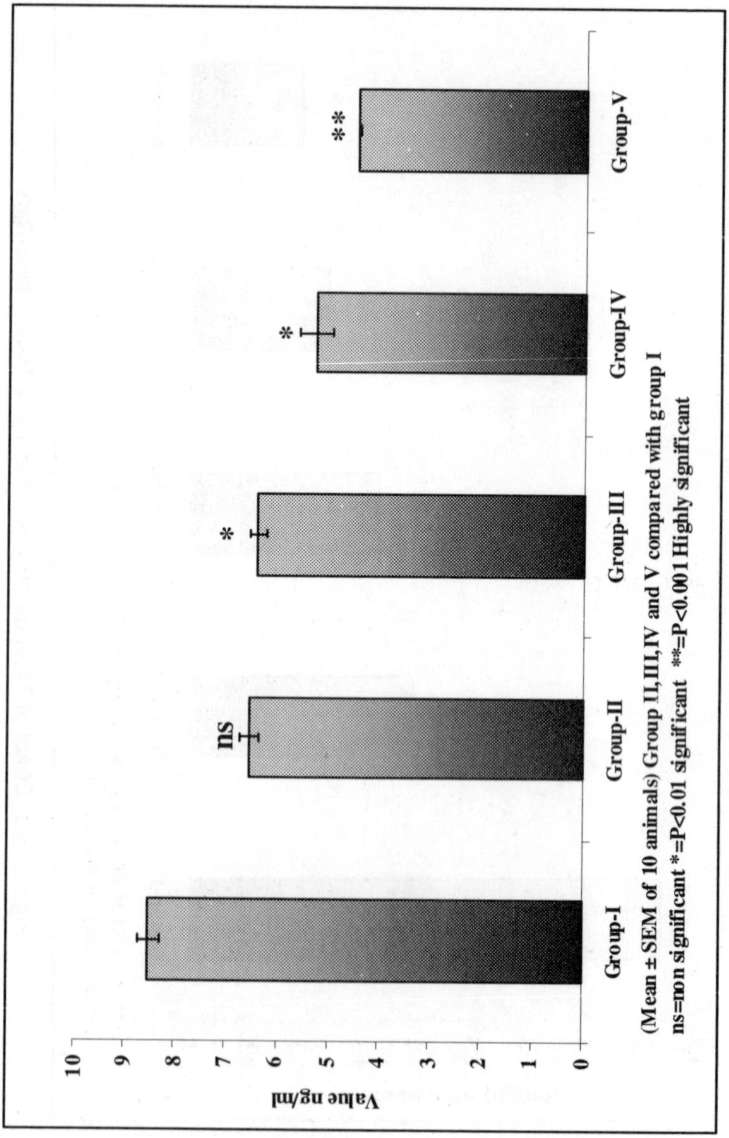

(Mean ± SEM of 10 animals) Group II, III, IV and V compared with group I
ns=non significant *=P<0.01 significant **=P<0.001 Highly significant

Figure 10.2: Effect of Fluoride on Serum T3 in Male Albino Rats

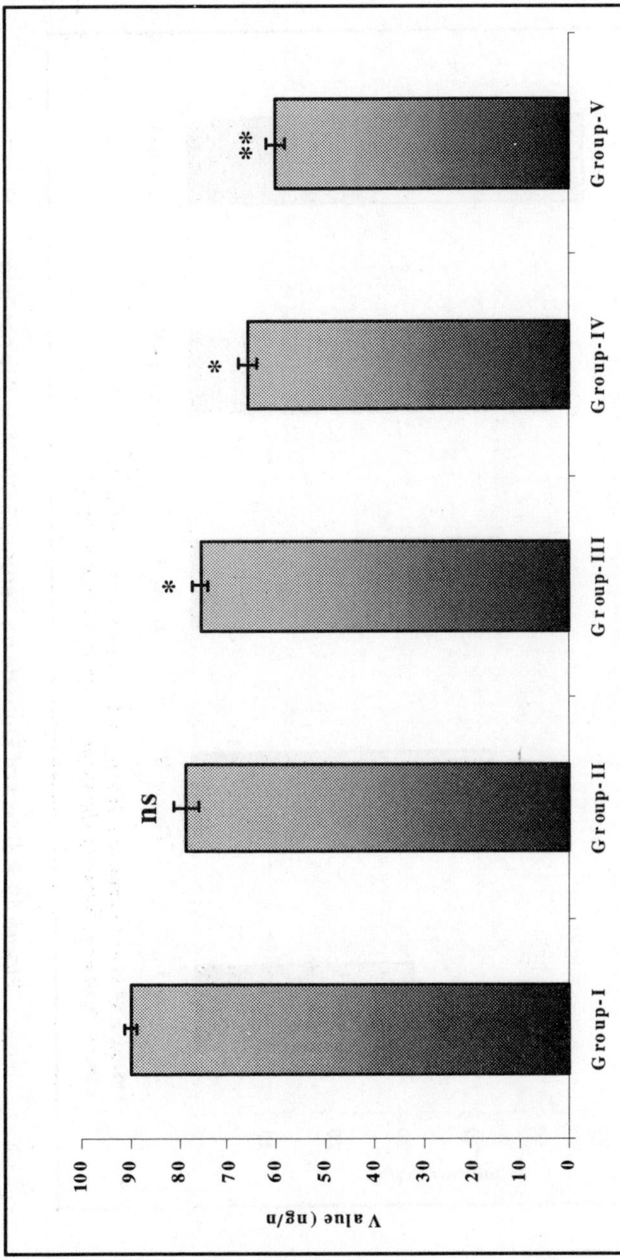

(Mean ± SEM of 10 animals) Group II, III, IV and V compared with group I
ns=non significant *=P<0.01 significant **=P<0.001 Highly significant

Figure 10.3: Effect of Fluoride on Serum T4 in Male Albino Rats

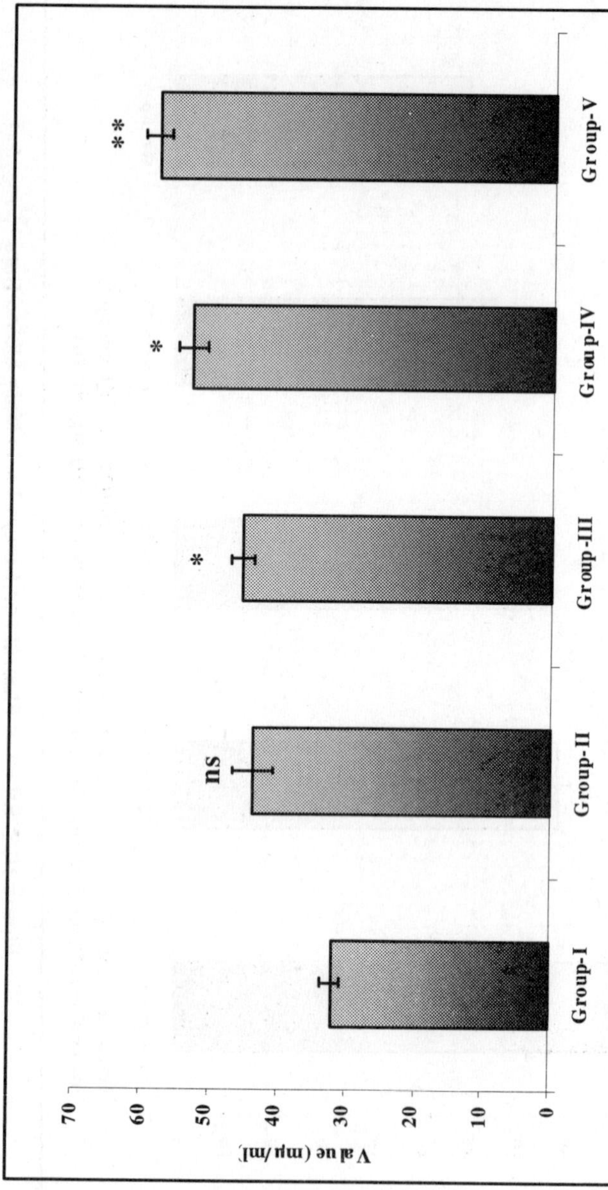

(Mean ± SEM of 10 animals) Group II,III,IV and V compared with group I
ns=non significant *=P<0.01 significant **=P<0.001 Highly significant

Figure 10.4: Effect of Fluoride on Serum TSH in Male Albino Rats

Fluoride is known to inhibit sperm motility. It has been demonstrated that bovine sperm treated with 30mM fluoride became immobile within two minutes[27]. Human spermatozoa lost their motility *in vitro* in the presence of 250mM NaF within two minutes incubation[28]. The decreased sperm density could be correlated with the testicular spermatogenic arrest following fluoride ingestion in mice, rats and rabbits[29–32]. The above mentioned alterations in sperm motility and density might be the outcome of the altered and hostile internal milieu of the epididymis of NaF treated rats since it is known that normal epididymal structure and its internal microenvironment are important for sperm maturation and for maintaining them in a viable, motile state[32–35].

Machalinska *et al*[36] found significant pathologic morphologic changes in the spleen of mice treated with fluoride. Spleen actively provides blood cell production throughout life. They showed that toxic damage to the spleen caused by sodium fluoride might therefore have marked negative effects on haematopoiesis. Eren *et al*[37] also found eosinophilia (5 per cent of peripheral blood leukocyte) in the fluorised group. Banupriya *et al*[38] also observed significant increase in the rats given 20 ppm fluoride in their drinking water. Level of blood sugar increased significantly in group III, IV and V. Increased blood sugar level may be due to disturbances in carbohydrate metabolism.

Level of blood urea was significantly increased at all dose level of fluoride exposure in rats during the study period. As in our findings here, Guzman *et al*[39] also found an increase in the urea content in the blood plasma of rats and mice treated intraperitoneally with Irloxacin, a fluorine containing antibiotic. Similar findings were reported by Monsour and Kruger[40] and Appleton[41].

SGPT and SGOT are markers of liver function. Drinking high-fluoride water over a long period can damage the liver. In the present study, elevated enzyme activities of SGPT and SGOT demonstrated liver damage in the fluorotic rats, in agreement with results of previous investigations[42–44].

Increase in alkaline phosphatase has been considered as an important factor in fluoride toxicology[45]. Fluoride induced cell injury in both osteoblasts and osteocytes initiate a repair response and results in increased SAP production in both of these cell populations[46–47]. Significant increase in Serum alkaline phosphatase concentration was also observed by Stanley *et al*[45] in an acute inhalation study of sodium fluoride in Wistar rats.

Fluoride inhibits protein synthesis *in vitro* and *in vivo*[48]. In the present study, the level of proteins in testes and accessory sex organs exhibited a significant decline in the NaF treated rats. This decrease might be due to impairment of protein metabolism/ synthesis. This decrease in the protein synthesis may be due to impairment of peptide chain initiation[49], decrease in mRNA transcription[50], and inhibition of DNA synthesis[51].

Cholesterol and its esters are involved in steroidogenesis. Cholesterol level increased significantly in the testes of all experimental groups. Cholesterol is most important precursor in synthesis of steroid hormones and its level is related to fertility of individuals[52]. Increased level of cholesterol may be due to decreased androgen production, which resulted in accumulation of cholesterol in testes, hence impaired spermatogenesis[53].

The increase in level of fructose in seminal vesicle after 180 days of NaF exposure supports an alteration in carbohydrate metabolism of fluorotic rats. As fructose has a vital role in providing energy to the sperm, it is evident that the increased fructose level might influence sperm metabolism. Chinoy and Sharma[24] has also reported significant increase in the fructose level in the seminal vesicle after NaF treatment for 30 days.

Ascorbic acid plays an important role in general oxidation-reduction process. In the present study ascorbic acid in adrenal gland was significantly increased in group V rats. Chinoy *et al*[54] found higher levels of ascorbic acid in the adrenal gland of male rats as a consequence of stress imposed by the fluoride.

Testosterone synthesis and production is the result of a series of complex biochemical interactions involving the hypothalamus, pituitary and the testes[55]. Zahvoronkov and Strochkova[50] found decreased amounts of rRNA and a decreased dry weight of Leydig cells of mice treated with fluoride. Narayana and Chinoy[12] reported a decrease in the Leydig cell diameter and the Leydig cell nuclear diameter in the testes of rats treated with fluoride. A study by Kumar and Susheela[31] also reported a decrease in Leydig cell and Leydig cell nuclear diameter in rabbits administered 10 mg NaF/kg body weight daily for a period of 23 months.

Rao and Susheela[56] have reported a decrease in the [sigma] 5-3-beta hydroxysteroid dehydrogenase levels in rabbits treated with fluoride. Das and Susheela[57] have reported decreased serum glucocorticoids in skeletal fluorosis patients and in rabbits treated with 10 mg NaF/kg/d for 18 months as compared to controls.

In the present study, levels of serum T3 and T4 decreased significantly as the concentration of fluoride increases from 8 ppm to 20 ppm while the concentration of serum TSH increased in a dose dependent manner. It has been known for a long time that fluoride mimics the action of the thyroid-stimulating hormone (TSH). It is generally believed that fluorine does not influence either thyroid function or structure at the amount (about 1ppm in water) used to prevent the dental caries[58]. However, if fluorine intake is extremely high such as in an endemic fluorosis area or in the cases when fluoride treatment is used, the secretion of T4 and T3 from the thyroid could be influenced. Yu[59] reported a decreased serum T4 level and increased TSH level in the residents of endemic fluorosis area. Bachinskii *et al*[60] compared the serum TSH and thyroid hormone levels in the area with high fluorine concentration in water (122±5 μmol/l, *i.e.* about 2.3 ppm) and a control area (52±5 μmol/l, *i.e.* about 1.0ppm) and found that the healthy people who lived in the high fluorine area tended to take up more iodine and had decreased T3 and increased TSH levels. Decreased T3 and/or T4 levels were also observed in animal experiments[61–62]. The results of the experiments showed that excessive fluorine intake increased serum T3 and T4 levels of iodine treated mice, especially in iodine deficiency conditions.

In conclusion: Fluoride ingestion adversely affects the reproductive organs as well as vital organs. Our results revealed that effects of fluoride toxicity are in dose dependent manner as the concentration of fluoride was increased the results became more serious. With the above study we can give some suggestions to prevent or cure the fluoride toxicity:

1. Regulatory agencies should collect water samples regularly and get them analyzed for different parameters.
2. People should be made aware about the quality of water currently in use, both for drinking purpose and agricultural uses.

3. Proper arrangements should be made for providing drinking water with allowable limits for fluoride.
4. Techniques should be made available for defluoridation of drinking water in individual households.
5. People should be made aware about the Dental, Skeletal and Non-skeletal fluorosis.

References

1. Chinoy NJ, Rao MV, Narayana MV and Neelakanta E (1991). Microdose vasal injection of sodium fluoride in the rat. Reprod Toxicol, 5(6): 505-512.
2. WHO (1984). Guidelines for drinking water quality. World Health Organization, Geneva.2: 249.
3. Handa BK (1975). Geochemistry and genesis of fluoride-containing ground waters in India. Ground Water, 13: 275-281.
4. Suma LS, Ambika SR and Prasad SJ (1999). Fluoride contamination status of groundwater in Karnataka. Curr Sci, 6: 730-734.
5. PHED (1991-1993). Survey, fluoride affected villages/habitation.
6. Bogin E, Abrams M, Avidar Y, Israeli B, and Dagan B (1976). Effect of fluoride on enzymes from serum, liver, kidney, skeletal and heart muscles of mice. Fluoride, 9(1): 42-46
7. Kaul RD and Susheela AK (1974). Evidence of muscle fiber degeneration in rabbits treated with sodium fluoride. Fluoride, 7(4): 177-181.
8. Susheela AK and Kharb P (1990). Aortic calcification in chronic fluoride poisoning: biochemical and electronmicroscopic evidence. Exp Mol Pathol, 53(1): 72-80.
9. Saralakumari D, Varadacharyulu NC and Ramakrishna Rao P (1988). Effects of fluoride toxicity on growth and lipids in liver, kidney and serum in rat. Arogya J Health Sci, 15: 24–29.
10. Carlson JR and Suttle JW (1996). Pentose phosphate pathway enzymes and glucose oxidation in fluoride fed rats. Am J Physiol, 210: 79-83.
11. Suketa Y and Terui Y (1980). Shizuoka Adrenal Function and Changes of Sodium and Potassium in Serum and Urine in Fluoride-Intoxicated rats. Fluoride, 13(1): 4-9.

12. Narayana MV and Chinoy NJ (1994). Effect of fluoride on rat testicular steroidogenesis. Fluoride, 27(1): 7-12.

13. Al-Hiyasat AS, Ahmed AM, Elbetieha B and Darmanib H (2000). Reproductive toxic effects of ingestion of sodium fluoride in female rats. Fluoride, 33(2): 79-84.

14. Ghosh D, Das SS, Maiti R, Jana D and Das UB (2002). Testicular toxicity in sodium fluoride treated rats: association with oxidative stress. Reprod Toxicol, 16(4): 385-390.

15. Prasad MRN, Chinoy NJ and Kadam KM (1972). Changes in succinate dehydrogenase levels in the rats epididymis under normal and altered physiological conditions. Fertil Steril, 23:186-190.

16. Montgomery R (1957). Determination of glycogen. Arch Biochem Biophys, 67:378-381.

17. Lowry OH, Rosenbrough NJ, Farr AL and Randall RJ (1951). Protein measurement with Folin-Phenol reagent. J Biol Chem, 192: 265-275.

18. Oser BL (1965). In: Hawk's physiological chemistry. (14th Ed.) McGraw Hill. New York, pp. 246.

19. Warren L (1959). The thiobarbituric acid assay of sialic acid. J Biol Chem, 234:1971-1975.

20. Mann T (1964). Fructose, polyols and organic acids. In: Biochemistry of semen and of the male reproductive tract. Methuen and Co. (London). pp. 237-249.

21. Be'langer A, Caron S and Picard V (1980). Simultaneous radio-immuno assay of progestins, androgens and estrogens in rat testis. J Steroid Biochem, 13(2): 185-190.

22. Chopra IJ, Soloman DH and Gnho RS (1971). A radioimmuneassay of thyroxin. J Clin Endocrinol, 33:865-867.

23. Hunt S and Mittwoch U (1984). Effects of gossypol on sperm counts in two inbred strains of mice. J Reprod Fert, 70(1): 341-345.

24. Chinoy NJ and Sharma A (1998). Amelioration of fluoride toxicity by Vitamins E and D in reproductive functions of male mice. Fluoride, 31(4): 203-216.

25. Patel KG, Bhatt HV and Chaudhury AR (2003). Alteration in thyroid after formaldehyde (HCHO) treatment in rats. Industrial Health, 41:295-297.

26. Zhao W, Zhu H, Yu Z, Aoki K, Misumi J and Zhang X (1998). Long-term Effects of Various Iodine and Fluorine Doses on the Thyroid and Fluorosis in Mice. Endocr, Regul, 32(2): 63-70.

27. Schoff PI and Lardy MA (1987). Effects of fluoride and caffeine on metabolism of ejaculated bovine spermatozoa. Biology of Reproduction, 37:1037-1046.

28. Chinoy NJ and Narayana MV (1994). *In vitro* fluoride toxicity in human spermatozoa. Reproductive Toxicology, 8(2): 155-159.

29. Kour K and Singh J (1980). Histological finding of mice testes following fluoride ingestion. Fluoride, 13(4): 160-162.

30. Chinoy NJ (1995). Role of fluoride in animal systems: A review. In: Toxicity and Monitoring of Xenobiotics.PP: 13-30.

31. Kumar A and Susheela AK (1995). Effects of chronic fluoride toxicity on the morphology of ductus epididymis and the maturation of spermatozoa of rabbit. Int J Exp Pathol, 76(1): 1-11.

32. Chinoy NJ, Mehta D and Jhala DD (2006). Effects of fluoride ingestion with protein deficient or protein enriched diets on sperm function of mice. Fluoride, 39(1): 11–16.

33. Rajalakshmi M and Prasad MRN (1979). Contribution of the epididymis and vas deferens in maturation of spermatozoa. In: Talwar GP (Ed). Recent Advances in Reproduction and Regulation of Fertility. Elsevier, Amsterdam. pp.253-258.

34. Cooper TG (1986). The Epididymal Sperm Maturation and Fertilization. Springer-Verlag, New York: 281.

35. Kumar A and Susheela AK (1994). Ultrastructural studies of spermiogenesis in rabbit exposed to chronic fluoride toxicity. Int J Fertil Menopausal Stud, 39(3): 164-171.

36. Machalinska A, Wiszniewska B, Tarasiuk J and Machalinski B (2002). Morphological effect of sodium fluoride on hematopoetic organs in mice. Fluoride, 35(4): 231-238.

37. Eren E, Zturk M, Mumcu EF and Canatan D (2005). Fluorosis and its hematological effects. Toxicology and Industrial Health, 21:255–258.
38. Banu priya CAY, Anitha K, Murli Mohan E, Pillai KS and Murthy PB (1997). Toxicity of fluoride to diabetic rats. Fluoride, 30(1): 51-58.
39. Guzman A, Garcia C and Demestre I (1999). Acute and subchronic toxicity studies of the new quinolone antibacterial agent irloxacin in rodents. Arzneimittelforschung. 49: 448-456.
40. Monsour PA and Kruger BJ (1985). Effect of fluoride on soft tissues in vertebrates (a review). Fluoride, 18(1): 53-61.
41. Appleton J (1995). Changes in the plasma electrolytes and metabolites of the rat following acute exposure to sodium fluoride and strontium chloride. Arch Oral Biol, 40:265-268.
42. Kessabi M, Boudarine B, Braun JP and Lamnouer D (1983). Serum biochemical effects of fluoride in sheep in the darmous area. Fluoride, 16(4): 214-219.
43. Chinoy NJ and Memon MR (2001). Beneficial effects of some vitamins and calcium on fluoride and aluminium toxicity on gastrocnemius muscle and liver of male mice. Fluoride, 34(1): 21-33.
44. Guo XY, Sun GF and Sun YC (2003). Oxidative stress from fluoride-induced hepatotoxicity in rats. Fluoride, 36(1): 25-29.
45. Stanley VA, Ramesh N, Kumar T, Pillai KS and Murthy PBK (1998). Acute inhalation of sodium fluoride in wistar rats. Ad Bios, 17(1): 33-40.
46. Farley JR, Wergedal JE and Baylink DJ (1983). Fluoride directly stimulates proliferation and alkaline phosphatase activity of bone-forming cells. Science, 222:330-332.
47. Marie PJ and Hott M (1986). Short-term effects of fluoride and strontium on bone formation and resorption in the mouse. Metabolism, 35:547-551.
48. Shashi A (2003). Histopathological investigation of fluoride-induced neurotoxicity in rabbits. Fluoride, 36(2): 95-105.

49. Godchaux W and Atwood KC (1976). Structure and function of initiation complexes, which accumulate during inhibition of protein synthesis by fluoride ion. J Biol Chem, 251:292-301.

50. Zahvoronkov AA and Strochkova LS (1981). Fluorosis: geographical pathology and some experimental findings. Fluoride, 14(4): 182-191.

51. Holland RI (1979). Fluoride inhibition of protein and DNA synthesis in cells *in vitro*. Acta Pharmacol Toxicol, 45:96-101.

52. Eik-Nes KB and Hall PF (1962). Isolation of Dehydroepiandrosterone C^{14} from dogs infused with cholesterol $_4C^{14}$ by the spermatic artery. Proc Soc Exp Biol Med, III: 280-283.

53. Bedwal RS, Edwards MS Katoch M, Bahuguna A and Dewan R (1994). Histological and biochemical changes in testis of zinc deficient BALB/c strain of mice. Ind J Exp Biol, 32:243-247.

54. Chinoy NJ, Sharma M and Michael M (1993). Beneficial effects of ascorbic acid and calcium on reversal of fluoride toxicity in male rats. Fluoride, 26(1): 45-56.

55. Susheela AK and Jethanandani P (1996). Circulating testosterone levels in skeletal fluorosis patients. J Toxicol Clin Toxicol, 34(2): 183-189.

56. Rao K and Susheela AK (1979). Effect of sodium fluoride on adrenal gland of rabbit. Studies on ascorbic acid and delta 5-3-beta hydroxysteroid dehydrogenase activity. Fluoride, 12(2): 65-71.

57. Das TK and Susheela AK (1991). Chronic fluoride toxicity and pituitary-adrenal function. Environ Sci, 1:57-62.

58. Buergi H, Siebenhuner L, Miloni E (1984). Fluorine and thyroid gland function: a review of the literature. Klinische Wochenschrift, 62: 564-569.

59. Yu YN (1985). Effects of chronic fluorosis on the thyroid gland. Chinese Med J, 65:747-749.

60. Bachinskii PP, Gutsalenko OA, Naryzhniuk ND, Sidora VD and Shliakhta AI (1985). Action of the body fluorine of healthy persons and thyroidopathy patients on the function of hypophyseal-thyroid the system. Probl Endokrinol, 31(6): 25-29.

61. Hara K. (1980). Studies on fluorosis, especially effects of fluoride on thyroid metabolism. Koku Eisei Gakkai Zasshi, 30(1): 42-57.

62. Guan ZZ, Zhuang ZJ, Yang PS, Pan S. (1988). Synergistic action of iodine-deficiency and fluorine-intoxication on rat thyroid. Chin Med J (Engl), 101(9): 679-684.

Environmental & Occupational Exposures (2010) *Pages 258–269*
Editors: **Sunil Kumar & R.R. Tiwari**
Published by: **DAYA PUBLISHING HOUSE, NEW DELHI**

Chapter 11

Impact of Fluoride on Male Reproduction

M.H. Trivedi, R.J. Verma and Neha P. Sangai*

Department of Zoology,
University School of Sciences,
Gujarat University, Ahmedabad

Trace elements are a group of chemicals, which play a dual role in many systems. They are essential and beneficial for human health at minute concentrations, but exert toxic effects if concentration exceeds the permissible limits. Fluoride is an essential trace element that helps in mineralization, development and functions of bone and teeth. At very low level it has been found to help in preventing dental caries as well as to cure osteoporosis. However, excessive ingestion of fluorine and its compounds leads to a crippling disease 'Fluorosis' because of its profound affinity for calcified tissues. Incidence of fluorosis has been recognized in many countries including U.S.A., Italy, India, Japan, Spain, Holland and several African and South American countries. The disease is widespread in India, and millions of people in 15 out of 26 states are affected, due to drinking high amount of fluoride contaminated water. The adversely affected States are Andhra Pradesh, Punjab, Haryana, Rajasthan, Uttar Pradesh, Gujarat, Tamil Nadu, Bihar, Madhya

* E-mail: ramtejverma2000@yahoo.com

Pradesh, Maharashtra, Orissa, Karnataka, West Bengal, Kerala and Delhi.

Fluoride is component of fluoroapatite, fluorite and cryolite. Irrespective of its primary source, the element is ultimately dispersed in the environment and is found in the atmosphere, soil and water. Therefore, it reaches to the living organisms by mentioned sources. Fluoride can enter into body mainly by oral route and toxicokinetic studies revealed that the absorbed fluoride in the human body is distributed between blood, soft organs and the skeleton. The half-life of fluoride in blood and soft organs is few hours and skeleton has a relatively longer half-life of mostly about eight years[1,2].

The term 'reproductive toxicity' is defined as any adverse effect on any aspect of male or female sexual function or fertility, or on the developing embryo or foetus, or postnatally, which would interfere with production or development of a normal offspring which can be reared to sexual maturity, capable in turn of reproducing the species. Sexual function and fertility' refers to effects on the male and female sexual behavior and gonads. This includes any effects on spermatogenesis or oogenesis through puberty to conception and on development of the fertilized ovum up to the stage of implantation in the uterine wall. 'Developmental toxicity" includes adverse effect on embryofoetal development from the stage of implantation through parturition and postnatal development to the stage of puberty. Examples include reduced intrauterine embryofoetal growth and developmental retardation, organ toxicity, death, abortion, structural (teratogenic) defects resulting in congenital malformations, and functional defects such as impaired postnatal mental or physical development. It may also include adverse effects on lactation that could interfere with normal postnatal development, either by altering the quality or quantity of milk produced, or by passage of chemicals into the milk to affect neonatal development.

In this chapter, we will consider the toxic effects of fluoride on male reproductive organs of different animal models, and the possible mechanism of action. The ameliorative effect of different antidote on fluoride intoxicated animals is also incorporated at the end.

There are limited published reports in the literature on reproductive toxicity of fluoride in men. However, two Russian studies showed that chronic occupational exposure to fluoride-contaminated compounds might affect reproductive function. Men who had worked in the cryolite industry for 10-25 years demonstrated clinical skeletal fluorosis showed decrease in circulating testosterone and compensatory increase in follicle-stimulating hormone (FSH) when compared with controls. Of the exposed men, those exposed to cryolite for 16-25 years had increased luteinzing hormone (LH) levels as compared with men exposed for 10-25 years[3].

Barot[4] has conducted a well planned study in North Gujarat, India. The author has analyzed water samples collected from different localities in Ahmedabad city showing fluoride concentration in the range of 0.5–0.72 ppm with a mean of 0.64±0.013 ppm in water. Survey conducted in 53 villages (forty in Mehsana district and thirteen in Banaskantha district) revealed wide variation in the levels of fluoride from a minimum of 1 ppm to a maximum of 6.53 ppm having a mean of 2.81±0.179 ppm. Fluoride levels in the serum of fluoride affected individuals also varied considerably and a large number of people showed significantly high amount of fluoride as compared to control population. The results revealed that FSH activities were not altered significantly in the afflicted individuals. These results might elucidate that folliculogenesis might not be affected. Serum testosterone level indicated significant decline in case of fluorotic individuals. It might be due to impaired steroidogenesis or else alteration in hormone receptor interaction since it is known that phospholipids especially phosphatidylinositol which is involved in hormone receptor action was reduced in testis and epididymis of animal intoxicated from fluoride.

In another study, one group of individuals exposed to 3–27 mg/day was compared with another group of individuals exposed to fluoride at lower doses; 2-13 mg/day. A significant increase in FSH ($p<0.05$) and reduction of inhibin-B, free testosterone and prolactin in serum ($p<0.05$) were noticed in the high fluoride group. Author has observed significant negative partial correlation between urinary fluoride and serum levels of inhibin-B ($r=0.333, p=0.028$) in the low fluoride group. Furthermore, author has also observed a significant partial correlation between a chronic exposure index for fluoride and the serum concentration of inhibin-B ($r=0.163$) in the high fluoride group. It was concluded that population exposed to high fluoride content induces a subclinical reproductive effect that can be explained by a toxic effects of fluoride in both Sertoli cells and gonadotrophs[5]

Araibi *et al.*[6] in their study added fluoride at 0, 100, or 200 mg/kg along with "standard" rat diet. After 60 days, blood was collected from some of the rats for determination of testosterone concentration and the microscopic examination of the testes were conducted. The fertility of the remaining rats was tested by mating them with normal females for 4 days. The number of pregnancies and offspring was reduced significantly in the 200-mg/kg group but not in the 100 mg/kg group. The litter sizes did not differ among any of the groups. The authors commented that the treated rats showed "less interest toward females." However, food and water intakes, body-weight changes, and activity levels were not reported by the authors were probably reduced in the 200 mg/kg group. If so, those effects might have been involved in the apparent loss of interest. The diameters of the seminiferous tubules were reduced slightly in both fluoride-treated groups. The thickness of the peritubular membranes was increased, the percentage of tubules with spermatozoa was reduced, and the serum testosterone level was lower in the 200 mg/kg group. These effects occur in the 100-mg/kg group.

Bataineh and Nusier[7] have studied the impact of 12 weeks ingestion of sodium fluoride on aggression, sexual behavior and fertility in adult male rats at 100 and 300 ppm in drinking water. The results revealed that body weight and absolute and relative testes weight were not affected, but the average weights of epididymis, ventral prostate, seminal vesicles and preputial glands decreased significantly. In addition, the treatment markedly diminished aggressive and sexual behavioral parameters such as lateralization, boxing bouts and ventral presenting postures. It also prolonged the time to the first mount, increased the intromission latency, decreased the number of intromissions, prolonged the post-ejaculatory interval and increased the number of fetal resorptions in female rats impregnated by these males, thereby reducing fertility.

A fertility effect of sodium fluoride in male mice was studied at different doses *i.e.* 100, 200 and 300 ppm in drinking water for 4 or 10 weeks. The results indicate low fertility rate in all three groups[8]. Kour and Singh[9] reported that male mice fed fluoride at a dose of 10, 500 and 1000 ppm showed lack of maturation and differentiation of spermatocytes in testis leading to alterations in spermatogenic process. These results were supported by detailed and systematic studies carried out by Chinoy and Sequeira[10]. A study undertaken by Chinoy *et al.*[11] confirmed that a single microdose vasal injection of NaF to rats also exhibited similar changes in testicular histoarchitecture affecting spermatogenic process. The electron microscopic studies also revealed changes in the structural integrity of testis by fluoride, affecting spermatogenic elements[12]. However, the Leydig cell and nuclear diameters as well as their morphology were not affected. In addition, testicular cholesterol and serum testosterone levels were under normal range in NaF treated mice[13]. Further, intermediate enzymes in androgen synthesis namely, 3 β and 17 β-hydroxysteroid dehydrogenases were unaffected by the treatment. Therefore, it is concluded that fluoride might not alter cholesterol synthesis as well as circulating androgen levels in short-term treatment. However, chronic exposure affects steroidogenesis[14]. Schoff and Lardy[15] reported that fluoride is a strong inhibitor of glycolysis and respiration process in spermatozoa. They became immobile within two minutes and their flagella acquired a linear, rod like conformation. In cauda epididymis, after fluoride treatment, confluence of tubules occurred resulting in larger tubules, decrease in epithelial cell height with denudation of cells in the lumen, which was devoid of sperm. These structural changes contributed towards alterations in cauda epididymal metabolism and function. This was evident by low adenosine triphosphatase (ATPase), protein and sialic acid levels[10]. In rabbit treated with fluoride, the cauda epididymal sperm showed low ATPase, acid phosphatase (ACPase) and succinate dehydrogenase (SDH) activities along with reduced protein. The electrolyte balance was severely affected with low Na^+ and K^+ but high calcium levels[16]. Experiments also revealed an inhibition of sperm acrosomal enzymes namely, hyaluronidase and acrosin[17]. The sperm of NaF treated rabbit when stained with silver nitrate (specific for acrosomal integrity) exhibited head to head agglutination deflagellation and loss of acrosome[11]. In rat, cauda epididymal sperms were deflagellated and damage to acrosome was apparent after fluoride treatment. Therefore, these alterations in sperm structure and metabolism are resulted of the hostile internal milieu of epididymis affecting sperm maturation which ultimately lead to a decline in sperm count motility and fertilizability and subsequently to a significant reduction in fertility after NaF treatment[11].

Vas deferens, which possesses absorptive, secretory and synthesizing ability, maintains the sperm in a viable state[18]. But, after fluoride treatment, the histoarchitecture of vas deferens indicated nuclear pycnosis in the region of the folds, clumping of stereocilia, increase in thickness of lamina propria and muscle coat as well as absence of sperms in the lumen[12,19]. The structural and functional integrity of the other accessory sex organs like seminal vesicle and ventral prostate gland were also adversely affected. These factors further added to a severe loss of sperm motility, ultimately manifested an impairment of fertility in treated mouse, rat and rabbit[11].

In vitro study on Ram semen incubated for 5 hr at 4 °C with different doses of fluoride *i.e.* 0.38, 1.9, 3.8 ppm revealed that sperm with intact acrosomes and the level of spermatozoa motility decreased significantly after incubation time is over. The authors have observed that both indices decreased significantly in the presence of NaF at concentration ranging from 0.1 -20 mg mol/L. The activities of androgen-dependent enzymes ACP, lactate deydrogenase (LDH) and gamma glutamyl transferase (g-GT)– decreased significantly when the ejaculate was treated with NaF at concentration of 20, 100, 2000 mgmol/L, but they returned to the intial value of the control at 0.1 mol/L (1900 ppm F). The activity of aspartate transaminase (ALT) displayed a large increase with the increasing lower fluoride concentration. These changes undoubtelly affect the physiological functions of sperm[20].

Chinoy and Mehta[21] have studied effects of protein supplementation and deficiency on fluoride-induced toxicity in reproductive organs of male mice. The results revealed that exposure of fluoride at 5, 10, 20 mg/kg body weight for 30 days and low protein diet caused significant decrease in protein levels in testes, cauda epididymis, and vas deferens, level of cholesterol in testis and glycogen in the vas deferens were significantly enhanced as compared to controls. As mentioned above, despite the fact that the normal circulating androgen levels were maintained during fluoride intoxication, the target organs whose structural and functional integrity is dependent on androgens, were adversely affected.

Lzquierdo *et al.*[22] studied the effect of environmentally relevant dosages of fluoride on the *in vitro* fertilization (IVF) capacity of spermatozoa and its relationship to spermatozoa mitochondrial transmembrane potential. Male Wistar rats were exposed to fluoride-containing water providing 5 mg fluoride ion/kg body weight mass/24 hr or to deionized water (control group) orally for 8 weeks. They have studied several sperm parameters in treated and untreated rats. Results revealed that spermatozoa from fluoride-treated rats exhibited 33 per cent decrease in SOD activity, accompanied by a significant 40 per cent increase in the generation of O_2, a significant 33 per cent decrease in mitochondrial transmembrane potential and a significant 50 per cent increase in lipid peroxidation relative to spermatozoa from the control group. Consistent with these findings were alterations of the plasma membrane of spermatozoa from fluoride-treated rats. In addition, the percentage of fluoride-treated spermatozoa capable of undergoing the acrosome reaction was decreased relative to control spermatozoa (34 vs. 55 per cent), while the percentage of fluoride-treated spermatozoa capable of oocyte fertilization was also significantly lower than in the control group (13 vs. 71 per cent). These observations suggest that subchronic exposure to fluoride causes oxidative stress damage and loss of mitochondrial transmembrane potential resulting in reduced fertility.

Liu *et al.*[23] have studied the effects of fluoride on the energy metabolism of the male reproductive system, The activities of LDH, SDH, ATPase, and ã-GT, along with sperm quality and testicular histology, were determined at week 6, 8, 10 and 12 in male offspring of rat exposed in their drinking water 150 mg/L sodium fluoride (NaF). Compared with control, LDH activities were significantly increased whereas SDH activities were decreased in the NaF group. They have also observed that ATPase and ã-GT activities were reduced. Sperm viability, density and abnormalities over the entire 12-week study period were altered.

Ghosh *et al.*[24] has reported that the toxic effect of fluoride on male reproductive organs is mainly associated with indicators of oxidative stress. The author has also observed significant diminution in the relative weight of the testis, prostate and seminal vesicle. Moreover epididymal sperm count was also decreased significantly at the 20mg/kg/day for 29 days to rat. Zhu *et al.*[25] has observed that NaF in drinking water at 150mg/L for 30 days cause significant decrease in sperm count and mobility, the increase of sperm and testicular lipid peroxidation (LPO) contents, ATPase activity decrease in epididymis in rats. Moreover glutathione peroxidase activities in testis and epididymis was also reduced.

Huang *et al.*[26] studied the effect and possible mechanisms of the action of fluoride on testis cell cycle and cell apoptosis in male mice. Sexually mature male Kunming mice were administrated with different doses *i.e.* 50, 100, 200, and 300 mg NaF/L in their drinking water for 8 weeks. At the end of the exposure periods, they have studied sperm quality, the percentage of G1/ G0 (Gap 1/Gap 0), S (synthesis), G2/M (Gap2/M, mitosis), and apoptosis rate in testicle cells measured using flow cytometry. Serum and testicular testosterone levels were determined with a radio immunoassay. Effects on sperm quality and oxidative stress were also observed. The results revealed that different dosages of NaF altered the changes in the testicular cell cycle. Compared to the control, the testicular cell cycle of mice drinking 50 or 100 mg NaF/L was not significantly affected ($P>0.05$). However, with the higher NaF concentrations of 200 and 300 mg/L, the percentage of cells in G1/G0 phase increased significantly ($P<0.01$), whereas those in S phase decreased significantly ($P<0.01$). On the other hand, the percentage of cells in G2/M phase was similar to that of the control. In the two higher NaF concentration groups, distinct cell apoptosis of testis was observed. Likewise, sperm quality and antioxidant defenses were significantly reduced and oxidative stress occurred, whereas these effects were only slight at the lower NaF concentrations. Serum and testicular testosterone levels were also significantly lower at 100, 200, and 300 mg NaF/L ($P<0.01$), compared with the control group.

Further studies by Huang *et al.*[27] had showed the effect of NaF on androgen receptor expression in male mice. At the end of this study computer imaging analysis were applied to examine the AR expression in the testis. As compared to control, expression of AR protein decreased significantly in 200 and 300 mg NaF/L groups. With quantitative real time PCR, they have also assessed the expression on AR-mRNA by culturing primary sertoli cells from immature mice with different concentration of fluoride (10-6, 10-5, 10-4, 10-3 mol/L) for 48 hours, resulting in a significant fluoride induced decline in the AR-mRNA level in the cells as compared to control. Finally the authors have concluded that decrease in AR protein and gene expression in testis is associated with impairment of reproductive function by NaF.

It is of interest to note that the toxic effects induced by fluoride were found to be reversible in reproductive organs after cessation of fluoride treatment. Therefore, the effects of fluoride were transient and reversible and thus functional sterility could be induced by fluoride in laboratory animals. However, efforts of scientists to investigate an ameliorative agents suggest that significant recovery takes place on co-treatment with vitamins C, E and C+D+E which is attributed to the action of these vitamins as free radical scavengers. Chinoy and Sharma[28] reported complete recovery from fluoride toxicity in reproductive functions in male mice on co-teatment with vitamin E and D alone and in combination. Wilde and Yu[29] opined that the toxicity of free radical is greater if fluoride can impair the production of free radical scavengers such as ascorbic acid and glutathione and this can be prevented by additional supplementation with vitamins C and E. The antidotal effect of vitamin E is by preventing the oxidative damage caused by fluoride, which increases peroxides free radicals of reactive oxygen species. Vitamin E channelizes the conversion of oxidized glutathione (GSSG) to reduced glutathione (GSH), which in turns helps compression of mono- and dehydroascorbic acid to maintain ascorbic acid levels[30].

Apart from this, ascorbic acid and calcium are known inhibitors of phosphodiesterase and would thereby enhance the c-AMP levels and help in the regain of sperm motility and fertility. Results also revealed for the first time that the combined treatment of ascorbic acid and calcium along with fluoride or during withdrawal period was more effective due to their synergistic action. Therefore, it is suggested that ascorbic acid and calcium are effective therapeutic agents, which help in amelioration of fluoride toxicity and should be tested in fluoride endemic population afflicted with fluorosis at least in children, as a precautionary step and to prevent the crippling disease.

References

1. W.H.O. (1970). Fluoride and Human Health. Geneva. World Health Organization. 364 (Monograph series No. 59).

2. Philippe, G., knud, J., and Ole M.J. (1985). Mortality and cancer morbidity after heavy occupational fluoride exposure. Ame. J. Epidemiol. 121(1); 57-64.

3. Tokar, V.I. and Savchenko, O.N. (1977). Effect of inorganic fluoride compounds on the functional state of the pituitary-testis system. Probal Endocrinol, 23 (4); 104-107.

4. Barot, V.V. (1998). Occurrence of endemic flurosis in human population of north Gujarat, India: human health risk. Bull. Environ. Contam. Toxicol., 61; 303-310.

5. Perez, O. and Martinaz, R. (2003). Fluoride induced disruption of reproductive hormones in man. Environ. Res., 93(1); 20-30.

6. Araibi AA, *et al.*(1989) Effect of high fluoride om the reproductive performance of the male rat. Journal of Biological Sciences Research 20:19-30.

7. Bataineh, H.N. and Nusier, M.K. (2006). Impact of 12 week ingestion of sodium fluoride on aggression, sexual behavior and fertility in adult male rats. Fluoride, 39(4); 293-301.

8. Elbetieha, A., Darmani, H. and Hiyasat, A. (2000). Fertility effects of sodium fluoride in male mice. Fluoride; 33(3); 128-134.

9. Kour, K. and Singh, J. (1980). Histological findings in mice testes following fluoride ingestion. Fluoride 13; 160-162.

10. Chinoy, N.J and Sequeria, E.(1989a) Fluoride induced biochemical changes in reproductive organs of male mouse. Fluoride, 22(2):78-85.

11. Chinoy, N.J.(1991). Effects of fluoride on physiology of animals and human beings. Ind J. Environ Toxicol. 1(1) 17-32.

12. Chinoy, N.J. and Sequeira E. (1989b). Effects of fluoride on the histoarchitecture of reproductive organs of male mouse. Reprod. Toxicol, 3(4):261-268.

13. Susheela, A.K. and Kumar, A. (1991). A study of effect of high concentrations of fluoride on the reproductive organs of male rabbits using light and scanning electron microscopy. J. Reproductive Fertillity., 92; 353-360.

14. Narayan, M.V. and Chinoy, N.J.(1994a). Effects of fluoride on rat testicular spermatogenesis. Fluoride 27 (1); 7-12.

15. Schoff, P.K. and Lardy,H.A.(1987). Effect of fluoride and caffeine on the metabolism and motility of ejaculated bovine spermatozoa. Biol Reprod (1987) 37(4): 1037-46.

16. Chinoy, N.J., Sequeira E and Narayana. M.V. (1991b). Effect of vitamin C and calcium on the reversibility of fluoride induced alterations in spermatozoa of rabbit. Fluoride 24 (1); 29-39

17. Narayan, M.V. and Chinoy, N.J.(1994). Reversible effects of sodium fluoride ingestion in spermatozoa of rat. Int. J. Fertil. Menopausal study 39;337-346.

18. Chinoy, N.J.(1985). Structure and physiology of mammalian vas deferens in relation to fertility regulation. J. Biosciences 7(2); 215-221.

19. Chinoy, N.J., Rao. M.V., Narayan, M.V. and Neelkanta, E. (1991a). Microdose vassal injection of sodium fluoride in the rat. Reproductive Toxicology. 5(6); 505-512.

20. Zakrzewska, H., Udata, J. and Blaszczyk, B. (2002). *In vitro* influence of sodium fluoride on rat semen quality and enzyme activities. Fluoride, 35(3);153-160.

21. Chinoy, N.J. and Mehta, D. (1999). Effect of protein supplementation and deficiency on fluoride induced toxicity in reproductive organs of male mice. Fluoride, 32(4); 204-214.

22. Lzquierdo, V.J.A., Sanchez, G.M. and Del Razo, L.M. (2008). Decreased *in vitro* fertility in male rats exposed to fluoride-induced oxidative stress damage and mitochondrial transmembrane potential loss. Fluoride, 41 (2); 171 (abstract).

23. Liu, H., Niu, R., Wang, J., He, Y. and Wang, J. (2008). Changes caused by fluoride and lead in energy metabolic enzyme activities in the reproductive system of male offspring rats. Fluoride, 41 (3); 184-191.

24. Ghosh, D., Das, S., Maiti, R. and Jana, D. (2002). Testicular toxicity in sodium fluoride treated rats: association with oxidative stress. Reproductive Toxicol., 16(4); 385.

25. Zhu, X.Z., Ying, C.J., Liu, S.H., Yang, K.D. and Wang, Q.Z. (2000). The primary study of antagonism of selenium on fluoride induced reproductive toxicity of male rat. China public health-article in China. 16 (8); 697-698

26. Huang, C., Niu, R. and Wang, J. (2007). Toxic effects of sodium fluoride on reproductive function in male mice. Fluoride 40(3); 162–168.

27. Huang, C., Yang H and Wang, J. (2008). Effect of sodium fluoride on Androgen Expression in male mice. Fluoride, 41(1):10-17.

28. Chinoy, N.J and Sharma, A.K (1998). Amelioration of fluoride toxicity by vitamins E and D in reproductive functions of male mice. Fluoride 31:203

29. Wilde, L.G and Yu, M.H. (1998). Effects of fluoride on superoxide dismutase (SOD) activity in germinating mung bean seedling. Fluoride 31:81.

30. Verma R J (2004) Impact of fluoride in mammals. Proc. Natl. Acad. Sci., India, 74:99-113.

Environmental & Occupational Exposures (2010) *Pages 270–303*
Editors: **Sunil Kumar & R.R. Tiwari**
Published by: **DAYA PUBLISHING HOUSE, NEW DELHI**

Chapter 12

Persistent Chemicals, Infertility and Endometriosis

Roya Rozati[1], *G. Simha Baludu*[2], *D. Srikant*[3] *and V. Srilaxmi*[3]

[1]*Research Director,*
MHRT Hospital and Research Centre,
H.No. 8-2-120/86/1/A, Road No # 3, Banjara Hills,
Hyderabad – 500 034, Andhra Pradesh
[2]*Maternal Health and Research Trust, Hyderabad*
[3]*Owaisi Hospital and Research Centre, Hyderabad*

ABSTRACT

Endometriosis is a gynaecological disorder characterized by the presence of ectopic endometrial glands and stroma. It affects approximately 15 per cent of women of childbearing age and is consistent with the estrogen dependent nature of the disease. Endometriosis is a complex gynecologic disorder that has long been recognized as showing heritable tendencies, with recurrence risks of 5-7 per cent for first-degree relatives. Familial and epidemiologic studies support that this disease is a genetic disorder of polygenic/multifactorial inheritance. Data indicating that a xenobiotic may affect multiple signaling pathways with data showing synergistic effects of multiple

* E-mail: drrozati@rediffmail.com

xenobiotics on estrogen-responsive genes reinforces the possibility that environmental xenobiotics although present at low concentrations may pose a threat to human health. This study for the first time from Indian subcontinent demonstrates that possibly Phthalate Esters and dioxins might have a role in aetiology of endometriosis. The women having higher concentration of PCBs, Dioxin and GSTM1 null (*0/*0) polymorphism might have an increased susceptibility of endometriosis.

Introduction

The interaction between man and environment is continuous and certainly, has influenced the process of evolution of the species. This interaction is, in certain cases, beneficial but hostile in many. Indeed, mankind has introduced elements in the environment that either pollute or modify environmental conditions with resultant negative effects on human health. Adverse environmental conditions not controlled or influenced by man can also affect human health and behavior. This is a continuously evolving process with some elements remaining fairly constant over a relatively long period of time (decades or centuries) and others rapidly progressing or undergoing change in a much shorter time frame owing to environmental disasters. Before attempting to evaluate the environmental influences on adult reproductive functions in the human male and female, it is necessary to provide the essential definitions to focus on the terms and the scope of the problem.

Environmental pollutants that have previously shown to be linked to endometriosis are polyhalogenated aromatic hydrocarbons (PHAH), a class of widespread environmental contaminants that includes polychlorinated dibenzo-p-dioxins (PCDDs), polychlorinated dibenzofurans (PCDFs), polychlorinated biphenyls (PCBs) and phthalate esters (PEs) [1,2]. The role of these chemicals in determining endocrine related diseases in humans, possibly a decrease of fertility, is still controversial[3].

Exposure to these persistent chemicals reportedly results in a variety of toxic effects in experimental animals, including immunologic, neurochemical, neurotoxic, carcinogenic, and endocrine changes[4, 5]. With the completion of the first draft of the human genome and the availability of cheaper and quicker genotyping technologies, there is a rapidly increasing interest in identifying genes and genetic polymorphisms that predispose women to increased risk of developing endometriosis[6,7]. Further, earlier studies have indicated a possible involvement of genetic component in endometriosis susceptibility[8].

However, the possible genetic predisposition of the individuals to endometriosis was observed with higher frequency around the industrial areas[9].

The compound 2, 3, 7, 8-tetrachlorodibenzo-p-dioxin (TCDD or dioxin), the most toxic halogenated aromatic hydrocarbon[10] is a ubiquitous contaminant of various industrial and combustion processes, including medical waste incineration. Dioxin is classified as a known human carcinogen[11], and concern about the reproductive toxicity of dioxin has been growing.

Exposure to Dioxin-TCDD and dioxin like PCBs is associated with endometriosis and this hypothesis was supported by experimental studies showing that exposure to these chemicals is associated with a dose dependent increase in the incidence and severity of endometriosis in rhesus monkeys[12,13]. While the results of human case control studies so far carried out are conflicting[14], but some epidemiological observations further support this hypothesis.

To understand how environmental factors contribute to fertility or infertility, it is first necessary to define "environment". Environment represents the external milieu by analogy with the well-defined concept of "internal milieu", introduced by the French physiologist Claude Bernard. Using this concept, the following definition has been proposed. Environment represents the totality of physical, chemical, biological and socioeconomic factors or conditions that constitute the external milieu surrounding the human organism (Table 12.1). The links and targets for environmental agents in man are represents in Table 12.2.

The GSTM1 gene located on chromosome 1p13.3[15], codes for cytosolic GST ì class enzyme, and has a deletion polymorphism that, when homozygote (GSTM1 null), results in the complete absence of functional gene product. An elevated frequency of inactive variant of the GSTM1 gene has been reported in endometriosis patients. In view of the controversies surrounding the environmental dioxins and polymorphisms in genes encoding detoxification enzymes and their association with endometriosis, the role of both these factors in the pathogenesis of endometriosis needs to be re-evaluated. To provide complete and quantitative evaluation of the impact of both dioxins and detoxification gene polymorphisms on the risk of endometriosis, we carried out the present study to establish whether women with endometriosis having more concentrations of dioxins, were more prone to carry polymorphisms comparing with control women free from the disease.

Table 12.1: Categories of Environmental Factors

Category	*Examples*
Physical	Light, temperature, altitude, radiation
Chemical	Natural or man-made
Biological	Viruses, microorganism
Behavioral	Stress, drug addiction
Socioeconomic	Nutrition, habituate occupation, hygiene education

Table 12.2: Links and Targets for Environmental Agents

Sl.No.	*System*	*Role*
1.	Nervous system	Target for all environmental factors that impact the neural control of reproduction.
2.	Endocrine system	Links environment to the human genome and controls reproduction.
3.	Immune system	Protects and adapts or affects cellular response to agents which can influence reproduction.
4.	Respiratory gastrointestinal skin	Route for entry/exit
5.	Receptors, enzymes, second messengers, genes	Ultimate targets for agents/ toxins affecting reproductive functions.

Stress, Nutrition and Behavioural Effects on Reproductive Functions

Defined by Selye[16] more than half a century ago, the term "stress" has been used to include a variety of responses elicited by noxious stimuli. Stress affects a large number of biological systems, including the reproductive system. Cultural, occupational and many other behavioral differences can modify or sensitize the stress response and the ensuing change in reproductive function.

Experimental data in animals and human suggest that chronic or severe stress leads to anovulation and amenorrhea in women[17] and to decrease in sperm count, motility and morphology[18, 19] in men. Stress affects the endocrine and other regulatory systems hence, the resulting effects of stress are usually not limited to changes in reproductive function. Nevertheless, there are some well-defined syndromes associated or induced by stress that result in abnormal reproductive functions. Moreover, the environmental chemicals and the neuroendocrine mechanism triggering the stress response, in addition to the chemical signals mediating these responses, are now better known.

Neuroendocrine Events during Stress

The hypothalamic-pituitary-adrenal (HPA) axis has been known to be involved in the stress response for many years[16]. The main players in this axis are corticotrophin-releasing hormone or factor (CRF), adrenocorticotrophin hormone (ACTH), and cortisol. In addition to CRF, several other brain neurotransmitters, such as vasopressin, oxytocin, β-endorphin, angiotensin II, epinephrine, norepinephrine, and serotonin among others, are known to be involved in mediating and integrating the response to stressful stimuli[20–22]. In many instances, activation or secretion of these hormones serves as a biochemical marker to measure the stress response. Secretion of CRF, vasopressin, and some of the amines into the pituitary portal vasculature leads to an increased activation of the corticotrophs in the anterior pituitary and to an enhanced release of ACTH and β-endorphin[20, 21]. The elevated levels of ACTH increase cortisol secretion from the adrenal gland, which leads to a number of adaptive changes in metabolic activity. Under chronic stress situations, changes in the steady-state levels of hormones and their metabolic clearance may occur, and part of the process of adaptation may compromise certain functions such as reproduction, in order to maintain other vital functions.

Enhanced CRF activity, *i.e.* increased release within the brain and into the pituitary portal circulation, leads to a suppression of gonadotropin secretion and, thereby, to decreased gonadal function. The intrinsic mechanism mediating this response involves a direct inhibition of the activity of the luteinizing hormone releasing hormone (LHRH) neurons that control gonadotropin secretion by CRF. CRF has been shown to shut down the electrical activity of the LHRH pulse generator in rhesus monkeys[23] and to decrease the release of LHRH in the hypophyseal portal circulation[24]. Decreased function or activity of the LHRH pulse leads to decreased gonadotropin secretion and disruption of the normal gonadotropin pulsatility pattern.

Stress and Female Infertility

Stress-related disorders in women:

1. Chronic anovulation
2. Psychogenic amenorrhea
3. Pseudocyesis
4. Stress-related eating disorders:
   (*a*) Anorexia nervosa
   (*b*) Bulimia
5. Menstrual dysfunction
6. Hyperprolactinemia and amenorrhea
7. Early pregnancy loss.

Chronic Anovulation

There is good evidence to support the fact that excessive emotional stress, alone or in combination with changes in eating and nutrition patterns and exercise, can cause chronic anovulation. This disorder usually falls under the classification of hypothalamic amenorrhea, but in reality, it represents a wide spectrum of reproductive disorders. Chronic anovulation associated with hypothalamic amenorrhea is frequently observed and detected, although the direct link to stress is not always easy to establish[17,23,24].

Psychogenic Amenorrhea

Psychologic distress is generally recognized as a contributing factors to infertility,[25] the incidence of this condition being high infertile couples. Psychologic amenorrhea is more common in women who have stressful lives and occupations, are usually under-weight, single, and have a history psychoactive drug use.

☆ Stress, diet, exercise, a frequent component of the triad (*i.e.* stress, diet and exercise) can clearly cause amenorrhea in women athletes[26]. Several other disorder including delayed onset of menarche, oligomenorrhea, anovulation, inadequate luteal phase, and secondary amenorrhea have been described in women athletes[27]. Menstrual cycle disorders associated with malnutrition and exercise is often reversible. Functional hypothalamic amenorrheas are commonly associated with a slow-down of the LHRH pulse generator and consequently of pulsatile gonadotropin secretion.

Stress and Male Infertility

Stress-Related Disorders in Men

1. Decreased sperm count
2. Decreased sperm motility
3. Altered sperm morphology
4. Impotence
5. Ejaculatory disorders
6. Decreased serum luteinizing hormone and testosterone.

Stress has been reported to decrease sperm count, motility, and morphology in men[18,19]. The other disorders such as impotence and retrograde ejaculation have been reported to be associated with psychological factors in male infertility. High levels of stress associated with a variety of occupational activities including business, combat or combat training have been reported to decrease plasma testosterone levels[18]. Emotional stress associated with the evaluation or treatment for infertility in affected couples has been associated with oligozoospermia, [19] and may contribute to the variations in semen quality observed during the evaluation.

Physical stress leads to low testosterone levels due to a reduction in LH pulse frequency. Decreases in gonadotropin and testosterone levels and gonadal atrophy have been reported in adult men as well as in adolescents following chronic malnutrition.

Therefore, it appears that in women and men, the influence of the triad of stress, diet, and physical activity can exert similar individual and, more often, complementary effects on the reproductive system leading to infertility. All these three factors mediate their effects by the activation of similar neuroendocrine pathways involving CRF, β-endorphin and the catecholaminergic systems (noradrenaline, adrenaline, and dopamine). These systems, in turn, control reproductive functions by interacting with the LHRH neuronal system as well as by modulating eating behavior and autonomic mechanisms involved in responses to exercise and metabolism.

Toxic Effects of Drugs or Chemicals on Gonadal Function

Centrally Acting Drugs

Decreased sperm motility has been demonstrated in morphine and heroin methadose addicts with 25 percent of the users exhibiting teratozoospermia[28]. Some cocanine addicts have higher than normal Prolactin levels. Cannabinoids are reported to depress leydig-cell function.

Heavy Metals

Lead intoxication (blood lead levels of 66-139μg/dl) cause clinical poisoning and appear to induce oligozoospermia and azoospermia in a substantial proportion of exposed individuals[28].

Nitrogen Sulfur Phosphorous Containing Compounds

Nitrogen inhibits spermatogenesis[28]. Chronic exposure to carbon disulphide (atmospheric levels of 120-240μg/m^3 for an average of 15 years) used in the viscose industry causes an increase in gonadotrophin levels among exposed workers[28].

Oestrogens, Environmental Pesticides, Infertility and Endometriosis

A decade ago, it was hypothesized that the reported adverse changes in male reproductive health could be explained by exposure to compounds with estrogenic (or other hormone disruptive) activity. Although this issue has been highly publicized, there has been little progress towards a realistic assessment of whether environmental estrogens pose a health risk to humans. Compounds within several major groups of chemicals including organochlorine pesticides, polychlorinated biphenyls, phenolic compounds and phthalate esters have been identified as being weakly estrogenic by *in vitro* and *in vivo* screening methods. Many of these compounds are widespread and persistent in the environment. They are likely to be present in the food chain, drinking water, plastics, households products and food packaging although which is the most important route of human exposure is unclear (Table 12.3). Bisphenol A [BPA: 2,2-bis (4-hydroxyphenyl) propoane] has been detected in liquid from canned vegetables[29] and in the saliva of patients with dental sealants[30]. Polychlorinated biphenyls (PCBs) are routinely detected in fish, wildlife, human adipose tissue, blood and breast milk[31-33].

The actual different diet habits of males and females are related to seasonal variation in the intake of PCDD/PCDF via food (self-produced foodstuffs and food originating from the contaminated area) (Figure 12.1). High consumption of contaminated food may results in a distinct difference in PCDD/PCDF levels compared to normal consumption habits.

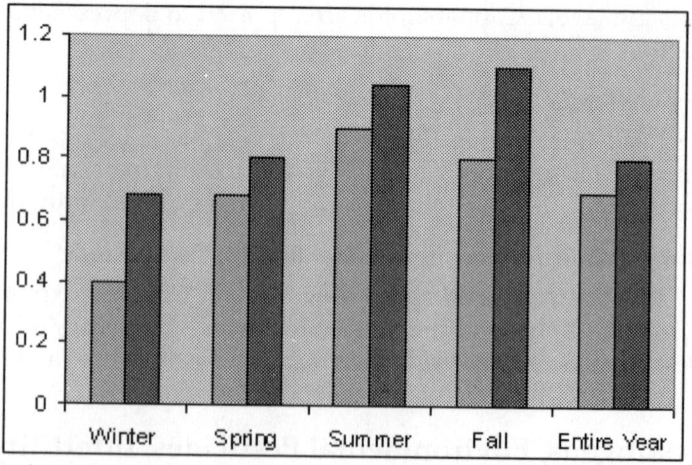

Figure 12.1: Mean Daily Intake of PCDD/PCDF by Season

The mean daily dietary intake of PCDDs/ PCDFs is about one fifth from milk and milk products, one fifth from water, eggs, meat and meat products, and one half from fish and fish products and the remaining ten percent is distributed among bread and cereals, vegetables and ready-to-serve meal (Figure.12.2). The daily

Table 12.3: Environmental Chemicals with Known Oestrogenic Effects *in vitro* (Adapted from KI Turner and RM Sharpe Review of Reproduction 1997; 2: 69-73)

Chemical	*Reproductive Effects*	*Human Exposure*	*Potential Routes of Exposure*
Organochlorine pesticides DDT, methoxychlor, dieldrin, Kepone	Well documented for wildlife and laboratory animals	High, especially in the 1940s-1960s	Ubiquitous in the environment; food contamination
Industrial chemicals Polychlorinated biphenyls: 3,4,3',4'-tetrachlorobiphenyl Alkylphenolic compounds: Nonylphenol, octylphenol	Well documented for wildlife and laboratory animals Poorly documented; adverse effects in aquatic species	High, especially in the 1940s-1960s Unknown also present in drinking water	Ubiquitous in the environment; food contaminationSurfactants; used in most plastics;Household products, food packaging, some cosmetics, shampoos, spermicides.
Phthalate esters, butylbenzyl phthalate, di-n-butyl phthalate	Reasonably well-documented effects on laboratory animals at high doses	High	Used in plastics, PVC and many other products; present in food packaging, drinking water, household products
Bisphenol-A and its derivatives	No published data	Unknown	Used in polycarbonate plastics, acrylic resins, Xeroxing, dentures and in the lacquer coating of food cans; some food packaging.
Food additives Butylated hydroxyanisole	No obvious effects from toxicity data	Moderate	Food antioxidant
Phytoestrogens Isoflavones; genistein, daizen coumestans: coumesterol	Well-documented effects in animals; some evidence in humans	High (very high on a soy-rich diet)	Many natural foods, especially soy products: many processed foods (soy): soy- formula infant milk.

consumption of low-level contaminated food leads to the accumulation of PCDDs/PCDFs in humans. In addition to exposure to man-made chemicals, the consumption of plant-derived estrogens in foodstuffs poses a potential risk to human health as phytoestrogens are more potent estrogens and their intake by some infants is likely to be considerable.

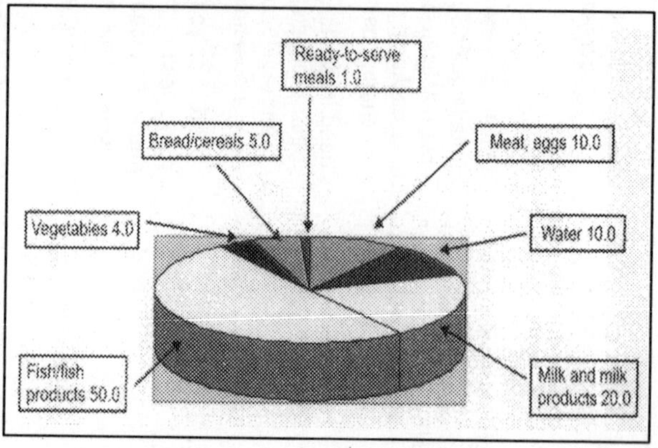

Figure 12.2: Mean Daily Intake of PCDDs/PCDFs of Humans in India (Previous study)

A certain group of women develop endometriosis implies that there is increased susceptibility to development of disease in certain cases. Individual's susceptibility is influenced not only by genetic background but also by the interaction of genes with environmental factors. Dioxin- TCDD have been implicated as involved in the development of endometriosis[34].

Materials and Methods

This is a prospective case-control study, which recruited women undergoing infertility treatment at three collaborating centers (BMMHRC: Bhagwan Mahavir Medical Hospital and Research Centre, MHRT: Maternal Health and Research Trust and OHRC: Owaisi Hospital and Research Centre) of Reproductive Medicine Hyderabad, which receives cases from all over the region of Andhra Pradesh, India. A proforma to obtain information on the with general, obstetric and gynecological details including age at menarche, length of menstrual cycle, associated symptoms, duration and amount of blood loss, duration of infertility, and socio-demographic details like age, body mass index (BMI) and limited information on diet was used for this study. The ethical committee of our institute approved the research protocol for this study. Informed consent was obtained from all the participants in this study.

The case group consisted of 224 women of Indian origin who were diagnosed by laparoscopy and found to have pelvic endometriosis. The severity of the disease was staged according to the revised American Society for Reproductive Medicine classification of endometriosis[35]. Endometriosis was staged as minimal (rASRM stage I) in 81, mild (rASRM stage II) in 47, moderate (rASRM stage III) in 67, and severe (rASRM stage IV) in 29 patients. All women were infertile (primary infertility in 71.8 per cent of cases and secondary infertility in 28.1 per cent of cases) with duration of infertility was 5.4 yr SD (3.8) and their mean age 26.2 yr SD (4.2) with the following clinical symptoms: dyspareunia (34 per cent) and dysmenorrhoea [mild (28 per cent); moderate (4 per cent); severe (3 per cent)]. In the remaining 31 per cent of cases were asymptomatic. All the patients were menstruating regularly and none of them had received hormonal treatment for at least 3 months prior to laparoscopy.

We selected two control groups. Group I comprised 127 women who attended the same hospital for other gynaecological pathology (*e.g.* fibroids, tubal defects, polycystic ovaries, idiopathic infertility and pelvic inflammatory disease) but were laparoscopically confirmed to be without endometriosis. All the patients in the control group I were also infertile (primary infertility 75.5 per cent; secondary infertility 24.5 per cent) with mean age 27.4 yr SD (4.7) and mean duration of 5.6 yr SD (3.7) years of infertility. The following symptoms were also present in the women in control group I: dyspareunia (17 per cent) and dysmenorrhoea [mild (26 per cent); moderate (6 per cent); severe (0 per cent)]. In the remaining 51 per cent of women there was none of these symptoms. Control Group II consists of 103 women with mean age 27.1 yr SD (3.4) who attended the same hospital for laparoscopic tubal sterilisation with proven fertility and no evidence of endometriosis and other gynaecological disorders. All the women in this group were asymptomatic. The entire case and control groups were living in urban areas and no history of any occupational exposure to reproductive toxicants. They also did not smoke or consume alcohol.

In a separate genetic study heparinised blood samples were collected from all the 97 cases and 102 controls (total=199) for DNA isolation. 6-10 ml of blood was collected from each patient in a vacuum system tube, transported in a cooling pail, and centrifuged (2500 g for 15 min) within 24 hours after collection. The serum (3-5 ml) was pooled and kept frozen at–20°C until the Phthalate Esters, PCBs and Dioxins were analyzed. Serum was isolated from Phthalate Esters 49/127 endometriosis and 38/128 control cases, PCBs 41/127 endometriosis and 47/128 control cases and Dioxins 37/127 endometriosis and 43/128 control cases blood samples for GC analysis.

GSTM1 Genotyping

Genomic DNA was extracted from peripheral blood by the method routinely used in our laboratory[36]. The pellet was washed with 300ml of 70 per cent ethanol, air-dried and DNA was stored at –20°C in hydrated form in Tris -EDTA buffer (Tris HCl–10mM, EDTA–1mM) until analysis was undertaken.

GSTM1 genotyping for deletion status for each participant was carried out by PCR by using a MJ Research Minicycler (Waltham, USA) to amplify the specific GSTM1 gene Exon 7 by using the following primers forward: 5^1-GAA CTC CCT GAA AAG CTA AAG C-3^1 and reverse: 5^1- GTT GGG CTC AAA TAT ACGG TGG-3^1 (MWG-Biotech AG Ltd, Banglore), which produced a 219 bp product based on the published sequence of Hur *et al.*, 2004[37]. Positive and negative controls were included in the study and GSTM1 null genotypes were confirmed by amplification of a 340bp fragment in exon 7 of the CYP1A1 gene as an internal positive control.

PCR was performed in a final volume of 25 ml, consisting of DNA 0.5ml, 0.5ml dNTP Mix (10mM; MBI-Fermentas), 2.5ml $MgCl_2$ (25 mM), 0.5ml Taq polymerase (3U/ml) (Banglore Genei Pvt Ltd), 2.5ml of 10x reaction buffer (15mM), 0.5ml of each forward and reverse primers and sterile water (17.5ml). Amplification was performed with an initial denaturation at 95°C for 5 min, followed by 35 cycles of denaturation at 94°C for 30sec, annealing at 55.2°C for 30sec and elongation at 72°C for 30sec, and final elongation of 72°C for 10 minutes. The amplified PCR products were electrophoresed on 2 per cent agarose gel, with ethidium bromide to visualize the DNA bands using UV transilluminator. Gel documentation and analysis were carried out using Chemi Imager, Alpha Innotech Corporation, USA. If the study subject is null (*0/*0) for the gene, no PCR product is present.

The extraction of PEs and Dioxin using gas chromatography (GC) was divided into 5 phases. Extraction of PEs was performed by the method described by Bruce et al[38] with modifications by Rozati et al[39]. The concentrated organic phases in phase four were pooled and dried under nitrogen gas. The sample was then re-suspended in hexane and then injected into the gas chromatograph. GC analysis carried out as per the instructions of the suppliers from Germany[40], and in-house modifications done at Hetero Research Foundation on GC-2010 series gas chromatograph (Shimadzu, Japan), equipped with a capillary column injection port.

Estimation of PCBs by Gas Chromatography with Flame Ionization Detector (GC FID)

Serum was separated from the heparinized blood samples within in 24 hours after collection by centrifugation (2,500 x *g* for 15 minutes). The Serum (4–5 mL) was pooled and kept frozen at -20°C until PCBs were analyzed. All solvents used were of analytical grade purity (HPLC grade; Qualigens, Ltd., Mumbai, India). Eight standard PCB congeners mix (PCB Mix 525, Supelco, Bellefonte, PA) were selected at a concentration 500 µg/mL in hexane of each PCB. Gas chromatography for the extraction of PCBs was divided into five phases. Extraction PCBs was performed by the method described by Burce *et al.*, 1994[38], with modifications by Rozati *et al.*, 2002[39]. The concentrated organic phases in phase four were pooled and dried under nitrogen gas. The sample was resuspended in hexane and then injected for gas chromatography. Gas chromatography analysis was carried according to the method given by Supelco (1998)[40], and in-house modifications done at Hetero Research Foundation on the GC-2010 series gas chromatograph (Shimadzu, Kyoto, Japan).

Results

Table 12.4 shows the reproductive history of the three study groups. Despite comparable ages at menarche more women (34 per cent) with endometriosis reported pain during intercourse compared to the control I (17 per cent) women. No significant difference in age, body mass index (BMI), age at menarche and duration of infertility were observed in between these groups.

Table 12.4: Reproductive History Among Cases and Control Groups

Characteristic	Endometriosis (n=224)	Control I (n=127)	Control II (n=103)
Age in years [a]	26.2 (4.2)	27.4 (4.7)	27.1 (3.4)
Body mass index (kg m^{-2}) [a]	24.1 (2.2)	23.5 (1.2)	23.9 (2.2)
Age at menarche (years) [a]	12.4 (1.1)	12.5 (1.0)	12.6 (1.1)
Duration of infertility (years)	5.4 (3.8)	5.6 (3.7)	NA
Primary infertility [n (per cent)]	161(71.8)	96(75.5)	NA
Secondary infertility [n (per cent)]	63(28.1)	31(24.5)	NA

Data are presented as mean (SD); $p< 0.05$ considered statistically significant;
a: Represents not significant in between the groups; NA: Not Applicable.

Table 12.5 shows that significant differences in the concentrations of phthalate esters were observed between women with and without endometriosis [study group: DnBP: 0.44 SD (0.41); BBP: 0.66 SD (0.61; DnOP: 3.32 SD (2.17) and DEHP: 2.44 SD (2.17)) $\mu g ml^{-1}$; control group I: DnBP: 0.08 SD (0.14); BBP: 0.12 SD (0.20); DnOP: 0 and DEHP 0.50 SD (0.80) $\mu g ml^{-1}$; control group II: DnBP: 0.15 SD (0.21); BBP: 0.11 SD (0.22); DnOP: 0 and DEHP: 0.45 SD (0.68) $\mu g ml^{-1}$].

Correlation analysis of serum concentrations of PEs with the different severity of endometriosis was computed to determine their strength of association. The correlations were strong, and statistically significant for all four compounds (DnBP: r= +0.73; P<0.0001, BBP: r= +0.78; P<0.0001, DnOP: r= +0.57; P<0.0001, DEHP: r= +0.44; P<0.0014).

Women with endometriosis showed significantly higher concentrations of dioxin when compared with the control group. We found the correlation between the concentration of difference in the severity of endometriosis was strong and statistically significant at p<0.05 for concentration of Dioxin-TCDD: r= + 0.36, p<0.0001(Table 12.6).

Table 12.5: Phthalate Ester Concentrations in Endometriosis and Two Control Groups

Groups	*DnBP (μg/ml)*	*BBP (μg/ml)*	*DnOP (μg/ml)*	*DEHP (μg/ml)*
Control group I	0.08 (0.14)	0.12 (0.20)	0	0.50 (0.80)
Control group II	0.15 (0.21)	0.11 (0.22)	0	0.45 (0.68)
Study group	0.44 (0.41)	0.66 (0.61)	3.32 (2.17)	2.44 (2.17)
C_1 Vs study group;				
t value	5.13	5.13	-9.52	5.22
p value	[b]<0.0001	<0.0001	<0.0001	<0.0001
C_2 Vs study group;				
t value	3.01	3.94	-6.97	4.10
p value[b]	0.004	0.0002	<0.0001	0.0001
C_1 Vs C_2;				
t value	1.55	0.21	–	-0.24
p value[a]	0.13	0.84	–	0.81

Data are presented as mean (SD); C_1: control group I; C_2: Control group II.

$p < 0.05$ considered statistically significant.

a: Not significant in between the groups; b: Significant in between the groups.

Table 12.6: Concentration of Dioxin-TCDD in Control and Different Stages of Endometriosis

Congener	*Control Group (n=91); μg/ml*	*Case Group Stages (n=86); μg/ml*				*Correlation Coefficient (r)*
		I (n=35)	*II (n=27)*	*III (n=14)*	*IV (n=10)*	
TCDD	0.0001± 0.0006	0.000± 0.001	0.002± 0.009	0.005 ± 0.013	0.013± 0.022	+0.36*

The correlation between the concentrations of Dioxin-TCDD in different stages of endometriosis were statistically significant at $P < 0.05$.

The frequencies of GSTM1 null (*0/*0) genotypes were 26.8 per cent in the cases, and 14.7 per cent in the controls. Significant association was found between the endometriosis and GSTM1 null mutation (P=0.037). The GSTM1 (*0/*0) null polymorphism may increase the risk of endometriosis development with an odds ratio of 2.12(95 per cent CI =1.045–4.314) (Table 112.7).

GSTM1 null (*0/*0) polymorphism with the different severity of endometriosis was computed to determine their strength of association. The correlations were strong and statistically significant for all four compounds (PCB1: r = +0.5388, P<0.0001; PCB5: r = +0.6753, P<0.0001; PCB29: r = +0.6471, P<0.0001; and PCB98: r = +0.4357, P<0.0001; GSTM1: r = +0.9439, P=0.05) (Table 12.8).

Discussion

In confirmation with over earlier report[41] there is a significant association between PCBs and PEs with endometriosis. Now in the present study we established an association between PCBs and GSTM1 null genotype and their possible impact in developing endometriosis in south Indian women, which is the first report from the Indian subcontinent. All of our patients had lived in the same area over a long period of time, no history of professional exposure to reproductive toxicants. We assume that they were exposed to similar amounts of environmental toxicants.

The mode of inheritance of endometriosis is mysterious, but the disease is thought to be a "multiplex phenotype," similar to diabetes or asthma, in which two or more (perhaps more than a dozen) genes are involved. Interaction of these genes with an environmental component such as PHAHs (including PCBs and dioxin).

Our results support the report of Cobellis[42], who reported higher concentrations of DEHP in women with endometriosis compared to women without disease.

In spite of the high prevalence of endometriosis all over the world, researchers have been unable to determine its aetiology. The combination of sex steroids, growth factors, environmental factors and impaired immune response has been implicated in the initiation of endometriosis, although the exact mechanism by which ectopic endometrium attaches to the peritoneum has not yet been identified. The mode of inheritance of endometriosis is mysterious, but the disease is thought to be a "multiplex phenotype," similar to diabetes or asthma, in which two or more (perhaps more than a dozen) genes are involved.

Table 12.7: Frequencies of GSTM1 Null Gene Polymorphism in Women with and without Endometriosis

Gene	*Endometriosis*					*Controls (n=102)*	*OR*	*95 per cent CI*
GSTM1	*Stage 1*[a] *(n=37)*	*Stage II*[a] *(n=33)*	*Stage III*[a] *(n=16)*	*Stage IV*[a] *(n=11)*	*Total (n=97)*			
Null (per cent)	4 (10.8)	6 (18.1)	8(50)	8 (72.7)	26(26.8)	15(14.7)	2.12	1.04–4.31
Non-null (per cent)	33(89.1)	27 (81.8)	8(50)	3 (27.2)	71(73.1)	87(85.2)		(P=0.03)**

a: Stages classified according to revised American Fertility Society's (rAFS) of endometriosis.

**: Two-tailed Fishers exact test. $P<0.05$ considered statistically significant.

Table 12.8: PCBs Concentrations in Different Stages of Endometriosis and Control Group

Congener	*Endometriosis (n=41)*				*Control Group (n=47)*	*r-value*
	Stage I (µg/ml)	*Stage II (µg/ml)*	*Stage III (µg/ml)*	*Stage IV (µg/ml)*		
PCB-1 (co-planar)*	0.23±0.26	0.42±0.28	0.60±0.27	0.84±0.56	0.05±0.14	+0.5388
PCB-5 (co-planar)*	0.10±0.12	0.24±0.21	0.62±0.39	0.75±0.43	0.01±0.06	+0.6753
PCB-29 (co-planar)*	0.13±0.15	0.29±0.31	0.50±0.34	0.99±0.54	0.02±0.08	+0.6471
PCB-98 (Non-coplanar)*	0.03±0.10	0.11±0.18	0.34±0.32	0.26±0.31	0.00±0.03	+0.4357

Data are represented as mean ±SD. $P<0.05$ is considered statistically significant.

* Significant between the groups. r=Correlation coefficient.

Gene appears to contribute to the susceptibility of endometriosis is the gene for *GSTM1*. The GSTM1 protein serves as both a detoxification enzyme and more relevant to the hormonal problem of endometriosis as an intracellular binding protein for hormones and drugs. Two functionally active alleles of the *GSTM1* gene (*GSTM1*1* and *GSTM1*2*, earlier termed **A* and **B*), and one null allele in which the gene is deleted (*GSTM1*0*) have been described so far. Curiously, the *GSTM1*1/*2* genotype has been reported as having the highest GSTM1 enzymic activity, whereas both the *GSTM1*1/*1* and *GSTM1*2/*2* homozygotes exhibit decreased GSTM1 enzyme activity.

In addition to its function as an intracellular protein for binding sex hormones, GSTM1 has been shown to have a high specificity for detoxifying a number of PHAH reactive metabolites of Phase I detoxification reactions thereby facilitating their elimination from the body. Therefore, individuals with the GSTM1 null (*0/*0) genotype could be at increased risk for toxicity caused by various PHAHs as a result of an enzymatic defect in detoxification by GSTM1. We assume that environmental PCBs and Xenoestrogens may stimulate the activity of genes coding for detoxification. So, analysis of GST gene status, particularly discovery of GSTM1 null (*0/*0) mutation might have a predictive and pathologic importance.

The higher concentration of Dioxin-TCDD in the serum of women with endometriosis compared with controls possibly suggests an association of these factors with the occurrence of endometriosis. We strongly believe that there might be an association between GSTM1 null mutation and endometriosis patients who were having higher concentrations of Dioxin-TCDD compared with control group. According to our observation we found that patients in stage III and IV having GSTM1 null mutation, have higher concentrations of Dioxin-TCDD when compared to patients in stage I and II and control group. This indicates that GSTM1 null mutation might play an important role in the prognosis of disease from stage I to IV.

Xenoestrogens and Infertility

Xenoestrogens are man-made chemicals that are estrogenic in nature with adverse effects on reproduction in wildlife and humans[43, 44].

In recent years evidence indicated that exposure to environmental toxicants possessing estrogenic activity resulted in endometriosis. Results of animal studies and cell culture experiments, suggested that it is biologically plausible for environmental toxicants to affect the pathobiology of endometriosis[45].

Recent research in animals and humans indicates a potential association between exposure to dioxins, endometriosis, and disruption of the immune system. Studies have shown that rhesus monkeys exposed to dioxins with elevated serum levels of certain toxic coplanar PCBs and an increased total serum toxic equivalency had a high prevalence of endometriosis, and the severity of disease correlated with serum concentrations of PCB77. Dioxin-exposed animals with endometriosis showed long-term alterations in immunity associated with elevated levels of dioxin and specific coplanar dioxin-like congeners[46].

Following the publication of this experimental report, several epidemiological studies in humans have examined the incidence of endometriosis following a known environmental exposure to TCDD or correlated incidence of disease to the body burden of TCDD or dioxin like polychlorinated biphenyls (PCBs)[47]. Of particular note, an increased incidence of endometriosis was identified among infertility patients in Belgium, a country in which high levels of TCDD have been documented in breast milk[47, 48].

Additionally, developmental exposure to environmental toxicants can result in epigenetic modification of critical genes[49], including those that regulate the complex endocrine-immune interface within the adult reproductive tract. Whereas inflammatory processes are a normal part of endometrial physiology, environmental toxicants that modify either acute or systemic inflammatory processes could negatively affect reproductive success and potentially contribute to disease. Importantly, the offspring of mice in previous study described[50] exhibited altered PR expression and disrupted fertility for at least three generations without additional toxicant exposure[51], suggesting that an inheritable, epigenetic alteration had occurred.

Male Infertility

Several studies have reported adverse effects such as oligozoospermia and azoospermia amongst male workers exposed to xenoestrogens and pesticides. We carried out a study at Maternal Health and Research Trust and Mahavir Hospital and Research Centre on twenty-one infertile men with oligozoospermia (sperm count <20 million/ml) and without evidence of and obvious etiology and 32 controls with normal semen analysis. We observed that PCBs were present in the seminal plasma of infertile men but absent in controls and the concentration of PEs was significantly higher in infertile men compared with controls. Ejaculate volume, sperm count, progressive motility, and fertilizing capacity were significantly lower in infertile men compared with controls. The highest average PCB and PE concentrations were found in urban fish eaters followed by rural fish eaters, urban vegetarians and rural vegetarians. The total motile sperm counts in infertile men were inversely proportional to their xenoestrogen concentrations and were significantly lower than those in respective controls. In conclusion, PCBs and PEs may be instrumental in the impairment of semen quality in infertile men without an obvious etiology[39].

The possible mechanisms and physiological pathways via which maternal oestrogens could cause impaired development and descent of testis and other abnormalities of the reproductive tract are depicted in Figure 12.3 and the hormonal control of the fetal testicle is illustrated in Figure 12.4.

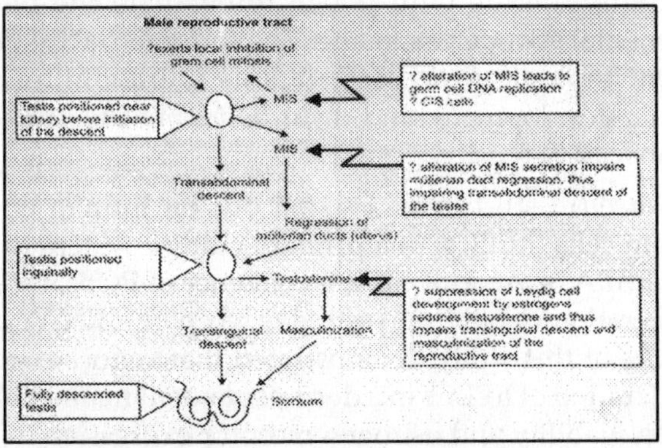

Figure 12.3: Possible Mechanisms and Physiological Pathways via which Material Oestrogens could Cause Impaired Development and Descent of Testis and Other Abnormalities of the Reproductive Tract (The Lancet 1993:1392-1395)[32]
(Points at which oestrogens derived from the mother could exert an adverse effect are indicated by bold lines and arrows)

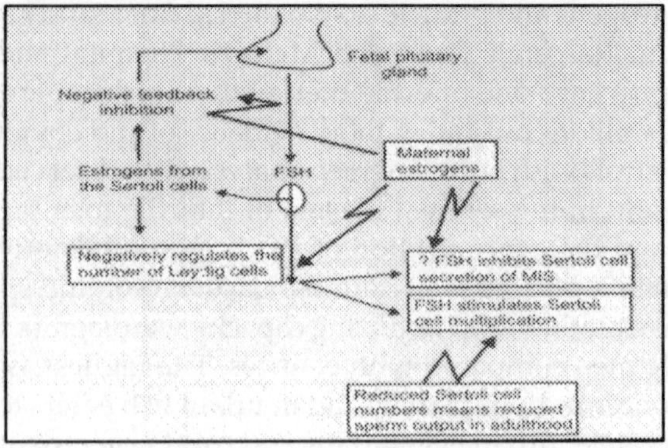

Figure 12.4: Hormonal Control of the Fetal Testicles (The Lancet 1993; 341:1392-1395)[32]
(Points at which estrogens derived from the mother could exert an adverse effect are indicated by bold lines and arrows)

Female Infertility

Xenoestrogens and the Endometrium

The endometrium is the main target for estrogens besides the breast, the pituitary, and the hypothalamus, and is thus a representative tissue with which to evaluate the relevance of environmental estrogen exposure. The endometrial tissue is vital to important biologic processes such as implantation and early embryonic development, and disturbances in the function of this organ can lead to reduced fertility.

An *in vitro* study was carried out on human endometrial epithelium cells (hEECs) in a primary culture system to assess the impact of BPA or Aroclor 1254, a congener of PCBs, by examining cell proliferation viability and estrogen receptor mRNA expression[52]. The results of this study demonstrated that xenoestrogens inhibit the proliferation of hEECs in a dose-dependent manner but have no impact on viability and estrogen receptor expression in a primary culture system. This suggests that the impact of xenoestrogens on hEECs may lead to reduced fertility. Wolfgang *et al.*, in 2000 reported that nonchlorinated environmental estrogens do not build up cumulative tissue concentration in the endometrium. The risk of reduced fertility because of ambient levels of environmental estrogens in the endometrium is negligible[43].

It has been reported that among the residues of environmental endocrine modulators, the DDT metabolite-p, p'-DDE, which is an androgen receptor antagonist of the flutamide type, was present in the highest concentration in the endometrium.[53] one of the sensitive targets of the anti-androgen compound is prenatal sexual differentiation during embryonic and fetal development.[54] Abnormalities observed in the reproductive track of the male alligators in Lake Apopka, Florida after a DDT spill[55] can be explained more plausibly by the antiandrogenic effects of p,p' DDE than by the estrogenic effects of o,p' DDT or other environmental estrogens. Thus, antiandrogens deserve more attention in the future.

Organochlorine Exposure and Endometriosis

In another case-control study,[56] exposure to organochlorines during adulthood, more specially to polychlorinated biphenyls and chlorinated pesticides, was not associated with endometriosis in the general population. Rier *et al.*[57] may have provided the strongest evidence linking endometriosis to organochlorine exposure. In dioxin-exposed monkeys the incidence of endometriosis was associated with the dioxin exposure and the severity of the disease was dependent upon the dose administrated ($p < 1.001$) even 10 years after the termination of dioxin treatment. Data published by Steel *et al.*[58] indicates that the half-life of polychlorinated biphenyls (Aroclor 1260-like mixture) in humans is approximately 10 years. Therefore, the polychlorinated biphenyl concentration measured in plasma lipids of women in their thirties most likely reflects the exposure to polychlorinated biphenyls during adult life. If exposure during puberty and in early infancy (modulated by breastfeeding or in utero) played a key role in the development of endometriosis, this would not be captured in the measurements obtained during adulthood. However, the influence of early exposure to organochlorines on the pathogenesis of endometriosis remains largely unknown.

In conclusion, it is important to known that exposure to organochlorines, specially polychlorinated biphenyls or chlorinated pesticides is not a significant risk factor for endometriosis in the general population.

Pesticides and Infertility

Consumption Pattern of Pesticides in India:

Unfortunately, 40 per cent of all pesticides used in India belong to the organochlorine class of chemicals, while an additional 30 per cent of the pesticides used belong to the organophosphate group (Figure 12.5).

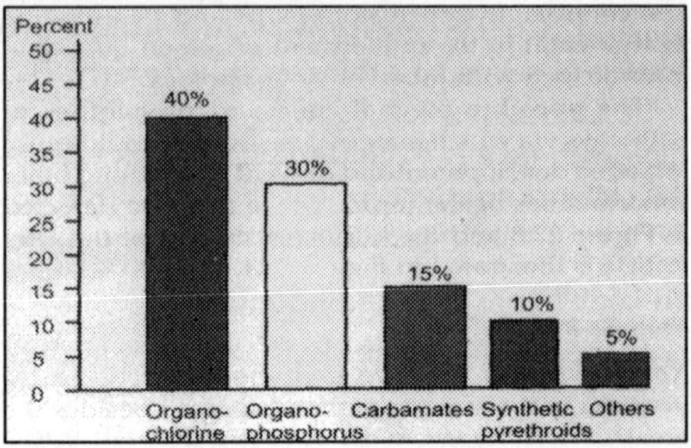

Figure 12.5: Consumption Pattern of Pesticides in India

Monocrotophos, phorate, phosphamidon, ethion,methyl parathion and dimethoate are some of the highly hazardous pesticides that are being continuously and indiscriminately used in India. While most of these chemicals are banned in other countries, the rest are awaiting risk assessment reports before appropriate action can be taken.

The DDT, HCH, Aldrin and Endosulfan were banned in the US and many other countries as early as in the 70s, but they are still being used in India. In fact, DDT, HCH and malathion account for 70 percent of the total pesticides banned in India continue to flow into the market despite government notifications. The small farmers prefer them because they are cost-effective, are easily available and display a wide spectrum of bioactivity.

Risk Assessment of Environmental Oestrognes

Figures 12.6A and B represents the present status and the correct pathway for an assessment of the risk of environmental estrogens in humans.

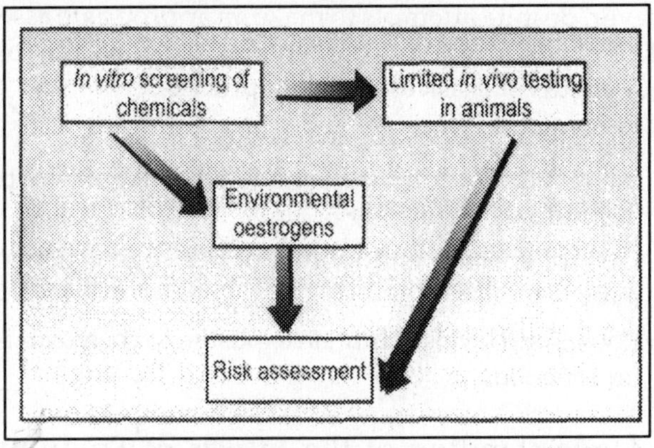

A: Present status on the risk assessment of environmental oestrogens

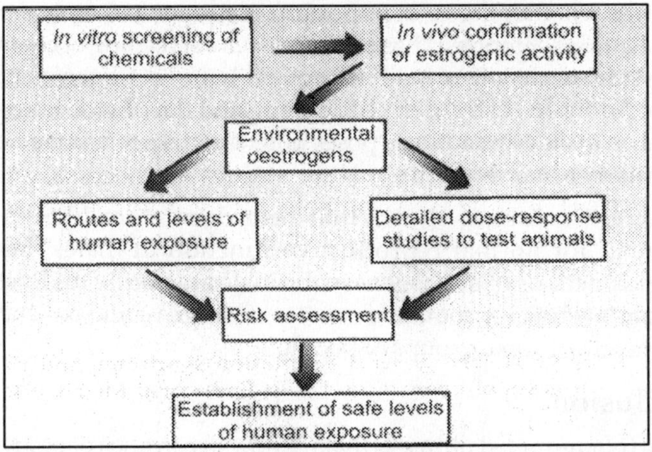

B: The correct pathway for risk assessment of environmental oestrogens

Figure 12.6: Contrast Between (A) The present understanding of the risk that environmental oestrogens pose to human health and (B) The complete risk assessment process (Turner KJ, Sharpe RM. Environmental oestrogens-Present understanding. Reviews of Reproduction 1997; 2:69-73)

However, despite attempts to make an appropriate assessment of the risk of exposure to environmental oestrogens, the following factors may hinder the risk assessment process:

1. More than one oestrogen receptor
2. Interactions (additivity, synergism, antagonism) between individuals chemicals
3. Lack of specific endopoints of oestrogens action in the male
4. Routes and levels of human exposure to chemicals is poorly understood.

Current Understanding of the Effects of Environmental Oestrogens on Humans

The list of environmental oestrogens is incomplete. It is therefore, unknown whether the most important oestrogenic chemicals have been identified. Emphasis has been on *in vitro* screening of chemicals for oestrogenecity. This may not equate with oestrogenic activity *in vivo*. Addition of soy- derived protein (and the phytooestrogens) to food on a widespread scale poses potential risks to human health, particularly to some infants.

Recent evidence shows that oestrogenic are likely to be important for normal reproductive function in males, but the biological actions of oestrogens in the male are poorly understood. A certain level of exogenous exposure to oestrogen could be beneficial to the health of some groups of people.

Conclusion

An often-quoted phrase is that we now live in a sea of oestrogens and there is clearly some truth in this. Data indicating that a xenobiotic may affect multiple signaling pathways with data showing synergistic effects of multiple xenobiotics on estrogen-responsive genes[59] reinforces the possibility that environmental xenobiotics although present at low concentrations may pose a threat of human health.

In the interim, all manner of changes in childhood growth age at puberty and incidence of hormone modulators disease/disorders like breast and prostatic cancer, undescended testicles, polycystic ovarian disease, endometriosis have occurred in humans.

While there may be a rational explanation for these changes that have little or nothing to do with exposure to hormones, when we know that "estrogens" can arguably affect all of these parameters, it is surely inappropriate to dismiss the possible involvement of environmental oestrogens just because we have no data. As we all are fond of saying "absence of evidence is not evidence of absence".

There is a general agreement that the original hypothesis suggesting that human exposure to compounds with oestrogenic (or other hormone- disruptive) activity could be responsible for reported adverse changes in male reproductive health (increase in testicular cancer, decline in sperm counts, and increase in testicular/genital malformations)[60] is biologically plausible. However, little progress has been made towards confirming or refuting this hypothesis over a decade. Therefore, further studies are necessary to further understand the role of the environmental estrogens in men and women with various reproductive health problems.

There are enormous uncertainties in assessing what might be a safe level of exposure to hazardous man-made chemicals, especially when they persist in the body for long periods. This is due in part to the lack of toxicity data and exposure data for the vast majority of chemicals people are exposed. It is difficult to suggest that exposure to a certain chemical at a certain concentration will cause a particular adverse effect. The best way to prevent this ongoing chemical contamination and the threat to future generations is to prevent the manufacture and use of chemicals that are found in elevated concentrations in biological fluids such as blood and breast milk.

The genetic study results suggest that women having GSTM1 null (*0/*0) polymorphism might have an increased susceptibility to endometriosis.

Acknowledgements

The authors are grateful to Hetero Drugs Ltd, for providing us the necessary financial assistance and equipments for carrying out this investigation. We thank Bhagwan Mahavir Medical Research Centre and MHRT, Centre for Infertility Management, Hyderabad, India for providing us the samples and for their entire support throughout this study. The authors thank Dr. Kamal Kiran, Kamineni Hospitals, Hyderabad, India for helping us in the statistical analysis.

References

1. Pauwels A, Schepens PJC, Hooghe TD, Delbeke L, Dhont M, *et al.*, The risk of endometriosis and exposure to dioxins and polychlorinated biphenyls: a case-control study of infertile women. Human Reproduction 2001; 16: 2050-2055.
2. Rier S, Foster, W.G. Environmental dioxins and Endometriosis. Toxicology Sci 2002; 70: 161-170.
3. Golden RJ, Noller KL, Titus-Ernstoff L, Kaufman RH, Mittendorf R, *et al.*, Environmental endocrine modulators and human health: an assessment of the biological evidence. CRC Critical Reviews in Toxicology 1998; 28:109-227.
4. Safe SH. Endocrine disruptors and human health-Is there a problem of update. Environ Health Perspect. 2000 Jun; 108(6): 487-93.
5. Kodavanti PRS, Ward TR, Derr-Yellin EC, Mundy WR, Casey AC, Tilson HA. Congener-specific distribution of PCBs in brain regions, blood, liver, and fat of adult rats following repeated exposure to Aroclor 1254. Toxicol Appl Pharmacol 1998; 153:199–210.
6. Zondervan K, Cardon L, Kennedy S Development of a Web site for the genetic epidemiology of endometriosis. Fertil Steril 2002a; 78:777–781.
7. Kennedy S. Genetics of endometriosis: a review of the positional cloning approaches. Semin Reprod Med 2003; 21:111–118.
8. Simpson JL, Bischoff FZ. Heritability and molecular genetic studies of endometriosis. Hum Reprod Update 2000; 6:37–44.
9. Kennedy S, Hadfield R, Mardon H. and Barlow D. Age of onset of pain symptoms in non-twin sisters concordant for endometriosis. Hum. Reprod 1996; 11: 403-405.
10. Warner M, Eskenazi B, Mocarelli P, Gerthoux PM, Samuels S, Needham L, Patterson D, Brambilla P. Serum dioxin concentrations and breast cancer risk in the Seveso Women's Health Study. Environ Health Perspect. 2002 Jul; 110(7): 625-8.
11. Eskenazi B, Mocarelli P, Warner M, Samuels S, Vercellini P, Olive D, Needham LL, Patterson DG Jr, Brambilla P, Gavoni N, Casalini S, Panazza S, Turner W, Gerthoux PM. Serum dioxin

concentrations and endometriosis: a cohort study in Seveso, Italy. Environ Health Perspect. 2002 Jul; 110(7): 629-34.

12. Rier SE, Martin DC, Bowman RE, Dmowski WP, Becker JL. Endometriosis in rhesus monkeys (Macaca mulatta) following chronic exposure to 2,3,7,8-tetrachlorodibenzo-p-dioxin. Fundam Appl Toxicol. 1993 Nov; 21(4): 433-41.

13. Rier SE, Turner WE, Martin DC, Morris R, Lucier GW, Clark GC. Serum levels of TCDD and dioxin-like chemicals in Rhesus monkeys chronically exposed to dioxin: correlation of increased serum PCB levels with endometriosis. Toxicol Sci. 2001 Jan; 59(1): 147-59.

14. Rier S, Foster WG. Environmental dioxins and endometriosis. Toxicol Sci. 2002 Dec;70(2):161-70.

15. Pearson WR, Vorachek WR, Xu SJ, Berger R, Hart I, *et al.*, Identification of class-mu glutathione transferase genes GSTM1-GSTM5 on human chromosome 1p13. Am J Hum Genet 1993; 53:220–233.

16. Selye H. The general-adaptation-syndrome and the diseases of adaptation. South Med Surg. 1951 Oct; 113(10): 315-23.

17. Barnea ER, Tal J. Stress-related reproductive failure. J *In vitro* Fert Embryo Transf. 1991 Feb;8(1): 15-23.

18. McGrady AV. Effects of psychological stress on male reproduction: a review. Arch Androl. 1984; 13(1): 1-7.

19. Moghissi KS, Wallach EE. Unexplained infertility. Fertil Steril. 1983 Jan; 39(1): 5-21.

20. Negro-Vilar A, Johnston C, Spinedi E, Valença M, Lopez F. Physiological role of peptides and amines on the regulation of ACTH secretion. Ann N Y Acad Sci. 1987; 512:218-36.

21. Plotsky PM, Cunningham ET Jr, Widmaier EP. Catecholaminergic modulation of corticotropin-releasing factor and adrenocorticotropin secretion. Endocr Rev. 1989 Nov; 10(4): 437-58.

22. Axelrod J, Reisine TD. Stress hormones: their interaction and regulation. Science. 1984 May 4; 224(4648): 452-9.

23. Berga SL, Mortola JF, Girton L, Suh B, Laughlin G, Pham P, Yen SS. Neuroendocrine aberrations in women with functional

hypothalamic amenorrhea. J Clin Endocrinol Metab. 1989 Feb; 68(2): 301-8.

24. Biller BM, Federoff HJ, Koenig JI, Klibanski A. Abnormal cortisol secretion and responses to corticotropin-releasing hormone in women with hypothalamic amenorrhea. J Clin Endocrinol Metab. 1990 Feb;70(2):311-7.

25. Wright J, Allard M, Lecours A, Sabourin S. Psychosocial distress and infertility: a review of controlled research. Int J Fertil. 1989 Mar-Apr;34(2):126-42.

26. Cumming DC, Rebar RW. Exercise and reproductive function in women. Am J Ind Med. 1983; 4(1-2): 113-25.

27. Seifer DB, Collins RL. Current concepts of beta-endorphin physiology in female reproductive dysfunction. Fertil Steril. 1990 Nov; 54(5): 757-71.

28. Vermeulen A. Environment, human reproduction, menopause, and andropause. Environ Health Perspect. 1993 Jul; 101 Suppl 2:91-100.

29. Brotons JA, Olea-Serrano MF, Villalobos M, Pedraza V, Olea N. Xenoestrogens released from lacquer coatings in food cans. Environ Health Perspect. 1995 Jun; 103(6): 608-12.

30. Olea N, Pulgar R, Pérez P, Olea-Serrano F, Rivas A, Novillo-Fertrell A, Pedraza V, Soto AM, Sonnenschein C. Estrogenicity of resin-based composites and sealants used in dentistry. Environ Health Perspect. 1996; 104(3): 298-305.

31. Asplund L, Svensson BG, Nilsson A, Eriksson U, Jansson B, Jensen S, Wideqvist U, Skerfving S. Polychlorinated biphenyls, 1,1,1-trichloro-2,2-bis(p-chlorophenyl)ethane (p,p'-DDT) and 1,1-dichloro-2,2-bis(p-chlorophenyl)-ethylene (p,p'-DDE) in human plasma related to fish consumption. Arch Environ Health. 1994 Nov-Dec; 49(6): 477-86.

32. Brock JW, Burse VW, Ashley DL, Najam AR, Green VE, Korver MP, Powell MK, Hodge CC, Needham LL. An improved analysis for chlorinated pesticides and polychlorinated biphenyls (PCBs) in human and bovine sera using solid-phase extraction. J Anal Toxicol. 1996 Nov-Dec; 20(7): 528-36.

33. Colborn T, vom Saal FS, Soto AM. Developmental effects of endocrine-disrupting chemicals in wildlife and humans. Environ Health Perspect. 1993 Oct; 101(5): 378-84.

34. Zeyneloglu HB, Arici A, Olive DL. Environmental toxins and endometriosis. Obstet. Gynaecol clin North Am 1997; 24:307-329.

35. American fertility Society (1985) Revised American Fertility Society classification of endometriosis. Fertil. Steril., 43, 351-352.

36. Alluri RV, Mohan V, Komandur S, Chawda K, Chowdary JR, Hasan Q. MTHFR C677T gene mutation a risk factor for arterial stroke: A hospital based study. Eur J Neurology 2005; 12(1): 40-4.

37. Hur SE, Ji Young Lee, Hye-Sung Moon, Hye Won Chung. Polymorphisms of the genes encoding the GSTM1, GSTT1 and GSTP1 in Korean women: no association with endometriosis. Mol Hum Reprod 2004; 11(1): 15–19

38. Burse VW, Groce DE, Caudill SP, Korver MP, Phillips DL, McClure PC *et al.*, Determination of polychlorinated biphenyl levels in the serum of residents and in the homogenates of sea food from the New Bedford, Massachusetts area: a comparison of exposure sources through pattern recognition techniques. Sci Total Environ 1994; 144:153–77.

39. Rozati R, Reddy PP, Reddanna P, Mujtaba R. Role of environmental estrogens in the deterioration of male factor fertility. Fertil Steril 2002; 78:6.

40. Supelco (1998) Data Sheet No. W710100, PCB MIx 525, Cat. No. 48246, Sigma-Aldrich Co.

41. Reddy BS, Rozati R, Reddy S, Shankarappa, Reddy P, Reddy R. High plasma concentrations of polychlorinated biphenyls and phthalate esters in women with Endometriosis: a prospective case control study. Fertility and Sterility 2006; 85:775–9.

42. Cobellis L, Latin G, DeFelice C, Razzi S, Paris I, Ruggieri F, Mazzeo P and Petraglia. High plasma concentrations of di- (2-ethylhexyl)-phthalate in women with endometriosis. Hum. Reprod, 2003; 18, No.7: 1512-1515,

43. Daston GP, Gooch JW, Breslin WJ, Shuey DL, Nikiforov AI, Fico TA, Gorsuch JW. Environmental estrogens and reproductive health: a discussion of the human and environmental data. Reprod Toxicol. 1997 Jul-Aug; 11(4): 465-81.

44. Sonnenschein C, Soto AM. An updated review of environmental estrogen and androgen mimics and antagonists. J Steroid Biochem Mol Biol. 1998 Apr;65(1-6):143-50.

45. Lee MS, Hyun SH, Lee CK, Im KS, Hwang IT, Lee HJ. Impact of xenoestrogens on the growth of human endometrial epithelial cells in a primary culture system. Fertil Steril. 2003 Jun; 79(6): 1464-5.

46. Foster WG. Endocrine toxicants including 2,3,7,8-terachlorodibenzo-p-dioxin (TCDD) and dioxin-like chemicals and endometriosis: is there a link? J Toxicol Environ Health B Crit Rev. 2008 Mar; 11(3-4): 177-87.

47. Heilier JF, Nackers F, Verougstraete V, Tonglet R, Lison D, Donnez J. Increased dioxin-like compounds in the serum of women with peritoneal endometriosis and deep endometriotic (adenomyotic) nodules. Fertil Steril 2005; 84:305–12. [PubMed: 16084869]

48. Porpora MG, Ingelido AM, di Domenico A, Ferro A, Crobu M, Pallante D, *et al.*, Increased levels of polychlorobiphenyls in Italian women with endometriosis. Chemosphere 2006; 63:1361–7. [PubMed: 16289286]

49. Heindel JJ, McAllister KA, Worth L Jr, Tyson FL. Environmental epigenomics, imprinting and disease susceptibility. Epigenetics 2006; 1:1–6. [PubMed: 17998808]

50. Bruner-Tran, KL.; Yeaman, GR.; Eisenberg, E.; Osteen, KG. Developmental Dioxin Exposure in Mice Alters Uterine DNA Methylation Patterns and Protein Expression in Adult Animals and Leads to an Endometriosis-like Phenotype. 63rd Annual Meeting of the American Society of Reproductive Medicine; Washington, DC. 2007.

51. Nayyar T, Bruner-Tran KL, Piestrzeniewicz-Ulanska D, Osteen KG. Developmental exposure of mice to TCDD elicits a similar uterine phenotype in adult animals as observed in women with

endometriosis. Reprod Toxicol 2007; 23:326–36. [PubMed: 17056225]

52. Sonnenschein C, Soto AM. An updated review of environmental estrogen and androgen mimics and antagonists. J Steroid Biochem Mol Biol. 1998 Apr; 65(1-6): 143-50.

53. Kelce WR, Stone CR, Laws SC, Gray LE, Kemppainen JA, Wilson EM. Persistent DDT metabolite p, p'-DDE is a potent androgen receptor antagonist. Nature. 1995 Jun 15; 375(6532): 581-5.

54. Imperato-McGinley J, Sanchez RS, Spencer JR, Yee B, Vaughan ED. Comparison of the effects of the 5 alpha-reductase inhibitor finasteride and the antiandrogen flutamide on prostate and genital differentiation: dose-response studies. Endocrinology. 1992 Sep; 131(3): 1149-56.

55. Guillette LJ Jr, Gross TS, Masson GR, Matter JM, Percival HF, Woodward AR. Developmental abnormalities of the gonad and abnormal sex hormone concentrations in juvenile alligators from contaminated and control lakes in Florida. Environ Health Perspect. 1994 Aug; 102(8): 680-8.

56. Lebel G, Dodin S, Ayotte P, Marčoux S, Ferron LA, Dewailly E. Organochlorine exposure and the risk of endometriosis. Fertil Steril. 1998 Feb; 69(2): 221-8.

57. Rier SE, Martin DC, Bowman RE, Dmowski WP, Becker JL. Endometriosis in rhesus monkeys (Macaca mulatta) following chronic exposure to 2,3,7,8-tetrachlorodibenzo-p-dioxin. Fundam Appl Toxicol. 1993 Nov; 21(4): 433-41.

58. Steele RW, Dmowski WP, Marmer DJ. Immunologic aspects of human endometriosis. Am J Reprod Immunol. 1984 Jul-Aug; 6(1): 33-6.

59. Arnold SF, Klotz DM, Collins BM, Vonier PM, Guillette LJ Jr, McLachlan JA. Synergistic activation of estrogen receptor with combinations of environmental chemicals. Science. 1996 Jun 7; 272(5267): 1489-92.

60. Sharpe RM, Skakkebaek NE. Are oestrogens involved in falling sperm counts and disorders of the male reproductive tract? Lancet. 1993 May 29; 341(8857): 1392-5.

Environmental & Occupational Exposures (2010) ***Pages 304–337***
Editors: **Sunil Kumar & R.R. Tiwari**
Published by: **DAYA PUBLISHING HOUSE, NEW DELHI**

Chapter 13

Occupational and Environmental Exposure to Chemicals and Reproductive Outcome

Sunil Kumar[1]*, Shagufta Shaikh[1], A.K. Gautam[1], V.V. Mishra[2] and H. Doshi[3]

[1]*Division of Reproductive and Cytotoxicology, National Institute of Occupational Health (ICMR)*
[2]*Department of Obstetrics and Gynecology, Institute of Kidney Disease, Ahmedabad – 380 016*
[3]*Civil Hospital, Ahmedabad – 380 016*

ABSTRACT

A growing body of scientific evidence point to the extreme sensitivity of embryos, fetuses and infants to the effects of persistent environmental/ occupational chemicals, which passed to them from their mothers directly and /or indirectly through father. Both father, and the mother, can pass on genetic defects to their offspring. Paternal / maternal exposure to some of these chemicals affects the gamete structure and function, which also have significant implication for the adverse effect on the pregnancy or out come.

The available data points that some of the organochlorine chemicals such as DDT, metals like lead, industrial pollutants

* E-mail: sunilnioh@yahoo.com

like dioxin, some of the organic solvent had adverse effect on reproduction and pregnancy out come. The data available supports the hypothesis that, in general, workingwomen have a higher risk of adverse reproductive outcomes, even though the data are limited. Studies are needed to find out the effects of those reproductive toxicants on human on priority basis, which have been proved to be toxic in animal studies.

Introduction

A large number of mutagenic or potentially toxic chemicals are in use in various industries or produced for various industrial or domestic uses and workers/ end users may be exposed to these chemicals. Exposures to environmental pollutants remain a major source ofhealth risk throughout the world, though risks are generally higher in developing countries, where poverty, lack of investment in modern technology and weak environmental legislation combine to cause high pollution levels[1]. Human beings are exposed to low levels of several thousands of man-made chemicals during their routine activities, occupation and through the food chain. Further, most of the chemicals in the workplace have not been evaluated for reproductive toxicity, and thus poses exposure potential to workers/ population. In reproductive toxicity both sexes are involved and impairments is not only restricted to the exposed individual but it could also be manifested in their progeny. Disruption of ovarian and hypothalamic pituitary function due to exposure to pollutants might affects women's reproductive and endocrine health. It is known that fetus is vulnerable to minutest concentration of toxic chemicals as compared to adult. Thomas and Colborn[2] reported that levels of exposure that cause no apparent effects in adults might cause irreversible harm to the developing foetus and newborn. Foetus is more susceptible to damage from a toxic insult of a given size than an adult because the fetus is growing at a rapid rate and is immature in a number of functional aspects[3]. It has been reported that neonates have a reduced capacity for metabolism and elimination of xenobiotics that may enhance chemical toxicity. Furthermore, the brain, reproductive organs and immune system have critical postnatal periods of maturation where they appear highly sensitive to toxic effects and may lead to permanent structural or functional organ changes. In the elderly, a combination of reduced organ function, disease and use of pharmaceuticals contributes to enhanced chemical sensitivity. In addition, there is a high degree of functional polymorphism in biotransforming enzymes. Such polymorphisms have been shown to contribute to inter individual variability in chemical response[4]. The parental exposure to persistent chemicals might be responsible for various reproductive impairments in the exposed individual itself and also the adverse reproductive outcome as these chemicals affects the gamete, foetus, and young one and later may be visible in adulthood or in progeny.

Material and Methods

This chapter is based on the available data on maternal and paternal occupational or environmental exposure and reproductive outcome. The chapter is divided in to different section on the basis of chemical groups. In the present chapter, emphasis has been given on parental exposure and reproductive outcome covering mainly human studies pertaining to exposure to chemicals and reproductive impairments. The data are summarized in Tables 13.1–13.2.

Exposure to Metals and Pregnancy Outcome

The most common routes of exposure to metal occur by dermal absorption, inhalation, or through diet. Metals enter the food chain often by way of bio-concentration in the environment and some metals like mercury bio-accumulated in the tissues of aquatic organisms. Some of the living beings are exposed to higher doses of these metals, through occupational or accidental exposure or through contaminated soil, water and food. Experimental studies indicated that both male and female reproductive system is vulnerable to the effects of some of the metals, such as lead, cadmium and mercury are having toxic effects on reproduction as well as reproductive outcome which depend upon dose, duration, and timing of exposure. However data pertaining to reproductive out come in human are less documented. There are reports on exposure of pregnant women to metals especially lead and adverse pregnancy out comes. Exposure to lead for women of childbearing age can have adverse effect on their offspring. It is known that lead deposited in the bone can be mobilized from bone during pregnancy and also transfer from mother to the fetus. Borja-Aburto *et al.*[18] evaluated the risk of spontaneous abortion from low or moderate lead exposures, and reported that mean blood lead levels were 12.03 μg/dL for cases (spontaneous abortion) and 10.09 μg/dL for controls. Odds ratios

Table 13.1: Maternal Exposure and Reproductive Outcome

Chemicals/ Physical Agents	*Workers/Subjects*	*Reported Effects*
Metals		
Mercury	Women workers in a lamp factory	Higher rates of menstrual disorders, sub fecundity and adverse pregnancy outcome[5].
	Dental Assistant	Less fertile[6]
	Women occupationally exposed to metallic mercury	Labour complication (late toxicosis of pregnancy, spontaneous abortions, duration of parturition and haemorrhage during parturition[7]
Lead	Cohort of pregnant women in Mexico City.	Increased spontaneous abortion[8]
	High blood Pb level in women	Associated with pre-term delivery, spontaneous abortion[9]
	Lead exposed mothers	Low birth weight and neural tube defects[10]
Cadmium	Women from area with high amount of soil Cd and Pb	Preterm infants with high Cd in blood[11]
	Maternal exposure to Cd	The rate of preterm deliveries increases and height and weight of newborn infants lower of mothers with higher urinary Cd[12]
	Maternal and cord blood Cd levels measured at delivery	Birth weight is inversely correlated with maternal and cord blood Cd concentrations[13]
Arsenic	Moderate arsenic exposures from drinking water (<50 μg/L) during pregnancy	Reduction in birth weight [14]

Contd...

Table 13.1–Contd...

Chemicals/ Physical Agents	*Workers/Subjects*	*Reported Effects*
Pesticides		
Multiple chemical/ pesticide exposure	Female gardeners	Casual association of cryptorchidism with occupation among sons of female gardeners[15]
Multiple pesticide exposure	Grape garden workers	Higher Abortion[16]
Exposed to pesticides during first trimester of pregnancy	Women Exposed to pesticides	Small for gestational age[17]
Maternal pesticide exposure	In indoor gardening	Spontaneous abortion
Maternal serum DDE level		Increased risk of spontaneous abortion[18] and increased risk of pre-term delivery[19]
Women farm operator	Correlated with timing of pesticide use on the farm	Moderate increases in risk of early abortions for preconception exposures to phenoxy acetic acid herbicides, triazines, and any herbicide. For late abortions, preconception exposure to glyphosate, thiocarbamates, and the miscellaneous class of pesticides was associated with elevated risks. Post conception exposures associated with late spontaneous abortions[20]

Contd...

Table 13.1–Contd...

Chemicals/ Physical Agents	*Workers/Subjects*	*Reported Effects*
Maternal exposure to pesticides	Maternal residual exposure to pesticides in an agricultural district in Poland.	Maternal exposure to synthetic pyrethroids associated with decrease in birth weight[21]
Exposure to pesticides	Mother involved in agricultural activities	Increased risk for congenial malformations[22]
Solvents		
2-bromo propane	Workers at an electronic company	Ovary dysfunction accompanying amenorrhea[23]
Carbon di dulphide	Workers of synthetic fibres factory	Early menopause and reduction of serum concentration of estrone, estradiol, progesterone, 17–hydroxyprogesterone[24]
	Carbon disulfide (CS_2) exposure	Menstrual disorders, pregnancy complications and spontaneous abortions[25]
	Community based study	No relationship between CS_2 concentration and miscarriage[26]
Organic solvent in petrochemical industry	Couples employed in petrochemical industry	Maternal exposure reduced birth weight[27]
Ethylene glycol ether	In semiconductor manufacturing	Female sub fertility[28]
Toluene	Printing industry workers	Reduced fecundity[29]

Table 13.2: Paternal Exposure and Reproductive Outcome

Chemicals/ Physical Agents	*Workers/Subjects*	*Reported Effects*
Metals		
Mercury		
Elemental mercury exposure	Male workers exposed to elemental mercury	No association between paternal mercury exposure and any reproductive outcome[30]
Urinary mercury	Exposed men's wives.	Urinary mercury concentration of 50 μgm/L or more was associated with the relative risk for spontaneous abortion[31]
Lead		
Low-to-moderate lead exposures		Increase risk for spontaneous abortion Picciotto[32]
Pre-conception employment in a high lead exposure job	Male employee of Lead and Zinc smelter	Elevated risk of stillbirth or birth defect but no association with spontaneous abortions[33]
Study on time to pregnancy	Wives of men monitored for lead	Limited support for the hypothesis that paternal exposure to lead is associated with decreased fertility[34]
DDT	DDT applicators in anti- Malaria campaign	The still birth rate elevated and the male /female ratio decreased[35]
Paternal agricultural work		Increases the risk of fetal death from congenital anomalies[36]

Contd...

Table 13.2–Contd...

Chemicals/ Physical Agents	*Workers/Subjects*	*Reported Effects*
DDT	Workers involved in anti-malaria campaign	No association with spontaneous abortion and sex ratio but higher risk for birth defect[37]
Solvent		
CS_2	Male workers exposed to CS_2 in a viscous rayonindustry	Higher miscarriage among the wives of the workers exposed to CS_2[38]
Organic solvent	Paternal exposure	Association paternal exposure to organic solvents and congenital malformations[39]

for spontaneous abortion comparing 5-9, 10-14, and >=15 μg/dL with the referent category of <5 μg/dL of blood lead were 2.3, 5.4, and 12.2, respectively, demonstrating a significant trend ($p = 0.03$). A mean blood lead level of 22.52 mg/dL among pregnant women with various adverse outcomes such as pre-term delivery, stillbirth and spontaneous abortion as compared to 19.4 mg/dL in normal delivery cases was also reported from India[9].

Various investigators have also reported lead induced male mediated adverse reproductive out come. Sallmen *et al.*[40] conducted a study within the wives of men biologically monitored for inorganic lead and mentioned that the odds ratio of congenital malformation for paternal lead exposure was increased non-significantly. They concluded that because of the small numbers and low participation, this study offers limited support for the hypothesis that paternal lead exposure is associated with congenital malformation. Lin *et al.*[41] examined the relationship between paternal occupational lead exposure and low birth weight/prematurity and found that there were no statistically significant differences in birth weight or gestational age between exposed and control groups. However, workers who had elevated blood lead levels for more than 5 years had a higher risk of fathering a child with low birth weight or prematurity than did controls. The risks of low birth weight and prematurity increased with the duration of exposure to lead. Picciotto[32] reported that low-to-moderate lead exposures might increase the risk for spontaneous abortion at exposures comparable to U.S. general population levels during the 1970s and to many populations worldwide today; these are far lower than exposures encountered in some occupations. Earlier Alexander *et al.*[33] reported that the risk of a stillbirth or birth defect was elevated for paternal pre-conception employment in a high lead exposure compared with a low-lead-exposure job. However, no association was found between pre-conception lead exposure and spontaneous abortion. Markku *et al.*[34] conducted a retrospective study on time to pregnancy among the wives of men biologically monitored for lead. The findings provide limited support for the hypothesis that paternal exposure to lead is associated with decreased fertility. All births in Norway during 1970-1993 with possible maternal or paternal occupational lead exposure were compared with a reference population of offspring of parents without occupational lead exposure. Offspring of lead exposed mothers had an increased risk of low birth weight and neural tube defects. Effects on birth weight and gestational age showed significant dose-response associations. Offspring of lead exposed fathers had no increased risks of any of the analyzed reproductive outcomes[10]. Srivastava *et al.*[42], determined the lead and zinc levels in mothers and neonatal blood, in cases with normal and IUGR babies. They reported that there was a weak but significant relationship between cord blood lead levels and birth weight. Joffe *et al.*[43] studied retrospectively current workers in lead using industries, and in non-lead using industries, with time to pregnancy as the outcome variable. Three exposure models were studied: 1) short term (recent) exposure; 2) total duration of work in a lead using industry; and 3) cumulative exposure. No consistent association of time to pregnancy with lead exposure was found in any of the exposure models, although reduced fertility was observed in one category each in models 2) and 3).

Epidemiological studies of paternal exposure to mercury have yielded conflicting results[30,31,44]. A retrospective cohort study was conducted among men who had worked with elemental mercury and exposure was determined from urinary mercury measurement records. No association was found between paternal mercury exposure and any reproductive outcome, including fertility, spontaneous abortion, major malformations, or childhood illness[30]. However, Cordier *et al.*[31], reported that a urinary mercury concentration of 50 μ gm / L or more was associated with the relative risk of 2.26 for spontaneous abortion in the men's wives. A study carried out among women workers exposed to mercury vapour in a lamp factory indicated that exposed women had higher rates of menstrual disorders, sub fecundity and adverse pregnancy outcome[5]. Further, women occupationally exposed to metallic mercury showed a correlation between length of service and concentration of mercury vapour with labour complication (late toxicosis of pregnancy, spontaneous abortions, duration of parturition and haemorrhage during parturition)[7]. Study carried out among the dental assistants also indicated that women who prepared 30 or more amalgams/ week and who had 4 or more poorer mercury hygiene practices had a fecundability score of only 63 per cent as compared to unexposed hygienists[6]. Earlier Sikorski *et al.*[45] also reported that dental work might represent an occupational hazard with reference to reproductive processes. However, a survey among the female dentists in United States suggests little, if any alterations in the risk of spontaneous abortions for female dentists working with amalgam and nitrous oxide[46].

Cadmium (Cd) is a known environmental pollutant, a major constituent of tobacco smoke and has no known beneficial effect. Based on animal studies Cd has been linked to a wide range of detrimental effects on reproduction. There are other metals such as chromium may have adverse effect on pregnancy out come but the data are inadequate to support the hypothesis. Laudanski *et al.*[11] found that the mean blood concentration of Cd in mothers delivered of preterm infants was higher than that of women who went to full term in an area with high amounts of lead and cadmium in the soil. Henson and Chedrese[47], mentioned that Cd^{2+} exposure during pregnancy has been linked to decreased birth weights and premature birth, with the enhanced levels of placental Cd^{2+} resulting from maternal exposure being associated with decreased progesterone biosynthesis by the placental trophoblast. The stimulatory effects of Cd^{2+} on ovarian progesterone synthesis, as revealed by the results of studies using stable porcine granulosa cells, appear centered on the enhanced conversion of cholesterol to pregnenolone by the cytochrome P450 side chain cleavage (P450scc). However, in the placenta, the Cd^{2+}-induced decline in progesterone synthesis is commensurate with a decrease in P450scc. Potential mechanisms by which Cd^{2+} may affect steroidogenesis include interference with the DNA binding zinc (Zn^{2+})-finger motif through the substitution of Cd^{2+} for Zn^{2+} or by taking on the role of an endocrine disrupting mechanism that could mimic or inhibit the actions of endogenous estrogens[47]. Nishijo et al[12] investigated the relationship between maternal exposure to Cd and pregnancy outcome. The rate of preterm deliveries of mothers with higher urinary Cd (2 nmol/mmol creatinine) was higher than that of mothers with lower urinary Cd (<2 nmol/mmol creatinine). The gestational age was significantly correlated with urinary Cd even after adjustment for maternal age. The height and weight of newborn infants of mothers with higher urinary Cd were significantly lower than those of the newborn infants of mothers with lower urinary Cd, but these decreases were ascribed to early delivery induced by Cd. A significant positive correlation was also found between maternal urinary Cd and Cd in breast milk. They concluded that maternal exposure to Cd seems to induce early delivery, which leads to a lower birth weight[12]. Salpietro *et al.*[13] measured at delivery, maternal and cord blood Cd levels and correlated with the birth weight of infants. They reported that Cd concentrations appeared to be the same order of magnitude both in cord and maternal serum, thus one could speculate that cadmium is transferred easily from the mother to the fetus through the placenta. They also found that birth weight is inversely correlated with maternal and cord blood Cd concentrations[13]. Zhang *et al.*[48] evaluated role of environmental exposure to cadmium on pregnancy outcome and fetal growth in cadmium polluted area in China. They reported that there was no significant association between cadmium exposure and birth weight. However, environmental exposure to cadmium significantly lowers neonatal birth height[48].

Some parts of the world have the higher level of arsenic in the ground water especially in Bangladesh and West Bengal, India. There are experimental reports on arsenic with reference to reproduction. However, data in human are scanty. Recently *Claudia et al*[14] *reported that* limited evidence suggests that arsenic may have adverse reproductive effects on human. They conducted a study in two Chilean cities [Antofagasta (40µg/L) and Valparaiso (<1µg/L)] with contrasting drinking water arsenic levels. The results indicated that Antofagasta infants had lower mean birth weight (-57g; 95 per cent confidence interval= -123 to 9). This suggests that moderate arsenic exposures from drinking water (<50 µg/L) during pregnancy are associated with reduction in birth weight[14].

It is known that some of the metals transfer from mother to fetuses and might have endocrine disruptive effects. Ong *et al.*[49] reported that lead absorbed by the pregnant mother is readily transferred to the developing fetus. Organic mercury also readily crosses the placenta[50]. Available studies indicated that metal like Pb, Hg and Cd could transfer from mother to offspring. The mechanism by which the heavy metals affect the female reproduction and pregnancy out come is not fully understood. Gerhard *et al.*[51], suggested that the hypothalamic-pituitary-ovarian axis could be affected by the heavy metals either directly or indirectly through modifications of the secretion of prolactin, adrenocortical steroids or thyroid hormones. They further, suggested that heavy metal induced hormonal and immunological alterations might be important factors in the pathogenesis of repeated miscarriages[52]. Heavy metals might affect female reproductive organs and pregnancy out comes directly and indirectly through hormonal production and regulation and also via endocrine disrupting mechanism. Based on experimental studies Lindstrom *et al.*[53] and Foster *et al.*[54] reported that heavy metal induce modifications of neurotransmitters in the central nervous system and impair the pulsatile hypothalamic release of gonadotropin-releasing hormone (GnRH). Further, in the adrenal gland, heavy metals are deposited in the lipid rich cortex and block various enzymatic pathways, causing hyperandrogenemia or partial hypoandrenalism[55,56]. Klages *et al.*[57] reported hypo and hyper thyroidism could result from Pb and Cd exposure. Further, in the ovary itself, accumulation of heavy metals impairs the production of estradiol and progesterone in experimental animals[58,59]. These hormonal changes might be possible in human also due to environmental exposure to various persistent chemicals including heavy metals and pesticides. Thus heavy metals affect the female reproduction and their out come by their action at multiple sites. Earlier Silbergeld[60] reported that deficiency of calcium, iron or zinc facilitates intestinal absorption of Pb and also helps in mobilizing it from bones during pregnancy and lactation. Thus calcium, iron and zinc might have an important role in the metal toxicity. Some of the metals such as copper, zinc etc are trace element and important for growth and development. Copper deficiency during pregnancy has been associated with low birth weight[61]. Roungsipragran *et al.*[62] reported that maternal plasma zinc levels during antenatal care, labour and infant birth weight in the intrauterine growth retardation infant group were significantly lower than that in normal growth infants. Recently Rwebembera *et al.*[63] investigated the relationship between infant birth weight and maternal zinc levels and noted a relationship between low infant birth weight and zinc deficiency.

Exposure to Pesticides and Pregnancy Outcome

Application of pesticides in agriculture has increased many folds worldwide in an effort to increase agriculture production and for vector control. A large number of workers of both sexes are engaged in agricultural sector and are being exposed to various pesticides. A considerable number of family members even children and pregnant women are also exposed to these chemicals. There are reports that both maternal and paternal exposures to some of the pesticides have adverse effects on reproduction. Arbuckle *et al.*[20]

collected data on the identity and timing of pesticide use on the farm, lifestyle factors, and reproductive history from the farm operator and examined exposures separately for preconception and postconception (first trimester) and for early and late spontaneous abortions. They observed moderate increases in risk of early abortions for preconception exposures to phenoxy acetic acid herbicides, triazines, and any herbicide. For late abortions, preconception exposure to glyphosate, thiocarbamates, and the miscellaneous class of pesticides was associated with elevated risks. Post-conception exposures were generally associated with late spontaneous abortions. Hanke *et al.*[21] evaluated the influence of maternal residual exposure to pesticides on birth weight in an agricultural district in Poland. They found that maternal exposure to synthetic pyrethroids in the first or second trimester was associated with a small but statistically significant decrease in birth weight and postulated that the observed effect of pyrethroids exposure was related to a slower pace of foetal development corresponding to the small-for-gestational-age birth. Regidor *et al.*[36] reported that paternal agricultural work increases the risk of fetal death from congenital anomalies. The risk is also increased for fetuses conceived during the time periods of maximum use of pesticides. The higher risk of fetal death from the remaining causes of death in the offspring of agricultural workers seems unrelated to pesticide exposure. However, Hjollund *et al.*[64] found no increased risk of spontaneous abortion in IVF-treated women attributable to paternal agricultural application of pesticides and growth retardants.

Garcia *et al.*[22] conducted a study in Spain, to assess the relation between occupational exposure to pesticides, and the prevalence of congenital malformations. For the mothers who were involved in agricultural activities during the month before conception and the first trimester of pregnancy, the adjusted odds ratio was 3.16 primarily due to an increased risk for nervous system defects, oral clefts, and multiple anomalies. Paternal agricultural work did not increase the risk, although fathers who reported ever handling pesticides had an adjusted odds ratio of 1.49 mainly related to an increased risk for nervous system and musculoskeletal defects. The significance of this association at lower exposure levels found in the general population remains uncertain. Longnecker *et al.*[19] reported evidence about the adverse effects of DDT in human. They described a powerful association between DDE levels in mother's blood and likelihood of pre-term birth and also showed that contamination was linked to babie's size, with babies more likely to be small for their gestational age when born to mothers with higher DDE levels. Korrick *et al.*[18] also reported a potential increased risk of spontaneous abortion with maternal serum DDE level. Recently, Bruoker-Davis[65] found an association between congenital Cryptorchidism and fetal exposure to PCBs and possibly DDE.

Male-mediated spontaneous abortion other reproductive outcome is well described among animals, but less documented in humans. Recently, Salazar-Garcia *et al.*[37] assessed potential effects of human DDT exposure, through the reproductive history of 2,033 workers in the anti malaria campaign of Mexico. No significant association was found for spontaneous abortion or sex ratio. However, found an increased risk of birth defects associated with high occupational exposure to DDT. Garry *et al.*[66] reported a modest but significant increase in risk (1.6- to 2-fold) for miscarriages and/or fetal loss in the spouses of applicators who use fungicides and also a significant deficit in the number of male children. First-trimester miscarriages occur most frequently in the spring, during the time when herbicides are applied. Use of sulfonylurea (odds ratio = 2.1), imidizolinone (OR = 2.6) containing herbicides, and the herbicide combination Cheyenne (OR = 2.9) by male applicators was statistically associated with increased miscarriage risk in the spring. With regard to personal pesticide exposures, only women who engaged in pesticide application are at demonstrable risk (OR = 1.8) for miscarriage. They hypothesized that the overall reproductive toxicity observed in this population is, for the greater part, a male-mediated event. Savitz *et* al[67] evaluated the male farm activities in the period from 3 months before conception through the month of conception in relation to miscarriage, preterm delivery, and small-for-gestational-age births. Miscarriage was not associated with chemical activities overall but was increased in combination with reported use of thiocarbamates, carbaryl, and unclassified pesticides. Preterm delivery was also not strongly associated with farm chemical activities overall, except for mixing or applying yard herbicides. Combinations of activities with a variety of chemicals (atrazine, glyphosate, organophosphates, 4-[2,4-dichlorophenoxy] butyric acid, and insecticides) generated odds ratios of two or greater. No associations were found between farm chemicals and small-for-gestational-age births or altered sex ratio. Potashnik and Porath[68] reassessed testicular function and reproductive performance of production workers with dibromochloropropan -induced testicular dysfunction and reported that there was no increase in the rate of spontaneous abortions and congenital malformations among pregnancies conceived during or after exposure. A low prevalence of male infants conceived during paternal exposure was found as compared with the pre-exposure period (16.6 per cent versus 52.9 per cent; P<. 025).

Recent researches indicated a new form of reproductive effect through endocrine disruptive mechanism and a number of pesticides and their metabolites have been reported to have estrogenic activity, which affect the normal hormone function[69,70]. Very recently, Kumar[71] reviewed the data on occupational exposure associated with reproductive dysfunction and reported that evidence suggestive of harmful effects of occupational exposure on the reproductive system and related outcomes has gradually accumulated in recent decades, which is further compounded by the persistent environmental endocrine disruptive chemicals. Arbuckle and Sever[72] summarized studies that have examined associations between fetal deaths (both spontaneous abortions and stillbirths) and specific pesticides, as well as maternal and paternal employment in occupations with potential for exposure and mentioned that the data are suggestive of increased risks of fetal deaths associated with pesticides in general and maternal employment in the agricultural industry. Garcia[73] reviewed epidemiological studies on occupational exposure to pesticides, and risk of congenital malformations, it seems reasonable to conclude that, to date, there is inadequate evidence for either establishing a relationship between pesticides exposure in human beings and birth defects or for rejecting it. The information accumulated in recent years one can hypothesize that the pesticides such as DDT might have potential to affect the reproduction and pregnancy outcome. However, based on available data, despite limitations in exposure assessment, there is a clear need for well design epidemiological research that focuses on specific pesticide, with improved exposure assessment and particularly male mediated reproductive out come in relation to miscarriage and preterm delivery.

Exposure to Solvents and Pregnancy Outcome

Solvents are one of the most prevalent sources of chemical exposure. They are volatile, lipophilic in nature and people may be exposed through inhalation or dermal route. In view of lipid solubility, it is likely that most organic solvents pass through the placenta into the foetus and could be potential for adverse effect on offsprings. Finkova *et al.*[25] reported that carbon disulfide (CS_2) exposure might cause disturbances in the ovarian function of young females, resulting in menstrual disorders, pregnancy complications and spontaneous abortions. Pieleszek[24] studied the effect of CS_2 on menopause, concentration of monoamines, gonadotropins, estrogens and androgens in women working in a synthetic fibers factory and exposed to CS_2 chronically. Menopause was present in 16.59 per cent in the population chronically exposed to CS_2 as compared with 8.05 per cent in the normal population. Mean age at menopause was also lower in CS_2 exposed group. Further, serum concentration of estrone, estradiol, progesterone, 17-hydroxyprogesterone were significantly lower in women exposed to CS_2. However, no significant differences in the level of FSH or LH were noted between exposed and control groups[24]. Earlier, Heinrichs[74] and Wang and Zhao[75] also reported increased incidence of spontaneous abortion with exposure to CS_2. However, a community based study of spontaneous abortion, occupation, and air pollution observed no relationship between CS_2 concentration and miscarriage rates[26]. Further, male mediated reproductive impairments in female in the form of higher miscarriage among the wives of the workers exposed to CS_2 in a viscous rayon industry were also reported[38]. In an experimental study, an increase in sperm head shape abnormality and decrease in sperm count was observed in CS_2 exposed group[76].

Plenge-Bonig and Karmaus[29] examined the possible influence of exposure to toluene on fertility among workers of printing industry, low daily exposure to toluene in women seems to be associated with reduced fecundity. Xiao *et al.*[77] examined the effects on semen and sperm quality of workers exposed to benzene, toluene, and xylene in shoemaking, spray-painting, or paint manufacturing factories and suggested that the mixture could affect the quality of semen and sperm, which might be the main reason of the abnormal pregnancy outcome among the wives of workers exposed to benzene, toluene, and xylene. Bukowski[78] reviewed toluene-specific findings. Six occupational studies reported associations between toluene and spontaneous abortion, two between toluene and congenital malformation, and three between toluene and reduced fertility. The spontaneous abortion studies provided the most suggestive evidence for an association with toluene. He further suggested that the results of the occupational studies should be considered "hypothesis generating". In an another review of epidemiological studies carried out between 1989-1999 on adverse developmental effects of maternal occupational exposure to organic solvents suggested the possibility of a moderate increase in the risk of spontaneous abortion and congenital malformations, especially facial clefts, associated with maternal exposure to solvents[79].

Sallmen *et al.*[80] assessed whether paternal exposure to organic solvents is associated with decreased fertility. The workers were classified into exposure categories based on work description and the use of solvents, and on biological exposure measurements. The study provides limited support for the hypothesis that paternal exposure to organic solvents might be associated with decreased fertility. Paternal exposure to organic solvents is associated with an increased risk for neural tube defects but not spontaneous abortions[81]. Hooiveld et al[39] observed a positive association between paternal exposure to organic solvents and congenital malformations in offspring. A study conducted among biomedical research laboratories female personnel to estimate the fecundability (probability of conception of a clinically detectable pregnancy per cycle) indicated that work with organic solvents in general in laboratory work, gave a decreased adjusted fecundability ratio (FR) of 0.79. Moreover, work with acetone and use of viruses also showed decreased FRs. The results pointed some indications of reduced fecundability for work with specific agents in laboratories[82].

In a fertility study (time to pregnancy (TTP) for the first pregnancy) conducted among workers exposed to metal fumes and solvents in the Italian mint (stampers, founders, and other technical workers) and non-exposed administrative staff. The groups with the highest prevalence of pregnancy delay beyond 6 months were stampers (21 per cent) and solvents (21.5 per cent). Logistic regression did not show a significant association of these job exposures with pregnancy delay. The data are not consistent with the hypothesis that male exposure to solvents and metal fumes is associated with an increase in the TTP[83]. Elliott *et al.*[84] conducted a study to examine the risk of spontaneous abortion (SAB) in semiconductor industry female workers and found no evidence of an increased risk of SAB in the British semiconductor industry. McMartin *et al.*[85] reported that maternal exposure to organic solvents is associated with a tendency toward an increased risk for spontaneous abortion. Doyle *et al.*[86] investigated the association between spontaneous abortion and work within dry cleaning units in the UK where the solvent perchloroethylene is used. They reported that women who worked in dry cleaning shops at the time of their pregnancy or in the three months before having higher risk for spontaneous abortion than non-operators. Logman *et al.*[87] conducted a meta-analysis to assess the risks of spontaneous abortions (SAs) and major malformations (MMs) after paternal exposure to organic solvents. Forty-seven studies were identified; 32 excluded, left 14 useable studies. Overall random affects odds ratios were 1.30 for SA, 1.47 for MMs, 1.86 for any neural tube defect, 2.18 for anencephaly, and 1.59 for spina bifida. They concluded that paternal exposure to organic solvents is associated with an increased risk for neural tube defects but not SAs. The available data suggests that maternal exposures to organic solvents are having adverse effect on reproductive out come, but conflicting reports exist concerning paternal exposure and adverse pregnancy outcomes especially for spontaneous abortion.

Exposure to Phthalates and Pregnancy Outcome

Phthalate compounds are the most abundant man made chemicals, are used as plasticizers in the production of polymeric materials. Endocrine disruptive nature of some of the phthalate compounds mostly reported *in vitro* might pose possible threat to the reproductive system. There are indications, which suggest that women in industrialized countries now reach menarche earlier and may experience menopause later. Early breast development in Puerto Rican girls has been a long-standing mystery in public health. In a study that included 17,077 girls, Herman- Giddens *et al.*[88] reported that girls in the US are developing pubertal characteristics at younger ages than previously reported. They concluded that the possibility of increasing use of certain plastics and insecticides that degrade in to substances that have estrogen–related effects should be investigated in relation to the earliest onset of puberty. Recently Colon *et al.*[89] analyzed 41 serum samples from thelarche patients and 35 control subjects No pesticides or their metabolites residues were detected in the serum of the study or control subjects. Significantly high levels of phthalates [dimethyl, diethyl, dibutyl) and di- (2-ethylhexyl)] and its major metabolites mono- (2-ethylhexyl) phthalate were identified in 28 (68 per cent) samples from thelarche patients. Of the control subjects, only one showed significant level of di-isooctyl phthalate. The most dramatic difference was the concentration of DEHP (di-ethyl hexyl phthalate), a known anti-androgen which was about seven times in girls with premature thelarche that of control group[89]. High plasma concentration of polychlorinated biphenyls and phthalate esters were reported among women with endometriosis[90]. Reader may also refer the chapter 8 from the book. However, more studies are needed on the role of phthalate compound and reproduction.

Exposure to Other Chemicals/Complex Work Environment and Pregnancy Outcome

A large number of workers are also exposed to complex mixture of chemicals during occupations such as dry-cleaning industry, petrochemical industry, rubber industry etc. These exposures might also have some affect on reproductive outcome. Women are exposed to relatively high concentrations of the solvent perchloroethylene in the dry cleaning industry. A study among female workers revealed that exposure to perchloroethylene was associated with greater incidence of spontaneous abortion during the first 3 months of pregnancy compared to unexposed women[91]. Earlier study of Hemminki[92], also suggested a greater incidence of spontaneous abortion (10.14 per cent) after exposure to dry cleaning chemicals compared to the general population (5.52 per cent). A study from Italy also showed a four-fold increase in the percentage of spontaneous abortions in the dry cleaning industry[93]. But Ahlborg[94] study on workers in Sweden did not find an association between spontaneous abortion and exposure to perchloroethylene.

Wright *et al.*[95] reported that maternal exposure to total trihalomethane (TTHMs) was associated with small for gestational age and reductions in birth weight. There was no evidence of an association between preterm delivery and increased TTHM levels, but there were slight increases in gestational duration with TTHM concentrations. Bonde *et al.*[96] examined reproductive end points in a

Danish cohort of 10,059 metalworkers. The occurrence of reduced birth weight, preterm delivery, infant mortality, and congenital malformation was not increased among children at risk from paternal welding exposure in comparison with children not at risk. However, pregnancies preceding a birth at risk from paternal exposure to stainless steel welding were more often terminated by spontaneous abortion.

Vassilev *et al.*[97] investigated the association between outdoor airborne polycyclic organic matter (POM) and adverse reproductive outcomes and found associations between outdoor exposure to airborne POM and several adverse pregnancy outcomes. Townsend *et al.*[98], investigated whether paternal exposure to 2,3,7,8-tetrachlorodibenzo-p- dioxin (TCDD) or other polychiorinated dioxins might be associated with adverse pregnancy outcomes. A total of 737 conceptions, which resulted in 637 live births and 100 stillbirths and spontaneous abortions, were identified as having paternal exposure; 2031 conceptions, resulting in 1785 live births and 246 stillbirths and spontaneous abortions, were identified as having no paternal exposure to dioxin. Overall, no statistically significant associations were found between any exposure and pregnancy outcome, either before or after stratification by pertinent sets of up to nine covarlables. Irgens *et al.*[99] tested previously established hypotheses on associations of birth defects with paternal occupation on the basis of a Norwegian registry material. They reported that vehicle mechanics had an association with hypospadias–OR 5.19; painters had a non-significant association with spina bifida–OR 2.03 and printers with clubfoot–OR 1.61. Associations observed previously in offspring of fathers in large occupational groups such as teachers, drivers, electricity related occupations, sales related occupations and agricultural workers were not confirmed in this dataset.

Seidler *et al.*[100] studied the association between maternal occupational exposure to specific chemical substances (organic solvents, carbon tetrachloride, herbicides, chlorophenols, polychlorinated biphenyls, aromatic amines, lead and lead compounds, mercury and mercury compounds) and birth of small-for-gestational-age infants. The results suggest that leatherwork might be associated with the birth of infants small-for-gestational-age through exposure to chlorophenols and aromatic amines. In the polytomous logistic regression analysis, only the association between exposure to mercury and growth retardation reached statistical significance; however, the power of the study is limited. These findings suggest that maternal exposure to specific chemicals at work may be a risk factor for the birth of SGA infants. Savitz *et al.*[101] addressed potential reproductive hazards in textile manufacturing. Miscarriage cases were identified from medical records (280 interviewed cases): pre-term delivery cases and term, normal birth weight controls (454 and 605, respectively) were identified from area hospitals. Relative to women and men working in nonhazardous occupations, workers in the textile industry were not at increased risk of miscarriage or preterm delivery, with the possible exception of preterm delivery among women and men employed in sectors other than knitting and yarn mills and men employed in yarn mills. Inferred exposures to specific agents were also not associated with adverse pregnancy outcome. Subject to uncertainty in exposure assessment and nonresponse, these data indicate an absence of adverse effects of the textile workplace environment on these pregnancy outcomes. Hourani and Hilton[102] examined data provided by pregnant Navy women both maternal and paternal exposure. Self-reported exposures to heavy metals, pesticides, petroleum products, and other chemicals were associated with adverse live-birth outcomes at the bivariate level. Only a father's exposure to pesticides at work predicted an adverse live-birth outcome (pre-term delivery). Maternal exposures to reproductive toxicants may exert their influence through maternal health and/or pregnancy complications on pregnancy outcome. Friedler[103] reviewed the experimental and epidemiological investigations and documented the adverse consequences of an array of paternal exposures on the development of subsequent offspring. Male-mediated abnormalities have been reported after exposure to therapeutic and recreational drugs, to chemicals in the workplace and environment and to ionizing radiation. The mechanism in the etiology of paternally mediated adverse outcomes is poorly understood.

Exposure to Tobacco Smokes

It is known that smoking during pregnancy is harmful not only to smokers but also to the fetus. Jaakkola *et al.*[104] assessed the effects of prenatal exposure to environmental tobacco smoke on fetal growth and length of gestation. The exposure assessment was based on nicotine concentration of maternal hair sampled after the delivery, which measures exposure during the past 2 months (*i.e.*, the third trimester). The exposure categories were defined as high (nicotine concentration >= 4.00 mg/g), medium (0.75 to < 4.00 mg/g), and low as the reference category (< 0.75 mg/g). The risk of pre-term delivery was higher in the high and medium exposure categories compared with the reference category, and there was a 1.22 increase in adjusted OR with a 1 mg/g increase in hair nicotine concentration. The corresponding adjusted OR was 1.06 for low birth weight and 1.04 for small-for-gestational-age. Jensen *et al.*[105] recruited, Danish couples, lived with a partner, and had no children. The couples were enrolled when they discontinued birth control, and were followed for six menstrual cycles or until a clinically recognized pregnancy. The fecundability odds ratio for smoking women exposed *in utero* was 0.53 compared with unexposed nonsmokers. Fecundability odds ratio for nonsmoking women exposed *in utero* was 0.70 and that for female smokers not exposed in utero was 0.67. Exposure *in utero* was also associated with a decreased fecundability odds ratio in males (0.68), whereas present smoking did not reduce fecundability significantly. They suggested that it seems advisable to encourage smoking cessation prior to the attempt to conceive as well as during pregnancy.

Conclusion

Epidemiological studies have identified associations between various maternal and paternal exposures and abnormal reproductive outcomes, but the risk factors for the paternal contribution to abnormal reproductive outcomes remain poorly understood. Shi and Chia[106] reviewed studies on maternal occupational exposures and birth defects, and the limitations with these studies. Unfortunately, most reported associations between occupational exposures and adverse reproductive outcomes are equivocal and often controversial and many associations are only suggestive. Later they[107] reviewed epidemiological studies on paternal occupations and birth defects. There were several common paternal occupations that were repeatedly reported to be associated with birth defects. They mentioned that common weaknesses in most of the studies include inaccurate assessment of exposures, different classification systems, different inclusion criteria of birth defects, and low statistical power. They concluded that epidemiological studies, reported in the past decade, suggest that several common paternal occupations are associated with birth defects. Future studies could be focused on these specific, rather than general, occupational groups so that causative agents may be confirmed. The broad spectrum of alterations recorded in reproductive outcome associated with the exposure to a variety of unrelated agents suggests the need for a more focused effort and multidisciplinary approaches to find out the potential role of both male and female exposure to persistent chemicals and reproductive out come. Need for the reduction in work place exposure to reproductive toxicants and women also need extra protection at work place by virtue of their role as the carrier of the unborn child. The Information Education and Communication (IEC) about the reproductive toxicants and legislation about the protection of pregnant women or even men and women attempting for the pregnancy against exposure to such pollutants in work place will be useful in prevention of adverse reproductive outcome.

References

1. Briggs David (2003) Environmental pollution and global burden of disease. British Med Bull 68, 1-24.
2. Thomas KB, Colborn T (1992) Organochlorine endocrine disruptors in human tissue. In: Colborn T. and Clement C. (Eds), Chemically-induced alterations in sexual functional development: The Wildlife/Human connection. Princeton Scientific Publishing Co., Inc. Priceton, New Jersey: 365-394.
3. South West Environmental Protection Agency (1995) Environmental poisoning and the law. ISBN 0 951 6073 1 6.
4. Lindeman B, Soderlund EJ, Dybing E (2002) Factors contributing to inter individual variability in chemical toxicity. Tidsskr Nor Laegeforen 122, 615-618. (in Norwegian).
5. De Rosis F, Anastasio SP, Selvaggi, Beltrame A, and Moriani G (1985) Female reproductive health in two lamp factories: Effects of exposure to inorganic mercury vapour and stress factors. Br J Ind Med 42, 488-494.
6. Rowland AS, Baird DD, Weinberg CR (1994) The effect of occupational exposure to mercury vapour on the fertility of female dental assistants Occup Environ Med 51, 28-34.

7. Mishonova VN, Stepanova PA Zarudin V V (1980) Characteristics of the course of pregnancy and births in women with occupational contact with small concentrations of metallic mercury vapours in industrial facilities. Gig Truda Prof Zabol 24, 21-23.

8. Borja-Aburto Victor H, Hertz-Piccitto Irva, Lopez M Rojas, Farias Paulina Rios Camilo and Blanco Julia (1999) Blood lead levels measured prospectively and risk of spontaneous abortion. Am J Epidemiol 150, 590-597.

9. Saxena DK, Singh C, Murthy RC, Mathur N, Chandra, SV (1994) Blood and placental lead levels in an Indian city: a preliminary report. Arch Environ Health 49, 106-110.

10. Irgens A, Kruger K, Skorve AH, Irgens LM (1998) Reproductive outcome in offspring of parents occupationally exposed to lead in Norway. Am J Ind Med 34, 431-437.

11. Laudanski T. Sipowicz P, Modzelewski J, Bolinski J, Szamatowicz J, Razniewska G, Akerlund M (1991) Influence of high lead and cadmium soil content on human reproductive outcome. Int J Gynecol Obstet *36*, 309-315.

12. Nishijo M, Nakagawa H, Honda R, Tanebe K, Saito S, Teranishi H, Tawara K (2002) Effects of maternal exposure to cadmium on pregnancy outcome and breast milk. Occup and Environ Med 59, 394-397.

13. Salpietro CD, Gangemi S, Minciullo PL, Briuglia S, Merlino MV, Stelitano A, Cristani M, Trombetta D, Saija A (2002) Cadmium concentrations in maternal and cord blood and infant birth weight: healthy non-smoking women. J Perinatal Med 30, 395-399.

14. *Claudia Hopenhayn, Catterina Ferreccio, Browning, Steven R, Huang Bin, Peralta Cecilia; Gibb Herman, Hertz-Picciotto Irva* (2003) Arsenic exposure from drinking water and birth weight. Epidemiology. 14, 593-602.

15. Weidner I.S, Moller H, Jenson TK, Skakkebaek NE (1998) Cryptorchidism and hypospadias in sons of gardeners and farmers. Environ Health Perspect 106,793-795.

16. Rita P, Reddy PP, Venkataram R (1987) Monitoring of workers occupationally exposed to pesticides in grape gardens of Andhra Pradesh. Environ Res 44, 1-5.

17. Zhang J, Cai W, Lee, DJ (1992) Occupational hazards and pregnancy out comes. Am J Ind Med 21, 379-408.

18. Korrick SA, Chen C, Damokosh AI, Ni J, Liu X, Cho SI, Altshul L, Ryan L, Xu X (2001) Association of DDT with spontaneous abortion: a case-control study. Ann Epidemiol 11,491-496.

19. Longnecker MP, Klebanoff MA, Zhou H, Brock JW (2001) Association between maternal serum concentration of the DDT metabolite DDE and pre-term and small-for-gestational-age babies at birth. The Lancet, 358, 110-114.

20. Arbuckle Tye E, Lin zhiqui, MERY laslie S (2001)an exploratory analysis of the effect of pesticide exposures on the risk of spontaneous abortions in an Ontario farm population. Environ Health Pers 109, 851-857.

21. Hanke Wojciech, Romitti Paul, Fuortes Laurence, Sobala Wojciech, Mikulski Marek (2003) The use of pesticides in a Polish rural population and its effect on birth weight. Int Archives Occcup Environ Health 76, 614-620.

22. Garcia AM, Fletcher, Fernando G Benavides, Erigue Orts (1999) Parental agricultural work and selected congenital malformations. Am J Epidemiol 149, 64-74.

23. Kim YH, Jung KP, Hwang TY, Jung GTW, Kim HJ, Park JS, Jim JY *et al*. (1996) Hematopoietic and reproductive hazards of Korean electronic workers exposed to solvents containing 2-bromopropane. Scand J Work Environ Health 22,387-391.

24. Pieleszek A. (1997) The effect of carbon disulphide on menopause, concentation of monamines, gonadotropins, estrogens and androgens in women. Ann Acad Med Stetin 43: 255-267, in Polish.

25. Finkova A, Simko A, Jindrichova J, Kovarik J, Preiningerova O, Klimova A, Korisko F (1973) Gynaecological problems of women working in an environment contaminated with carbon disulphide. Cesk Gynekol. 38, 535-536.

26. Hemminki K, Niemi ML (1982) Community study of spontaneous abortions: Relation to occupation and air pollution by sulfur dioxide, hydrogen sulfide and carbon disulfide. Int Arch Occup Environ Health 51: 55-61.

27. Ha E, Cho SI, Chen D, *et al.* (2002) Parental exposure to organic solvents and reduced birth weight. Arch Environ Health 57, 207-214.

28. Chen PC, Hsieh GY, Wang JD, Cheng TJ (2002) Prolonged time to pregnancy in female workers exposed to ethylene glycol ethers in semiconductor manufacturing. Epidemiology 13, 191-196.

29. Plenge-Bonig A Karmaus W (1999) Exposure to toluene in the printing industry is associated with subfecundity in women but not in men. Occup and Environ Med, 56, 443-448.

30. Alcser KH, Brix KA, Fine LJ, Kallenbach R, Wolfe RA (1989) Occupational mercury exposure and male reproductive health. Am J Ind Med 15, 517-529.

31. Cordier S, Deplan F, Mandereau L, Hemon D (1991) Paternal exposure to mercury and spontaneous abortions. Br J Ind Med 48, 375-381.

32. Picciotto Irva-Hertz (2000). The evidence that lead increases the risk for spontaneous abortion. Am J Ind Med 38, 300-309.

33. Alexander BH, Checkoway H, Van Netten G, Kaufman JD, Vaughan TL, Mueller BA, Faustman EM (1996) Paternal occupational lead exposure and pregnancy outcome. Int J Occup Environ Health 2, 280-285.

34. Markku S, Lindbohm Marja-Liisa, Anttila Ahti, Taskinen Helena, Hemminki K (2000) Time to pregnancy among the wives of men occupationally exposed to lead. Epidemiology 11,141-147.

35. Cocco P, Fadda D, Ibba A, Melis M, Tocco MG, Atzeri S, Avataneo G, Meloni M, Monni F, Flore C (2005) Reproductive outcomes in DDT applicators. Environ Res 98,120-126.

36. Regidor E, Ronda E, García AM, Domínguez V (2004) Paternal exposure to agricultural pesticides and cause specific fetal death. Occup and Environ Med 61, 334-339.

37. Salazar-Garcia F, Gallardo-Diaz E, Ceron-Mireles P, Loomis D, Borja-Aburto VH (2004) Reproductive effects of occupational DDT exposure among male malaria control workers. Environ Health Perspect 112, 542-547.

38. Patel KG, Yadav PC, Pandya CB, Saiyed HN (2005) Male exposure mediated adverse reproductive outcomes in carbon disulphide exposed rayon workers. J Environ Biol 25, 413-418.

39. Hooiveld M, Haveman W, Roskes K, Bretveld R, Burstyn I, Roeleveld N (2006) Adverse reproductive outcomes among male painters with occupational exposure to organic solvents. Occup Environ Med 63, 538-544.

40. Sallmen M, Lindbohm ML, Anttila A, Taskinen H and Hemminki K (1992) Paternal occupational lead exposure and congenital malformations. J Epidemiol and Community Health 46, 519-522.

41. Lin Shao, Syni-An Hwang, Elizabeth G Marshall and Dave Marion (1998) Does paternal occupational lead exposure increase the risks of low birth weight or Prematurity? Am J Epidemiol 148, 173-181.

42. Srivastava S, Mehrotra PK, Srivastava SP, Tandon I, Siddiqui MKJ (2001) Blood lead and zinc in pregnant women and their offspring in intrauterine growth retardation cases. J Analytical Toxicol 25, 461-465.

43. Joffe M, Bisanti L, Apostoli P, Kiss P, Dale A, Roeleveld N, Lindbohm ML, Sallmen M, Vanhoorne M, Bonde JP, Asclepios (2003) Time to pregnancy and occupational lead exposure. Occup Environ Med 60, 752-758.

44. Antilla A, Sallmen M (1995) Effects of parental occupational exposures to lead and other metals on spontaneous abortion. J Occup Environ Med 37, 915-921.

45. Sikorski R, Juszkiewicz T, Paszkowski T, Szprengier-Juszkiewicz T (1987) Women in Dental Surgeries: Reproductive Hazards in Occupational Exposure to Metallic Mercury. Int Archives Occup Environ Health 59(6): 551-527.

46. Kaste LM (1997) Occupation and reproductive health of female dentists: the relationship to nitrous oxide and amalgam (mercury) with spontaneous abortion. Diss Abstr Int Sci 57, 7489 B.

47. Henson MC, Chedrese PJ (2004) Endocrine disruption by cadmium, a common environmental toxicant with paradoxical

effects on reproduction. Exp Biol Med (Maywood). 229(5): 383-392.

48. Zhang YA-Li, Zhao Yong-Cheng, Wang Ji-Xian, Zhu Hong-Da, Liu Qing-Fen, Fan YA-Guang, War Nai-Fen, Zhao Jin-Hui, Liu Hu-Sheng, Yang Ai-Ping, Fan Ti-Qiang (2004) Effect of environmental exposure to cadmium on pregnancy outcome and fetal growth: A study on healthy pregnant women in China. J Environ Science Health (part A) 39, 2507-2515.
49. Ong CN, Phoon WO, Law HY, Tye CY, Lim HH (1985) Concentrations of lead in maternal blood, cord blood and breast milk. Arch Dis Child. 60, 756-759.
50. Kuhnert PM, Boyette DD, Watson WJ, Cefalo RC (1992) Elemental mercury exposure in early pregnancy. Obstet Gynecol 79, 874-876.
51. Gerhard I, Monga B, Waldbrenner A, Runnebaum B (1998 a) Heavy metals and fertility. J Toxicol Environ Health Part A 54, 593-611.
52. Gerhard I, Waibel S, Daniel V, Runabout B. (1998 b) Impact of heavy metals on hormonal and immunological factors in women with repeated miscarriages. Human Reprod Update 4, 301-309.
53. Lindstrom H, Luthman J, Oskarsson A, Sundberg J, Olson L (1991) Effects of long-term treatment with methyl mercury on the developing rat brain. Environ Res 56,158-169.
54. Foster WG, McMahon A, Young Lai EV, Hughes EG, Rice DC (1993) Reproductive endocrine effects of chronic lead exposure in the male cynomolgus monkey. Reprod Toxicol 7, 203-209.
55. Gerhard I, Becker T, Eggert-Kruse W, Kling K, Runnebaum B (1991) Thyroid and ovarian function in infertile women. Human Reprod 6, 338-345.
56. Mgbonyebi OP, Smothers CT, Mrotek JJ (1994) Modulation of adrenal function by cadmium salts: 2. Sites Affected by $CdCl_2$ during unstimulated steroid synthesis. Cell Biol Toxicol 10, 23-33.
57. Klages K, Sourgens H, Bertram HP, Muller C, Kemper FH (1987) Lead exposure and endocrine functions: Impact on the hypophyseal-gonadal axis and the pituitary-thyroid system. Acta Endocrinol. Suppl. 283,17-18.

58. Wiebe JP, Barr KJ, Bunkingham KD (1988). Effects of prenatal and neonatal exposure to lead on gonadotropin receptors and steroidogenesis in rat ovaries. J Toxicol Environ Health 24, 461-476.

59. Piasek M, Laskey JW (1994). Acute cadmium exposure and ovarian steroidogenesis in cycling and pregnant rats. Reprod Toxicol 8, 495-507.

60. Sildbergeld EK. (1991) Lead in bone: implications for toxicology during pregnancy and lactation. Environ. Health Perspect. 91, 63-70.

61. Al-Rasnd RA, Spangler J (1977) Neonatal copper deficiency. N Engl J Med 235,841-843.

62. Roungsipragran R, Borirug S, Herabutya Y (1999) Plasma zinc level and intrauterine growth retardation: a study in pregnant women in Ramathibodi Hospital. J Med Assoc Thai 82,178-181.

63. Rwebembera Anant Ab-Bakari, Munubhi EKD, Manji KP, Mpembeni R Philip J (2006) Relation ship between infant birth weight <2000 g and maternal zinc levels at Muhimbili National Hospital, Dar Es Salaam, Tanzania. J Tropical Pediatrics 52, 118-125.

64. Hjollund NH, Bonde JP, Ernst E, Lindenberg S, Andersen AN, Olsen J (2004) Pesticide exposure in male farmers and survival of *in vitro* fertilized pregnancies. Human Reprod 19, 1331-1337.

65. Bruoker-Davis F, Wagner-Mahler K, Delattre I, Ducot B, Ferrari P[6], Bongain A[7], Kurzenne Jean-Yves, Mas Jean-Christophe, Fénichel P and the Cryptorchidism Study Group from Nice Area (2008). Cryptorchidism at birth in Nice area (France) is associated with higher prenatal exposure to PCBs and DDE, as assessed by colostrum concentrations. Human Reproduction 23, 1708-1718

66. Garry Vincent F, Harkins Mary, Lyubimov Alex, Erickson Leanna, Long Leslie (2002): Reproductive outcome in the women of the red river valley of the north. I. The spouses of the pesticide applicators: Pregnancy loss, age at menarche, and exposure to pesticides. J Toxicol and Environ Health Part A. 65, 769-786.

67. Savitz DA, Arbuckle T, Kaczor D, Curtis KM (1997) Male pesticide exposure and pregnancy outcome. Am J Epidemiol 146, 1025-1036.

68. Potashnik G Porath A: Dibromochloropropane(DBCP) (1995) A 17 year reassessment of testicular function and reproductive performance. J Occup Environ Med 37, 1287-1292.

69. Gray LE (1992) Chemical induced alterations of sexual differentiation a review of effects in human and rodents. In: Colborn T and Clement C. Chemically induced alterations in sexual and functional development: the wildlife and human connection. Princeton, New Jersey: *Princeton Scientific publishing, 203-223,* 1992.

70. Crisp TM, Clegg ED, Copper RL, Wood WP, Anderson DG, Baetcke KP, Hoffman JL, Morrow MS, Rodier DJ, Schaeffer JE, Tourt LW, Zeerman LW, Patel YM (1998) Environmental endocrine disruption: An effects assessment and analysis. Environ Health Persp 106 (Suppl.1), 11-56.

71. Kumar Sunil (2004) Occupational Exposure Associated with Reproductive Dysfunction. J Occup Health 46, 1-19.

72. Arbuckle Tye E, Sever Lowell E (1998) Pesticide exposure and fetal death: A review of the epidemiologic literature. Crit Reviewe Toxicol 28, 229-270.

73. García Ana M (1998) Occupational exposure to pesticides and congenital malformations: A review of mechanisms, methods, and results. Am J Ind Med 33, 232-240.

74. Heinrich WL (1983) Reproductive hazards of the workplace and home. Clin Obstet Gynecol 26: 429-436.

75. Wang YL, Zhao XH (1987) Occupational health of working women in China. Asia-Pacific J Public Health 1, 66-71.

76. Kumar S, Patel KG, Gautam AK, Agarwal K, Shah BA, Saiyed HN (1999) Detection of germ cell genotoxic potential of carbon di sulphide using sperm head shape abnormality test. Hum Exp Toxicol 18, 731-734.

77. Xiao G, Pan C, Cai Y, Lin H, Fu Z (1999) Effect of benzene, toluene, xylene on the semen quality of exposed workers. Chin Med J (Engl) 112, 709-912.

78. Bukowski JA (2001) Review of the epidemiological evidence relating toluene to reproductive outcomes. Regul Toxicol Pharmacol, 33, 147-56.

79. Saillenfait AM, Robert E (2000) Occupational exposure to organic solvents and pregnancy. Review of current epidemiologic knowledge Rev Epidemiol Sante Publique, 48, 374-388 (in French).

80. Sallmen M, Lindbohm ML, Anttila A, Kyyronen P, Taskinen H, Nykyri E Hemminki K (1998) Time to pregnancy among the wives of men exposed to organic solvents. Occup and Environ Med, 55, 24-30.

81. Floris J, Logman S, de Vries Laurens E, Hemels Michiel EH, Sohail Khattak, Einarson Thomas R (2005) Paternal organic solvent exposure and adverse pregnancy outcomes: A meta-analysis. Am J Ind Med 47, 37-44.

82. Wennborg H, Bodin L, Vainio H, Axelsson G (2001) Solvent use and time to pregnancy among female personnel in biomedical laboratories in Sweden Occup Environ Med 58, 225-231.

83. Figa-Talamanca I, Petrelli G, Tropeano R, Papa G, Boccia G (2000) Fertility of male workers of the Italian mint. Reprod Toxicol, 14(4), 325-30.

84. Elliott RC, Jones JR, McElvenny DM, Pennington MJ, Northage C, Clegg TA, Clarke SD, Hodgson JT, Osman J (1999) Spontaneous abortion in the British semiconductor industry: An HSE investigation. Health and Safety Executive. Am J Ind Med 36, 557-572.

85. McMartin KL, Chu M, Kopecky E, Einerson TR, Koren G (1998) Pregnancy outcome following maternal organic solvent exposure: a meta-analysis of epidemiologic studies. Am J Ind Med 34(3), 288-292.

86. Doyle P, Roman E, Beral V, Bnrookes M (1997) Spontaneous abortion in dry cleaning workers potentially exposed to perchloroethylene. Occup Environ Med, 54(12), 848-853.

87. Logman JF, de Vries LE, Hemels ME, Khattak S, Einarson TR (2005) Paternal organic solvent exposure and adverse pregnancy outcomes: a meta-analysis. Am J Ind Med, 47, 37-44.

88. Herman-Giddens ME, Slora EJ, Wasserman RC, Bourdony CJ, Bhapkar MV, Koch GG, Hasemeir CM (1997) Secondary sexual characteristics and menses in young girls seen in office practice: a study from the pediatric research in office settings network. Pediatrics 99, 505-512.

89. Colon D Caro, Carles J Bourding, Rasario O (2000) Identification of phthalats esters in the serum of young Puerto Ricen girls with premature breast development. Environ. Health. Perspect 108, 895-900.

90. Reddy BS, Rozati R, Reddy S, Shankarappa, Reddy P, Reddy R. High plasma concentrations of polychlorinated biphenyls and phthalate esters in women with Endometriosis: a prospective case control study. Fertility and Sterility 2006; 85:775–9.

91. Kyyronen P, Taskinen H, Lindbohm M-L, Hemminki K, Heinonen O (1989) Spontaneous abortions and congenital malformations among women exposed to tetrachloroethylene in dry cleaning. J Epidemiol and Community Health 43, 346-351.

92. Hemminki K, Franssila E, Vainio H (1980) Spontaneous abortion among female chemical workers in Finland. Int Occup Environ Health 45, 123-126.

93. Bosco MG, Figa-Talamanca I, Salerno S (1987) Health and reproductive status of female workers in dry-cleaning shops. Int. Arch. Occup Environ Health 59, 295-301.

94. Ahlborg G Jr. (1988). Adverse pregnancy outcome among women working in laundries and dry cleaning shops using perchloroethylene. In: Hogstedt C, Reuterwall C, ed. Progress in occupational epidemiology. Amsterdam: Elsevier Science Publishers BV (Biomed div) 173-176.

95. Wright J M, Schwartz J, Dockery D W (2003) Effect of trihalomethane exposure on fetal development. Occup and Environ Med; 60:173-180.

96. Bonde JP, Olsen JH, Hansen KS (1992) Adverse pregnancy outcome and childhood malignancy with reference to paternal welding exposure. Scand J Work Environ Health 18,169-177.

97. Vassilev Zdravko P, Mark G Robson, Judith B Klotz (2001) Outdoor exposure to airborne polycyclic organic matter and

adverse reproductive outcomes: A pilot study Am J Ind Med 40,255-262.

98. Townsend Jean C, Kenneth M Bodner, Vanpeenen PFD, Richard D Olson, Ralph K Cook (1982) Survey of reproductive events of wives of employees exposed to chlorinated dioxins. Am J Epidemiol 115, 695-713.

99. Irgens Agot, Krüger Kirsti, Skorve Anne Helene, Irgens M Lorentz (2000) Birth defects and paternal occupational exposure. Hypotheses tested in a record linkage based dataset. Acta Obstetricia et Gynecol Scandinavica 79, 465-470.

100. Seidler Andreas, Elke Raum MD, Arabin, Birgit, Hellenbrand Wiebke, Walter Ulla, Friedrich W. Schwartz (1999) Maternal occupational exposure to chemical substances and the risk of infants small-for-gestational-age. Am J Ind Med 36:213-222.

101. Savitz Brett KM, Baird NJ, Baird NJ, Tse CK (1996) Male and female employment in the textile industry in relation to miscarriage and pre-term delivery. Am J Ind Med 30, 307-316.

102. Hourani L, Hilton S (2000) Occupational and environmental exposure correlate of adverse live-birth outcomes among 1032 US Navy women. J Occop Environ Med 42(12), 1156-1165.

103. Friedler G, (1996). Paternal exposures: impact on reproductive and developmental outcome. An overview. Pharmacol Biochem Behav 55, 691-700.

104. Jaakkola JKK, Magnus P, Skrondal A, Hwang B-F, Becher G, Dybing E (2001) Fetal growth and duration of gestation relative to water chlorination: Occup Environ Med, 58, 437-442.

105. Jensen TK, Henriksen TB, Hjollund NH, Scheike T, Kolstad H, Giwercman A, Ernst E, Bonde JP, Skakkebaek NE, Olsen J (1998) Adult and prenatal exposures to tobacco smoke as risk indicators of fertility among 430 Danish couples. Am J Epidemiol 148, 992-997.

106. Shi LM, Chia SE (2001) A review of studies on maternal occupational exposures and birth defects, and the limitations associated with these studies Occup Med 51, 230-244.

107. Chia SE, Shi LM (2002) Review of recent epidemiological studies on paternal occupations and birth defects. Occup Environ Med 59,149-155.

Environmental & Occupational Exposures (2010) *Pages 338–369*
Editors: **Sunil Kumar & R.R. Tiwari**
Published by: **DAYA PUBLISHING HOUSE, NEW DELHI**

Chapter 14

Perspectives in Reproductive Toxicity of Heavy Metals

*S.V.S. Rana**

Professor and Head,
Department of Zoology, Ch. Charan Singh University,
Meerut –250 004

ABSTRACT

The information on reproductive toxicity of environmentally significant elements described in foregoing paragraphs reviews the effects of lead, cadmium, mercury, chromium, manganese, nickel and arsenic mainly on testes and ovary of experimental animals and man. Comparatively, much attention has been paid to testicular toxicity than ovarian toxicity. Nickel, chromium, manganese are poor reproductive toxicants whereas cadmium, lead and mercury are strong reproductive poisons. Their prevalence in work environment might result in serious reproductive problems in both sexes. Moreover, combined effects of trace elements with reference to reproduction have been poorly studied. Teratogenic effects of metals further need attention. Due to widespread contamination of environment by heavy metals, endocrinal disruption seems inevitable. Reproduction and development should be on the priority of toxicologists specially those dealing with health problems related to heavy metals.

* E-mail: sureshvs_rana@yahoo.com; sureshvs.rana@gmail.com

"Toxicity of metals", one of the oldest environmental problems has acquired new dimensions today. Mining activities specially in developing countries have led to increased exposure of general public to heavy metals through ambient air, drinking water, food and consumer products. High technology development has also resulted in new products that need more metals *i.e.*, electronics, fuel cells and car exhaust technology. e-waste, together with drug waste have as emerged serious new problems. The use of metals like gallium, indium, and germanium, which are used in semiconductors, has increased steadily over the last 25 years. The e-waste problem is further augmented by the export of electronic waste from developed to developing countries. Nanotechnology can also lead to unforeseen problems caused by consumer products and combustion of material based on nanoparticles.

Environmental health problems–as well as success stories in perspectives of toxicology of metals–have been highlighted in the EEA report on Environment and Health (2005). Adverse effects of metals on human reproduction and development continue to be a demanding challenge for researchers. It is often difficult to identify the metals involved, or their sources and wide range of adverse effects. Further, there are limited data on their mechanisms of action and damage. For most metals, there is little information about quantitative dose-response relationships and no-adverse-effect exposure thresholds. Furthermore, most published studies have considered effects of a single metal, with few studies addressing combined exposure to toxic and/or essential metals–which is typical for human exposure. The possibility of synergistic or antagonistic interactions of metals and other factors need much more attention.

Metals can produce a wide variety of adverse effects on reproduction and development, influencing fertility, intrauterine growth retardation, abortions, malformations, birth defects, and developmental effects, including those on the nervous system. Although considered severe in general, the relevance of these out comes is, however, differently perceived in various social, economic, and cultural contexts. Abortion or malformations are generally more easily identified, whereas subtle effects on fertility may be less obvious. There is also a worldwide tendency to delay parent-hood, thus lengthening the preconception period for potential exposure, with possible effects on both male or female reproductive ability, as well as increasing prenatal and early postnatal cumulative exposure to toxic metals.

Metals may affect reproduction or development directly, at relatively low doses, or act indirectly through systemic toxicity, generally at higher doses. The direct toxicity can be identified as a "critical effect" on reproduction or development. With regard to occupational and environmental exposures, in contrast to experimental conditions, it is difficult to correlate specific exposures to specific effects because of the complexity of such exposures and the need to measure metals at very low levels in biological specimens.

Recently, increasing interest has been shown in the mechanisms of action of heavy metals on reproduction and development, on endocrine disruption, and oxidative stress. Endocrine disruptors (EDs) have been defined as "exogenous chemical substances or mixtures able to alter the structure or function of the endocrine system and to cause adverse effects on organisms or their progeny[1]". The importance of EDs is related to the biological hypothesis that low-level exposure to certain chemicals may contribute to endpoints such as lowering of age at menarche, impairment of semen quantity and quality, decreasing male-to- female sex ratio at birth, increasing rates of hypospadias and testicular cancer, infertility spontaneous abortions, and structural and functional congenital malformations. However, linking specific exposures to effects is often difficult because of multiple exposures, the latency of effects, and the subtle nature of some outcomes[2–4]. Some effects of EDs may be receptor-mediated and may directly interact with cellular targets[5]. Cadmium, for example, may affect steroidogenesis by mimicking or inhibiting the actions of endogenous estrogens[6]. The experimental and human investigations on EDs were reviewed by Sharpe and Irvine[7]; they concluded that few definitive studies link reproductive disorders with exposure to environmental chemicals; this may either reflect the difficulty in obtaining such data or a genuine lack of effects.

The toxicity of several metals, including iron, copper, cobalt, and lead, may be mediated through oxidant or free-radical–based mechanisms, leading to oxidative stress. These metals increase the production of reactive oxygen species, decrease the levels of glutathione and other antioxidants (including selenium and zinc), affect the protective antioxidant enzymes by interfering with the metabolism of the specific metal(s) essential for the enzyme activity (such as Cu, Zn dependent superoxide dismutase, Se-dependent glutathione peroxidase, Fe-dependent catalase), enhance cell membrane lipid peroxidation, cause apoptosis, and contribute to oxidative DNA damage. Specific contribution of these mechanisms in reproductive toxicity of metals is far from being understood. Present review is an attempt to gather all necessary information for ready reference of a reproductive toxicologist.

General Structure and Function of the Male Reproductive System

Anatomically and functionally the male reproductive system can be separated into a number of units. The testes are responsible for sperm production within the seminiferous tubules and for steroidogenesis in the interstitial Leydig cells. The production of sperm from primitive stem cell spermatogonia, through spermatocytes and spermatids, is termed spermatogenesis.

The developing germ cells are arranged in orderly layers between the base and lumen of the tubule, thus forming the seminiferous or germinal epithelium. Each germ cell is enveloped by the cytoplasmic processes of the somatic Sertoli cells, which provide both structural and metabolic support to the germ cells. Four generations of germ cells develop simultaneously within the seminiferous epithelium and their synchronous development gives rise to specific cellular associations that follow each other in a precisely defined sequence. One unit of repetition of the sequence of cellular associations is termed a cycle of the seminiferous epithelium (often abbreviated to spermatogenic cycle), whereas the individual cellular associations are referred to as stages of the cycle. The number of stages in the cycle and the duration of the stages and of the cycle itself vary according to the species and the morphological criteria used. For example the spermatogenic cycle of the rat is divided into fourteen stages, whereas in the dog, eight stages are recognized. This scheme of morphological classification of spermatogenesis into cycles and stages has now been applied to most species, providing 'road maps' for histological evaluation of spermatogenesis[8] (Figure 13.1).

While it is imperative that the toxicological pathologist has a good working knowledge of the stages of the spermatogenic cycle, it is also necessary for the toxicologist to have an understanding of the

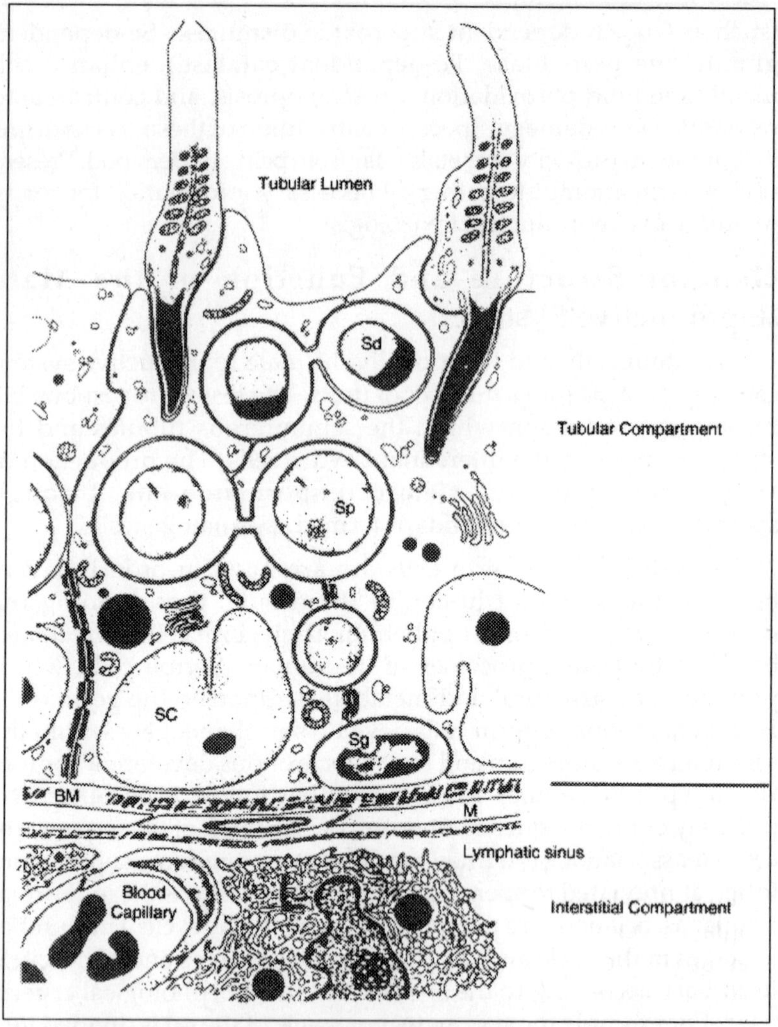

Figure 13.1: Morphology of a Mammalian Testes showing Cellular Composition of the Seminiferous Epithelium and the Interstitial Compartment

Sertoli cells (SC) cytoplasm envelops and separates layers of germ cells comprising spermatogonia (Sg), spermatocytes (Sp), round spermatids (Sd) and elongating spermatids. Myoid peritubular cells (M) surround the basal lamina of the tubule. In the interstitial compartment, testosterone secreting Leydig cells (L) surround blood capillaries and lymphatic sinuses.

dynamics and basic concepts of spermatogenesis of the species under study to be able to interpret the significance and likely consequences of toxicological disturbances. The reader is recommended to a number of comprehensive descriptions and reviews on spermatogenesis and guides for the histological recognition of the various stages of the cycle[8–10].

General Structure and Function of the Female Reproductive System

During embryonic development, the ovary forms from the mesoderm concomitant with the arrival of the primordial germ cells from the yolk sac into the gonadal ridge. In humans, germ cells arrive from the yolk sac to the gonadal ridge during the second month of gestation[11,12]. Upon contact with (or stimulation by) the germ cells, mesodermal derived cells of the gonadal ridge proliferate into primary and secondary sex cords surrounding the primordial germ cells to form follicles. It is still unclear whether the sex cords are derived from the coelomic mesothelium or arise from the mesonephros tubules, but evidence suggests the latter are a likely origin[13,14].

The sex cord cells immediately surrounding the oocyte are first to differentiate into granulosa cells, followed by differentiation of primary theca cells and fibroblasts to form the actual follicle. As follicles form, the germ cells undergo a series of mitotic divisions to increase cell number, and then undergo meiosis. In rodents, meiosis is synchronized and oocytes arrest at the diplotene stage of meiosis I about gestational day 17 to postpartum day 5[13]. In the human, meiosis is not synchronized, and mitosis and meiosis occur from gestational months 2 to 7 with arrest in the diplotene stage of meiosis I about gestational month 7[11–12]. The oocyte arrests in prophase I until conditioned to resume meiosis in preparation for fertilization.

Much of the knowledge of the growth of follicles has been derived from studies in the mouse or rat. Growth of follicles is initiated with the enlargement of the oocyte and subsequent proliferation and differentiation of the granulosa and thecal cells. These early growth phases appear to be independent of hypothalamic and pituitary signals; however, later stages of follicle growth and differentiation are dependent on hormonal signals[15]. Once growth is initiated, the oocyte rapidly increases in size[16]. Its maximum size is reached concurrently with the development of four granulosa cell layers (Figure 13. 2). Gonadotrophins begin to regulate granulosa cell growth and follicle stimulating hormone (FSH), binding to granulosa cells is associated with the cessation of growth of the oocyte[17]. FSH stimulates granulosa cell proliferation in small follicles whereas luteinizing hormone (LH) stimulates thecal cell proliferation[18]. As the number of granulosa cells increases in the follicles, the granulosa cells enter a period of rapid proliferation in which approximately 85–90 percent of them label with tritiated thymidine during a 24-hour infusion[19–20]. These granulosa cells have very low concentrations of classical oestrogen receptors and both FSH and oestradiol stimulate proliferation[21–22].

After this period of rapid proliferation, granulosa cells begin to differentiate and form a large antral space within the follicle. The granulosa cells have a high content of FSH receptors and are highly responsive to FSH[20,23,24]. These follicles also have high levels of classical oestrogen receptors[22] and androgen receptors[25]. However, they do not yet have aromatase cytochrome P-450 to convert androgens to oestrogens[26] and thus lack the ability to synthesize oestradiol *in vivo*. As these antral follicles continue to enlarge to form the pre-ovulatory or graafian follicle, the granulosa cells develop the capacity to aromatize androgens to oestrogens via aromatase cytochrome P-450. However, the granulosa cells are heterogeneous in their state of differentiation. For example, mural granulosa cells have aromatase cytochrome P-450 enzymes, and a greater abundance of LH receptors, whereas antral granulosa cells have a greater abundance of prolactin receptors.

Successful follicular maturation results in the release of the ovum; most follicles (approximately 80 per cent), however, degenerate. The process of follicular degeneration is referred to as follicular atresia and is characterized by granulosa cell death, which is morphologically and biochemically comparable to apoptosis. Thus, cell death is a common and normal histological feature in the ovary. Oocyte degeneration and fragmentation, and thecal cell apoptosis are also features of follicular atresia. However, most of the thecal cells from atretic follicles undergo hypertrophy, forming the interstitial tissue, which surrounds lacunae containing fragments of the oocyte and zona pellucida. Because hypertrophic interstitial cells are considered a primary source of ovarian androgens, follicular atresia represents an important physiological function in the ovary[27].

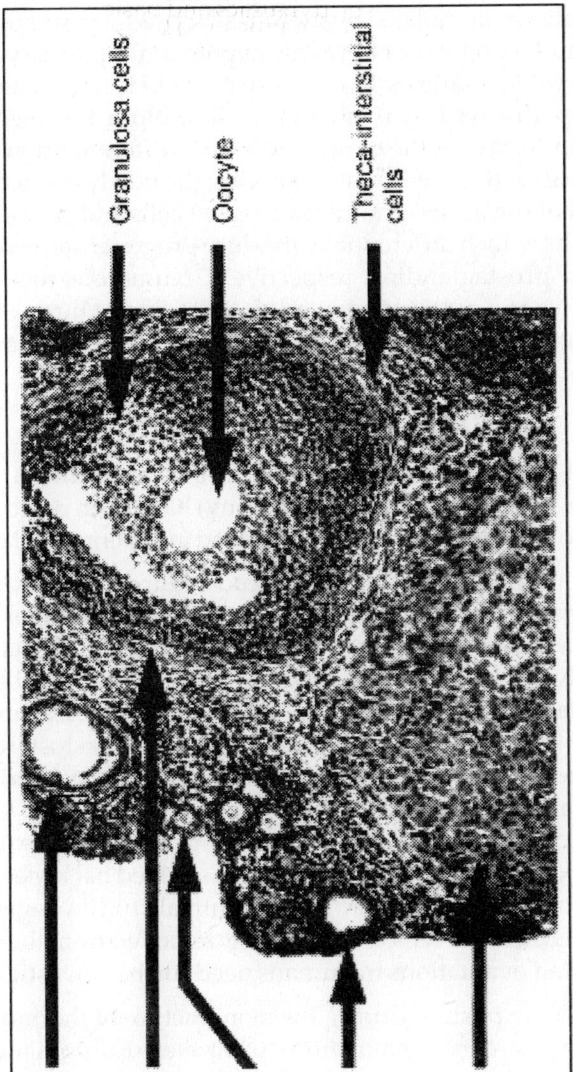

Figure 13.2: T.S. of Mammalian Ovary Showing Follicles in Various Stages of Development are Scattered Throughout

Ovulation is stimulated by the follicular production of oestradiol and the pituitary release of LH as the hypothalmic–pituitary-ovarian feedback system matures. In response to the LH surge, a new set of signaling pathways is activated in the granulosa and thecal cells, resulting in release of the ovum and a final differentiation into the Corpora Luteal (CL) cells[28]. In all species, the newly formed CL are composed of the 'large' granulosa-derived cells and 'small' thecal-derived cells, which differentially produce progesterone in response to LH and prostaglandins, respectively. Numerous neutrophils, lymphocytes and macrophages are also distributed throughout the corpora lutea and are likely to have a role in CL maintenance and regression.

General Toxicity of Heavy Metals

Metals (*e.g.* lead, mercury, cadmium, aluminium, cobalt, chromium, arsenic, lithium and antimony) have been noted to exert adverse reproductive effects in humans and in experimental animals.

More reports are available on lead-induced toxicity than on any other heavy metal. Historically, the fall of the Roman Empire has been attributed to lead poisoning[29]. Adverse effects on the reproductive capacity of men working in battery plants and exposed to toxic levels of lead have been reported[30]. In animals, lead exposure results in a dose-dependent suppression of serum testosterone and spermatogenesis[31,32]. Although testicular biopsies reveal peritubular fibrosis, vacuolation and oligospermia, suggesting that lead is a direct testicular toxicant[33], some mechanistic studies have revealed that lead exposure can disrupt the hormonal feed back mechanism at the hypothalamic-pituitary level[34]. Animal studies suggest that these effects can be reversed when lead is removed from the system. Such detailed evaluations in humans need further investigations.

Mercury exposure (during the manufacture of thermometers, thermostats, mercury vapour lamps, paint, electrical appliances and in mining) can alter spermatogenesis and has been found to decrease fertility in experimental animals. Boron (extensively used in the manufacture of glass, cements, soaps, carpets, crockery and leather products) has a major adverse reproductive effect on the testes and at the hypothalamic–pituitary axis in a manner similar to lead. Oligospermia and decreased libido were reported in men working in boric acid producing factories[35].

Cadmium, another heavy metal used widely in industries (electroplating, battery electrode production, galvanizing, plastics, alloys, paint pigments) and present in soil, coal, water and cigarette smoke, is a testicular toxicant[36]. In animal studies, cadmium has been shown to cause strain dependent severe testicular necrosis in mice[37]. Cadmium–DNA binding and inhibition of sulfydryl-containing proteins mediate cadmium toxicity directly or through transcription mechanisms, Cadmium can also induce the expression of heat shock proteins, oxidative stress response genes, and heme oxygenase induction mechanisms[38]. Further study is needed to delineate the specific gonadotoxic mechanisms involved. Clinical studies have associated cadmium exposure with testicular toxicity, altered libido and infertility.

Male Reproductive Toxicity of Specific Heavy Metals

Lead

A recent comprehensive review presents the relevant literature[39] on lead toxicity and therefore, the subsequently published reports are discussed here. Several studies amongst men occupationally exposed to lead have shown that blood lead levels equal to 400 µg/L were associated with significantly reduced semen quality with no significant effect[40,41].

Some data suggest that the reproductive effects of lead in man are reversible; a trend toward normalization was found in subjects treated with a lead-chelating agent[42,43] or after cessation of occupational lead exposure[44]. Recent data indicate that lead can adversely affect human semen quality even at blood lead levels <150µg/L[45–46]. Several experimental studies in rats, mice, rabbits, or monkeys have indicated that chronic lead exposure for at least 30 days, resulting in current blood lead levels equal to 400 µg/L, was associated with decreased intra-testicular or epididymal sperm counts, sperm production rate, sperm motility, and serum testosterone levels, although mainly without significant effect on male fertility, whereas several other studies have shown no significant reproductive effect at comparable blood lead levels[47]. A recent experimental study in rabbits[48] showed an estimated threshold for reduced sperm count at a blood lead level of 240 µg/L and even lower for several other semen characteristics (Figure 13.3).

With regard to possible mechanisms for a male-related transgenerational effect of lead, an *in vitro* study[49] has shown that lead can compete with or replace zinc in human protamine P2 (HP2), a zinc-containing protein that protects sperm DNA by binding to it during spermatogenesis. Exposure of HP2 to lead resulted in a dose-dependent decrease in the extent of HP2-DNA binding, although lead effects on sperm DNA also contributed to this effect. This may affect sperm chromatin integrity, thereby reducing sperm fertilizing capacity and causing sperm DNA damage.

The adverse effects of lead on the human reproductive function were first reported at the end of the 19th century. It was found that lead exerts direct toxic effects on male gonads and that the high fetal wastage rate observed was due to abnormal spermatogenesis. Lead is known to hamper the production and transport of sperms. The enhanced formation of reactive oxygen species plays a role in the pathogenesis of lead intoxication. Several pathogenic mechanisms have been proposed. First, ROS may be generated by auto-oxidation at a slightly alkaline pH, from the intracellular accumulation of aminolevulinic acid (ALA) and in particular from its enolaminic from[50]. Addition of 2-15 mM ALA to isolated mitochondria induces morphologic changes, loss of transmembrane potential and calcium efflux Secondly, it has been demonstrated that Pb induces lipid peroxidation when non-protein bound Fe^{++} is added to phospholipids liposomes. Third, Pb accelerates the conversion of oxyhemoglobin to methemoglobin with the production of superoxide radicals O_2 and H_2O_2. Several biochemical antioxidants (α-tocopherol and ascorbic acid) and (SOD, catalase and GSH-Px) can offset oxygen toxicity (Figure 13.4) *in vivo*[51]. Lead induced cellular toxicity can be partly ascribed to the impairment of mitochondrial respiration and partly to the uncoupling of oxidative phosphorylation. Mitochondria from lead-intoxicated animals show impaired respiration and reduced phosphorylative ability.

Mercury

A significant positive correlation between serum total testosterone, but not free testosterone, and cumulative mercury exposure were found in workers exposed to mercury vapor for an average of 10 years. No effect on fertility as assessed by the rate of live births was observed in male workers chronically exposed to mercury vapor (urinary mercury levels, 5.1-271.2 μg/g creatinine)[52].

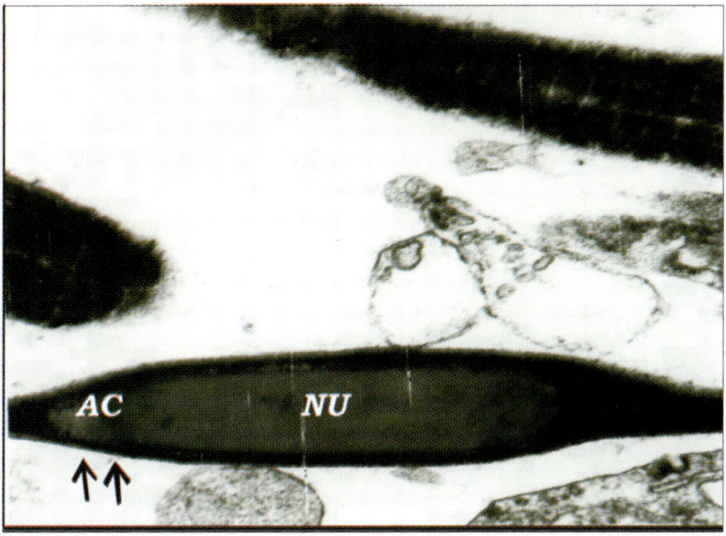

Figure 13.3: T.E.M. Observation on the Sperm of a Lead Treated Rat Shows a Sperm Head [AC: Acrosome; NU: Nucleus] (8600X)

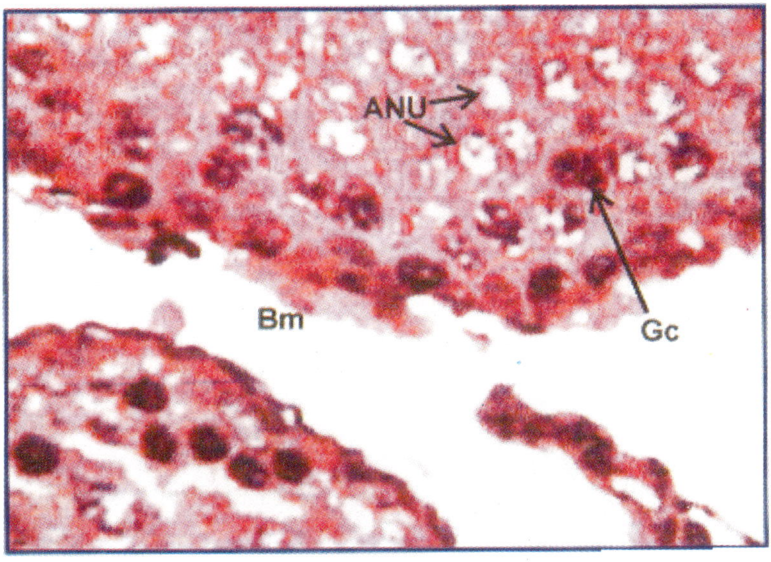

Figure 13.4: T.S. of Testis of a Rat Treated with Lead and GSH shows Seminiferous Tubules with Intact Chromatin in Germ Cells, but the Developing Spermatocytes are Apoptotic [ANU: Apoptotic Nucleus; Gc: Germ Cell; Bm: Basement Membrane]. (H/E 600X)

Exposure of mice to methylmercury or inorganic mercury (a single intraperitoneal injection of 1 mg Hg/kg body weight) resulted in adverse effects on spermatogenesis, testicular morphology and fertility, whereas DNA synthesis in spermatogonia was depressed by methylmercury and to a lesser extent, by inorganic mercury[53]. In rats, mice guinea pigs, and hamsters exposed to inorganic mercury (mercuricchloride, intraperitoneally, 1,2, or 5 mg/kg/day for 1 month), the highest doses caused testicular degeneration and cellular deformation of the seminiferous tubules and the Leydig cells in all species, whereas the lowest dosage caused testicular degeneration only in the hamster; partial degeneration was observed in the rat and mouse, and no change was noted in the guinea pig[54]. In mice exposed to inorganic mercury through drinking water (4 ppm mercuric chloride, for 12 weeks), degenerative testicular changes, decreased absolute and relative testicular weight, and decreased epididymal sperm count were found; a protective effect of zinc was reported[55]. Vitamin E, administered with mercuric chloride (1.25 mg/kg/day) by gavage for 45 days in mice, was protective against reduced epididymal sperm count, sperm motility and

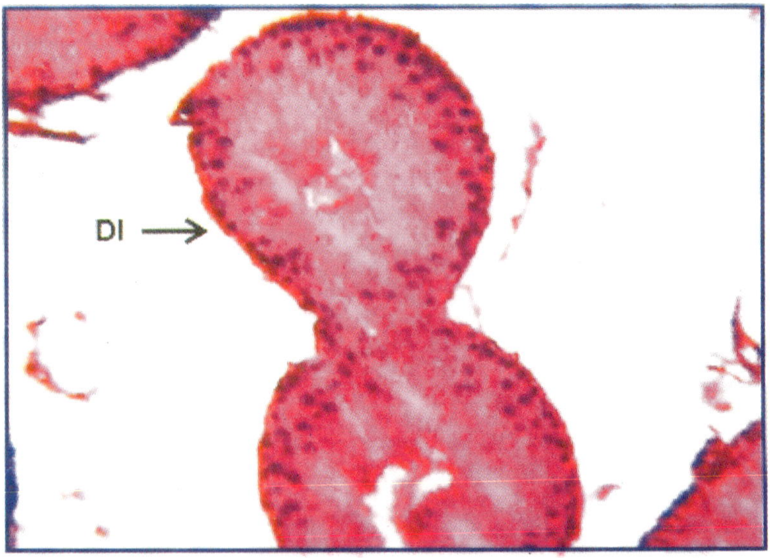

Figure 13.5: T.S. of Testis of a Rat Treated with Cadmium Shows that Cadmium can Force Seminiferous Tubule to Divide [DI: Dividing lobules]. (H/E 400X)

viability and resulted in lower concentrations of mercury in the testis, epididymis, and vas deferens[56].

Cadmium

The exquisite sensitivity of the mammalian testis to cadmium has been recognized for almost half a century. Studies by Parizek *et al.*[57] demonstrated that a single parenterally administered dose of cadmium salts, even at extremely low concentrations, leads to massive haemorrhagic necrosis of both testis and irreversible sterility. Although the time sequence of the injury differs according to the methods of administration[58] subcutaneous, intramuscular, intravenous and intraparitoneal routes, all result in characteristic testicular changes.

In men not occupationally exposed to cadmium, a significant increase in cadmium levels in blood and seminal plasma has been related to smoking habits (cigarette/years, or cigarettes/day)[41,58]. Published data on men with suspected infertility (including nonsmokers and smokers) showed a significant positive correlation between abnormal sperm morphology and blood cadmium levels[41,58,59] but not with seminal plasma cadmium levels[41]. An inverse correlation has been reported between testis size and blood cadmium[45], between sperm motility and blood cadmium[41], between semen volume and either blood cadmium[59] or seminal plasma cadmium[58,60], and between sperm concentration and sperm count with respect to blood cadmium levels[58,60]. In nonsmokers and nonconsumers of alcohol, a significant positive correlation was found between sperm DNA oxidative damage (8-OHdG level in sperm DNA) and the seminal plasma levels of both cadmium (range, 0.5-1.3 μg/L) and lead (range 5-14 μg/L) cadmium may contribute to sperm DNA oxidative damage and thereby affect semen quality[60]. A study of 297 Chinese men environmentally exposed to cadmium showed that increased chronic cadmium exposure can cause injury to the human prostate[61]. Other studies of cadmium–exposed male workers showed no significant effect of cadmium on reproductive endocrine function[62,63]. Many studies in experimental animals have shown that the mammalian testis is highly vulnerable to cadmium, which can cause germinal cell damage and testicular necrosis, possibly through a direct effect on the testicular vasculature, which may exert a secondary action by lowering testosterone production and thereby also affecting accessory genital organs, including the prostate. The acute effects reported in experimental animals injected with soluble cadmium salts include: decreased serum testosterone, a decreased size and weight of the testes, epididymis, vas deferens, prostate and seminal vesicles, decreased sperm production and motility, and suppressed libido and reproductive capacity[64–69].

A Synergistic effect of lead and cadmium on testicular injury in rats has been reported[70]. In contrast, a protective effect against male animals treated with zinc[67,70–72], selenium[73,74], or with sulfhydryl (-SH) containing compounds such as BAL, cysteine, glutathione, and metallothionein[66,75] has been reported.

Present light microscopical investigations revealed prolific apoptosis and occasional necrosis in seminiferous tubules. A number of dividing lobules were also observed. The nuclei of the basement membrane appeared normal but those of the developing spermatocytes showed marginalization of chromatin giving the nucleus a hollow appearance (Figure 13.5).

With electron microscopy, the initial alterations appear as clefts or vacuoles, some upto 500 mm in diameter, between endothelial cells[76]. These clefts enlarge and eventually split the cell junctions, exposing the subeptithelial structures. The loss of endothelial continuity is accompanied by infiltration of the interstitium by plasma fluids, as demonstrated by leakage of electron-dense tracers[76]. Eventually, the interepithelial gaps are plugged with platelets. The venuoles, capillaries and arterioles become occluded by agglutinated erythrocytes and platelets[77]. The primary effect of cadmium was on the germinal epithelium of the seminiferous tubules, and that toxic products of these degenerating cells secondarily damaged the intratesticular vasculature[67]. The fact that zinc, an essential metal in spermatogenesis, could prevent the manifestations of cadmium toxicity in the testis, indicated a direct containing enzymes or by inhibiting DNA synthesis by dividing spermatogonial elements[78,79]. It was speculated that the metal might act with both phosphate and nitrogen bases of DNA and alter the three-dimensional configurations of DNA necessary for replication and transcription. Studies have provided evidence that the initial insult of cadmium is on the endothelial cells of arterioles, venuoles and capillaries[80]. The interaction of cadmium with the endothelial cells has not been characterized at the molecular level. The clefts or vacuoles observed ultrastructurally separating endothelial cells originate between the cell junctions. An early decrease in electron density of the endothelial cytoplasm adjacent to the cell junction appears to accompany or precede the formation of intercellular clefts[81].

Manganese

Chronic dietary exposure of young rats to manganese (Mn_3O_4) for 224 days resulted in no effect on male fertility at manganese doses <1100 ppm, whereas at a dose of 3500 ppm decreased testicular weight, sperm count and serum levels of FSH and testosterone were noted together with general toxic effects[82]. In mice orally exposed to manganese acetate for 43 days, a significant decrease in sperm count and motility was observed at doses of 15.0 and 30.0 mg/kg/day, whereas there was no effect no fertility and testicular pathology[83].

Chromium

Animal exposure to high doses of chromium (III or VI) has been shown to adversely affect spermatogenesis. Chromium(IV) is considerably more toxic[84–86] and may involve oxidative stress. This is evidenced by increased lipid peroxidation in the testes, decreased sperm count, and increased abnormal sperm morphology of mice exposed to chromium (VI), each of which was partially preventable by the supplementation with the antioxidants, vitamin E and especially vitamin C[87].

Nickel

Experiments in animals have shown testicular toxicity involving oxidative stress after high doses of nickel. This is evidenced by increased lipid peroxidation, DNA damage, and apoptosis in the testes, morphological sperm head abnormalities, and decreased fertility in mice[88]; decreased DNA, RNA and total protein testes, and decreased sperm count and motility in rats[89]; and decreased absolute and relative weights of testes, epididymis, seminal vesicles and prostate gland, decreased sperm count and motility, and increased abnormal sperm morphology in mice[90]. Other reports provide some evidence that nickel may be essential for male reproduction in rat[91,92].

Arsenic

Exposure of mice and rats to high doses of inorganic arsenic can adversely affect spermatogenesis and can decrease testicular and accessory sex organ weights and serum levels of LH, FSH and testosterone[93,94]. Relative testicular weight but not of epididymal and accessory sex organ weights, a decrease in sperm count and motility, increase in abnormal sperm morphology and changes in the activities of testicular enzymes[95]. Exposure of mice to the same dose of sodium arsenite in the drinking water (4 ppm arsenic) for only 35 days produced no significant effects[93].

Female Reproductive Toxicity of Specific Heavy Metals

Lead

The investigation by Borja-Aburto *et al.*[96] on pregnant women environmentally exposed in Mexico City concluded that lead exposures in the range 100-250 μg/L could have adverse effects on pregnancy. Hertz-Picciotto[97] concluded that low-to-moderate exposures to lead can cause spontaneous abortions. In experimental animals, lead has been shown to reduce litter size, weight of offspring, survival rate, and to alter maturation of the female reproductive system or to interfere with function in the sexually mature animal[98]. Co-administration of estrogens, progesterone and lead prevented implantation failure. The normally occurring increase in estrogen and progesterone after implantation was not observed in lead-treated mice. These data suggest that lead interferes with ovarian steroid stimulation of the endometrium[99–102]. Mc Givern *et al.*[103] administered lead acetate in drinking water to Sprague-Dawley rat dams. Female offspring from lead-treated dams had significantly delayed vaginal opening, and 50 per cent of them exhibited prolonged and irregular periods of diestrous, accompanied by an absence of observable corpora lutea. Blood levels of approximately 350μg/L resulted in subclinical suppression of circulating LH and FSH and estradiol without producing overt effects on general health and menstruation[104].

Mercury

Earlier studies had noted menstrual cycle changes in women who were exposed to higher levels of mercury vapor in the workplace[105, 106]. A number of effects have been described in experimental animals exposed to mercury, including alterations in ovulation and estrous cycle. Mercury vapor exposure resulted in prolonged estrous cycles and alterations in progesterone and estradiol levels, but primarily in animals with weight loss; morphological changes in corpora lutea were also observed. However, no adverse pregnancy outcomes (rate or number of implantation sites) were observed[107]. Morphological alterations in the actuate nucleus of the hypothalamus were associated with changes in pituitary levels of FSH and LH in hamsters treated with mercuric chloride[108].

Cadmium

After acute and high-dose administration in rats, cadmium has been shown to affect various changes in the ovary and uterus or in persistent estrous and ovulation. These effects could be prevented by co-administration of selenium[109, 110].

Manganese

In rats, manganese exposure reduced the number of ovarian follicles and induced persistent corpora lutea[76]. In mice, exposure during gestation led to fetal growth retardation and encephaly[111].

Chromium

Murthy *et al.*[112] reported a number of reproductive effects (reduced number of follicles at different stages of maturation, reduced number of ova/mice, increased estrous cycle duration and histological alterations) in the ovaries of female mice exposed to potassium dichromate in drinking water for 20 days. In females of different species fed with potassium dichromate (VI), microscopic examination of the ovaries revealed no significant effects[113].

Nickel

In more recent animal studies, no effect was demonstrated on the length of the estrous cycle or microscopic structure of ovary in rats exposed to air concentrations of nickel sulfate, nickel oxide, or nickel subsulfide, ranging from 0.11 mg Ni/m^3, respectively[114–116]. Other studies on histological alterations in reproductive tissues of rats exposed to nickel or to nickel sulfate in drinking water also failed to show any relevant effect[117].

Arsenic

In the multigenerational experimental study by Schroeder and Mitchener[118], female rats continuously exposed to arsenate in drinking water did not show decreased fertility. Two other studies demonstrated that reproductive functions (included precoital internal, mating index, and fertility index) were not affected in female rats orally exposed to trivalent arsenic by gavage from 14 days before mating through gestation[119,120]. However, overt maternal toxicity (including death) was found at the same or lower doses as those leading to developmental effects[121–123].

Combined Toxicity of Heavy Metals

Since the initial discoveries that zinc administration was capable of preventing cadmium induced toxicity to testicular tissue, numerous workers have not only verified this original finding[115] but have shown that numerous other adverse effects caused by cadmium exposure may also be prevented by zinc administration. These protective effects of zinc occur in a number of species including mice rats[125] and hamsters[126] etc. It was reported that zinc may reduce or prevent cadmium toxicity by outcompeting it for key binding sites as well as by enhancing the synthesis of metal binding proteins to which cadmium binds, thereby preventing cadmium from reaching critical areas.

Protection against toxic effects of cadmium on the testes could be secured by concurrent injections of zinc[127] but also by feeding animals on selenium[128].

Recently Gunnarsson *et al.*[129] showed that pretreatment with zinc protected against Cd-induced testicular prostaglandin increase, a probable mechanism by which cadmium inhibits testosterone synthesis.

In a study in metal contaminated areas in China, interactions between cadmium and inorganic arsenic were demonstrated. Reproductive implications of concomitant exposure to cadmium and arsenic are not known at present. Interaction of lead with zinc[130], iron[131] and calcium[132] have been studied but role of these interactions in reproductive toxicity of lead is not known.

Influence of metals and metalloids on the toxicity of mercury has been extensively studied. Selenites have been shown to reduce the lethal effects of inorganic mercury in rat[133,134]. More recent studies by a number of investigators have examined the role of selenoproteins in mediating the binding and transport of mercury in blood and tissues. More recent studies[135, 136] have further examined the role of selenoprotein P in serum samples from miners with occupational exposure to mercury and porcine liver and kidney using pigs raised in an area of China with extensive mercury contamination. Effects of any such interaction on reproduction are not known.

Acknowledgements

I am thankful to my students Rajul Singh., Tanu Allen, Y. Verma, Anju Singh, Neetu Singh and Seema Sharma for helping me in the preparation of this article. Skillful assistance of Mr. Nitin Sharma is gratefully acknowledged.

References

1. Medical Research Council (1995). IEH Assessment on environmental oestrogens: Consequences to human health and wildlife. Pp. 105. University of Leicester, Leicester, England.
2. Davis, S.L. (1998). Environmental modulation of the immune system via the endocrine system. Domest. Anim. Endocrinol. 15(5): 283-289.
3. Kaplowitz PB, Slora EJ, Wasserman RC, Pedlow SE, Herman-Giddens ME. (2001). Earlier onset of puberty in girls: relation to increased body mass index and race. Pediatrics. 108(2): 347-353.
4. McKiernan JM, Goluboff ET, Liberson GL, Golden R, Fisch H. (1999). Rising risk of testicular cancer by birth cohort in the United States from 1973 to 1995. J. Urol. 162(2): 361-363.
5. Kavlock RJ, Daston GP, DeRosa C, Fenner-Crisp P, Gray LE, Kaattari S, Lucier G, Luster M, Mac MJ, Maczka C, Miller R, Moore J, Rolland R, Scott G, Sheehan DM, Sinks T, Tilson HA. (1996). Research needs for the risk assessment of health and environmental effects of endocrine disruptors: a report of the U.S. EPA-sponsored workshop. Environ. Health. Perspect. 104 Suppl. 4. 715-740.
6. Henson, M.C. and Chedrese, P.J. (2004). Endocrine disruption by cadmium, a common environmental toxicant with paradoxical effects on reproduction. Exp. Biol. Med. (Maywood). 229(5): 383-392.

7. Sharpe, R.M. and Irvine, D.S. (2004). How strong is the evidence of a link between environmental chemicals and adverse effects on human reproductive health? BMJ. 328(7437): 447-451.

8. Russell, L.D., Ettlin, R.A., Sinha Hikim, A.P. and Clegg, E.D. (1990). Histological and Histopathological Evaluation of the Testis. Cache River Press, Clearwater, FL, pp. 62-193.

9. Creasy, D.M. and Foster, P.M.D. (1991). Male reproductive system In *Handbook of Toxicologic Pathology*. W.M. Haschek and C.G. Rousseaux (eds.). Academic Press, San Diego, CA, pp. 829-887.

10. Hess, R.A. (1996). Stages: Interactive software on Spermatogenesis. Vanguard Productions Inc. PO Box 6595, Champaign, Illinois 61826-6595, USA.

11. Baker, T. (1972). Oogenesis and oavarian development. In Reproductive Biology. H. Balin and S. Glasser (eds). Excerpta Medica, Amsterdam.

12. Peters, H. and McNatty, K.P. (1980). The Ovary. Paul Elek, New York.

13. Byskov, A. (1974). Does the rete ovarii act as a trigger for the onset of meiosis? Nature. 252: 396-397.

14. Satoh, M. (1985). The histogenesis of the gonad in rat embryos. J. Anat. 143: 17-37.

15. Erickson, G.F. (1983). Primary cultures of ovarian cells in serum-free mecium as models of hormone dependent differentiation. Mol. Cell. Endocrinol. 29: 21-49.

16. Mandi, A.M. and Zuckerman, S. (1952). The growth of the oocyte and follicle in the adult rat. J. Endcorinol. 8: 126-132.

17. Richards, J.S., Ireland, J.J., Rao, M.C., Bernath, G.A., Midgley, A.R. and Reichert, L.E. (1976). Ovarian follicular development in the rat: Hormone receptor regulation by estrodiol, follicle stimulating hormone and luteinizing hormone. Endocrinology. 99: 1562-1570.

18. Wang, X., Roy, S.K. and Greenwald, G.S. (1991). *In vitro* DNA synthesis by isolated prenatal to pre-ovulatory follicles from the cyclic mouse. Biol. Reprod. 44: 857-563.

19. Pedersen, T. (1970). Cell kinetics in the ovary of the cyclic mouse. Acta Endocrinol. 64: 304-323.

20. Hirschfield, A.N. and Midgley, A.R. (1978). Morphometric analysis of follicular development in the rat. Biol. Reprod. 19: 597-605.
21. Goldenberg, R.L., Vaitukaitis, J.L. and Rose, G.T. (1972). Oestrogen and follicle stimulating hormone interactions of follicle growth in rats. Endocrinology. 90: 1492-1498.
22. Richards, J.S. (1975). Estradiol receptor content in rat granulose cells during follicular development: modification by estradiol and gonadotropins. Endocrinology. 97: 174-184.
23. Schwartz, N.B. (1974). The role of FSH and LH and their antibodies on follicle growth and on ovulations. Biol. Reprod. 10: 236-272.
24. Nimrod, A., Erickson, G.F. and Ryan, K.J. (1976). A specific FSH receptor in rat granulose cells: properties of binding *in vitro*. J. Endocrinol. 98: 56-64.
25. Zeleznik, A.J., Hillir, S.G. and Ross, G.T. (1979). Follicle stimulating hormone induced follicular development: and examination of the role of androgens. Biol. Reprod. 21: 673-681.
26. Erickson, G.F. and Hsueh, A.J.W. (1978). Stimulation of aromatase activity by follicle-stimulating hormone in rat granulose cells *in vivo* and *in vitro*. Endocrinology. 102: 1275-1282.
27. Welschen, R. (1973). Amounts of gonadotropins required for normal follicular growth in hypophy-sectiomized adult rats. Acta Endocrinol. 72: 137-155.
28. Richards, J.S. and Hedin, L. (1988). Molecular aspects of hormone action in ovarian follicular development, ovulation and luteiniztion. Ann. Rev. Physiol. 50: 441-463.
29. Gilfillan, S.C. (1965). Lead poisoning and the fall of Rome. J. Occup. Med. 7: 53-60.
30. Lancranjan, I., Popescu, H.I., Gavanescu, O., Klepsch, I. and Serbanescu, M. (1975). Reproductive ability of workmen occupationaly exposed to lead. Arch. Environ. Health. 30: 396-401.
31. Ewing, L., Zirkin, B.R. and Chubb, C. (1981). Assessment of testicular testosterone production and leydig cell structure. Environ. Health Perspect. 38: 19-27.

32. Foster, W.G., McMahon, A., Young-Lai, E.V., Hughes, E.G. and Rice, D.C. (1992). Reproductive endocrine effects of chronic lead exposure in the male cynomolgus monkey. Reprod. Toxicol. 7: 203-209.

33. Braunstein, G.D., Dahlgren, J. and Loriaux, D.O. (1978). Hypogonadism in chronically lead poisoned men. Infertility. 1: 33-35.

34. Sokol, R.Z. (1987). Hormonal effects of lead acetate in the male rat: mechanism of action. Biol. Reprod. 37: 1135-1138.

35. Weir, R.J. and Fisher, R.S. (1972). Toxicological studies on borox and boric acid. Toxicol. Appl. Pharmacol. 23: 251-262.

36. Friberg, L., Piscator, M. and Nordberg, G.F. (1974). Cadmium in the environment. 2nd Edn. CRC Press, Cleveland, OH, pp. 37-53.

37. King, L.M., Anderson, M.B., Sikka, S.C. and George, W.J. (1997). Murine strain differences in cadmium-induced testicular toxicity. The toxicologist. 36(2): 186.

38. Snow, E.T. (1992). Metal carcinogenesis: mechanistic implications. Pharmacol. Ther. 53: 31-65.

39. Apostoli P, Bellini A, Porru S, Bisanti L. (2000). The effect of lead on male fertility: a time to pregnancy (TTP) study. Am. J. Ind. Med. 38: 310-315.

40. Alexander BH, Checkoway H, Van Netten C, Kaufman JD, Vaughan TL, Mueller BA, Faustman EM. (1996b). Paternal Occupational Lead Exposure and Pregnancy Outcome. Int. J. Occup. Environ. Health. 2(4): 280-285.

41. Telisman S, Cvitkoviæ P, Jurasoviæ J, Pizent A, Gavella M, Rociæ B. (2000). Semen quality and reproductive endocrine function in relation to biomarkers of lead, cadmium, zinc, and copper in men. Environ. Health. Perspect. 108: 45-53.

42. Cullen MR, Kayne RD, Robins JM. (1984). Endocrine and reproductive dysfunction in men associated with occupational inorganic lead intoxication. Arch. Environ. Health. 39: 431-440.

43. Fisher-Fischbein, J., Fishbein, A., Melnick, H.D. *et al.* (1987). JAMA. 257-803-805.

44. Viškum S, Rabjerg L, Jørgensen PJ, Grandjean P. (1999). Improvement in semen quality associated with decreasing occupational lead exposure. Am. J. Ind. Med. 35: 257-263.

45. Jurasoviæ J, Cvitkoviæ P, Pizent A, Colak B, Telisman S. (2004). Semen quality and reproductive endocrine function with regard to blood cadmium in Croatian male subjects. BioMetals. 17: 735-743.

46. Telisman, S., Cvitkovic, P., Jurasovic, J. *et al.* (2003). 27th International Congress on Occupational Health. Iguassu Falls, Brazil.

47. Apostoli P, Kiss P, Porru S, Bonde JP, Vanhoorne M. (1998). Male reproductive toxicity of lead in animals and humans. ASCLEPIOS Study Group. Occup. Environ. Med. 55: 364-374.

48. Moorman WJ, Skaggs SR, Clark JC, Turner TW, Sharpnack DD, Murrell JA, Simon SD, Chapin RE, Schrader SM. (1998). Male reproductive effects of lead, including species extrapolation for the rabbit model. Reprod. Toxicol. 12: 333-346.

49. Quintanilla-Vega B, Hoover DJ, Bal W, Silbergeld EK, Waalkes MP, Anderson LD. (2000). Lead interaction with human protamine (HP2) as a mechanism of male reproductive toxicity. Chem. Res. Toxicol. 13: 594-600.

50. Hermes-Lina, M., Valle, V.G.R., Vercesi, A.E., Bechara, E.J.H. (1991). Damage to rat liver mitochondria promoted by δ-amino levulinic acid- generated reactive oxygen species. Connections with acute intermittent porphyria and lead poisoning. Biochem. Biophys. Acta. 1056: 57-63.

51. Pounds, J.G. and Rosen, J.F. (1986). Cellular metabolism of lead: a kinetic analysis in cultured osteoclastic bone cells. Toxicol. Appl. Pharmacol. 83: 531-545.

52. Lauwerys R, Roels H, Genet P, Toussaint G, Bouckaert A, De Cooman S. (1985). Fertility of male workers exposed to mercury vapor or to manganese dust: a questionnaire study. Am. J. Ind. Med. 7: 171-176.

53. Lee, I.P., and Dixon, R.L. (1975). Effects of mercury on spermatogenesis studied by velocity sedimentation cell separation and serial mating. J. Pharmacol. Exp. Ther. 194: 171-181.

54. Chowdhury, A.R., and Arora, U. (1982). Toxic effect of mercury on testes in different animal species. Indian. J. Physiol. Pharmacol. 26: 246-249.

55. Orisakwe OE, Afonne OJ, Nwobodo E, Asomugha L, Dioka CE. (2001). Low-dose mercury induces testicular damage protected by zinc in mice. Eur. J. Obstat. Gynecol. Reprod. Biol. 95: 92-96.

56. Rao, M.V. and Sharma, P.S. (2001). Protective effect of vitamin E against mercuric chloride reproductive toxicity in male mice. Reprod. Toxicol. 15: 705-712.

57. Parizek, J. and Zahor, Z. (1956). Nature (London). Effect of cadmium salts on testicular tissue. 177: 1036.

58. Chia SE, Xu B, Ong CN, Tsakok FM, Lee ST. (1994). Effect of cadmium and cigarette smoking on human semen quality. Int. J. Fertil. 39: 292-298.

59. Chia SE, Ong CN, Lee ST, Tsakok FH. (1992). Blood concentrations of lead, cadmium, mercury, zinc, and copper and human semen parameters. Arch. Androl. 29: 177-183.

60. Xu DX, Shen HM, Zhu QX, Chua L, Wang QN, Chia SE, Ong CN. (2003). The associations among semen quality, oxidative DNA damage in human spermatozoa and concentrations of cadmium, lead and selenium in seminal plasma. Mutat. Res. 534: 155-163.

61. Zeng X, Jin T, Jiang X, Kong Q, Ye T, Nordberg GF. (2004a). Effects on the prostate of environmental cadmium exposure–a cross-sectional population study in China. BioMetals. 17: 559-566.

62. Mason, H.J. (1990). Occupational cadmium exposure and testicular endocrine function. Hum. Exp. Toxicol. 9: 91-94.

63. McGregor, A.J. and Mason, H.J. (1990). Chronic occupational lead exposure and testicular endocrine function. Hum. Exp. Toxicol. 9: 371-376.

64. Laskey JW, Rehnberg GL, Laws SC, Hein JF. (1984). Reproductive effects of low acute doses of cadmium chloride in adult male rats. Toxicol. Appl. Pharmacol. 73: 250-255.

65. Lau IF, Saksena SK, Dahlgren L, Chang MC. (1978). Steroids in the blood serum and testes of cadmium chloride treated hamsters. Biol. Reprod. 19: 886-889.

66. Norberg, G.F. (1971). Effects of Acute and Chronic Cadmium Exposure on the Testicles of Mice, with special reference to protective effects of metallothionein. Environ. Physiol. Biochem. 1: 171-187.

67. Parizek, J. (1960). Sterilization of the male by cadmium salts. J. Reprod. Fertil. 1: 294-309.

68. Saksena, S.K. and Lau, I.F. (1979). Effects of cadmium chloride on testicular steroidogenesis and fertility of male rats. Endokrinologie. 74: 6-12.

69. Waalkes, M.P. and Rehm, S. (1994). Cadmium and prostate cancer. J. Toxicol. Environ. Health. 43: 251-269.

70. Saxena DK, Murthy RC, Singh C, Chandra SV. (1989). Zinc protects testicular injury induced by concurrent exposure to cadmium and lead in rats. Res. Commun. Chem. Pathol. Pharmacol. 64: 317-329.

71. Gunn SA, Gould TC, Anderson WA. (1966a). Loss of selective injurious vascular response to cadmium in regenerated blood vessels of testis. Am. J. Pathol. 48: 959-969.

72. Niewenhuis, R.J. (1980). Effects of cadmium upon regenerated testicular vessels in the rat. Biol. Reprod. 23: 171-179.

73. Jones, M.M., Xu, C., and Ladd, P.A. (1997). Selenite suppression of cadmium-induced testicular apoptosis. Toxicology. 116: 169-175.

74. Niewenhuis, R. and Fende, P. (1978). The protective effect of selenium on cadmium-induced injury to normal and cryptorchid testes in the rat. Biol. Reprod. 19: 1-7.

75. Gunn, S., Gould, T. and Anderson, W. (1966b). Protective effect of thiol compounds against cadmium-induced vascular damage to testis. Proc. Soc. Exp. Biol. Med. 122: 1036-1039.

76. Gabbiani, G., Badonnel, M., Matewson, S.M. and Ryan, G.B. (1974). Acute cadmium intoxication: early selective lesions of endothelial clefts. Lab. Invest. 30: 686-695.

77. Aoki and Hoffer, A. P. (1978). Re-examination of the lesions in rat testis caused by cadmium. Biol. Reprod. 18: 579-591.

78. Prohaska, J.R., Mowafy, M. and Ganther, H.E. (1977). Interactions between cadmium, selenium and glutathione peroxidase in rat testis. Chem-biol. Interactions. 18: 253-265.

79. Johnson, A.D. (1977). The influence of cadmium on the testis. In: A.D. Johnson, W.R. Gomes, and N.K. Van Demark. Eds. The testis. Academic Press, New York Pp. 565-577.

80. Gunn, S.A., Gould, T.C. and Anderson, W.A.D. (1963). The selective injurious response of testicular and epididymal blood vesicles to cadmium and its prevention by zinc. Amer. J. Pathol. 42: 685-702.

81. Fende, P.L. and Niewenhevis, R.J. (1977). An election microscopic study of the effects of cadmium chloride on cryptorchid testis of the rat. Biol. Report. 16: 298-305.

82. Laskey JW, Rehnberg GL, Hein JF, Carter SD. (1982). Effects of chronic manganese (Mn_3O_4) exposure on selected reproductive parameters in rats. J. Toxicol. Environ. Health. 9: 677-687.

83. Ponnapakkam TP, Bailey KS, Graves KA, Iszard MB. (2003). Assessment of male reproductive system in the CD-1 mice following oral manganese exposure. Reprod. Toxicol. 17: 547-551.

84. Ernst, E. (1990). Testicular toxicity following short-term exposure to tri- and hexavalent chromium: an experimental study in the rat. Toxicol. Lett. 51: 269-275.

85. Ernst, E., and Bonde, J.P. (1992). Sex hormones and epididymal sperm parameters in rats following sub-chronic treatment with hexavalent chromium. Hum. Exp. Toxicol. 11: 255-258.

86. Li H, Chen Q, Li S, Yao W, Li L, Shi X, Wang L, Castranova V, Vallyathan V, Ernst E, Chen C. (2001). Effect of Cr(VI) exposure on sperm quality: human and animal studies. Ann. Occup. Hyg. 45: 505-511.

87. Acharya UR, Mishra M, Mishra I. *et al.* (2004). Potential role of vitamins in chromium induced spermatogenesis in Swiss mice. Environ. Toxicol. Pharamcol. 15: 53-59.

88. Doreswamy K, Shrilatha B, Rajeshkumar T, Muralidhara (2004). Nickel-induced oxidative stress in testis of mice: evidence of DNA damage and genotoxic effects. J. Androl. 25: 996-1003.

89. Das, K.K. and Dasgupta, S. (2000). Effect of nickel on testicular nucleic acid concentrations of rats on protein restriction. Biol. Trace Elem. Res. 73: 175-180.

90. Pandey R, Kumar R, Singh SP, Saxena DK, Srivastava SP. (1999). Male reproductive effect of nickel sulphate in mice. BioMetals. 12: 339-346.

91. Nielsen, F.H., Yokoi, K. and Uthus, E.O. (2002). 7th International Symposium on Metal Ions in Biology and Medicine. 7: 29-33.

92. Yokoi, K., Uthus, E.O. and Nielsen, F.H. (2003). Nickel deficiency diminishes sperm quantity and movement in rats. Biol. Trace Elem. Res. 93: 141-153.

93. Pant N, Kumar R, Murthy RC, Srivastava SP. (2001). Male reproductive effect of arsenic in mice. BioMetals. 14: 113-117.

94. Sarkar M, Chaudhuri GR, Chattopadhyay A, Biswas NM. (2003). Effect of sodium arsenite on spermatogenesis, plasma gonadotrophins and testosterone in rats. Asian J. Androl. 5: 27-31.

95. Pant, N., Murthy, R.C. and Srivastava, S.P. (2004). Male reproductive toxicity of sodium arsenite in mice. Hum. Exp. Toxicol. 23: 399-403.

96. Borja-Aburto VH, Hertz-Picciotto I, Rojas Lopez M, Farias P, Rios C, Blanco J. (1999). Blood lead levels measured prospectively and risk of spontaneous abortion. Am. J. Epidemiol. 150(6): 590-597.

97. Hertz-Picciotto, I. (2000). The evidence that lead increases the risk for spontaneous abortion. Am. J. Ind. Med. 38(3): 300-309.

98. WHO (1977). Environmental Health. Criteria 3: lead. 160 pp. WHO, Geneva.

99. Jacquet, P. (1977). Early embryonic development in lead-intoxicated mice. Arch Pathol Lab Med. 101(12):641-3.

100. Wide, M. (1983). IN: Reproductive and Developmental Toxicity of Metals. (T.W. Clarkson, G.F. Nordberg, and P.R. Sagar, Eds.), pp. 343-356. Plenum Press, New York.

101. Wide, M. and Nilsson, O. (1977). Differential susceptibility of the embryo to inorganic lead during periimplantation in the mouse. Teratology. 16: 273-276.

102. Wide, M. and Wide, L. (1980). Estradiol receptor activity in uteri of pregnant mice given lead before implantation. Fertil. Steril. 34: 503-508.

103. Mc Givern R.F., Sokol R.Z. and Berman N.G. (1991). Prenatal lead exposure in the rat during the third week of gestation: long-term behavioral, physiological, and anatomical effects associated with reproduction. Toxicol. Appl. Pharmacol. 110(2): 206-215.

104. Foster, W.G. and Younglai, E.V. (1991). An immunohistochemical study of the GnRH neuron morphology and topography in the adult female rabbit hypothalamus. Am. J. Anat. 191(3): 293-300.

105. De Rosis F, Anastasio SP, Selvaggi L, Beltrame A, Moriani G. (1985). Female reproductive health in two lamp factories: effects of exposure to inorganic mercury vapour and stress factors. Br. J. Ind. Med. 42: 488-494.

106. Sikorski R, Juszkiewicz T, Paszkowski T, Szprengier-Juszkiewicz T. (1987). Women in dental surgeries: reproductive hazards in occupational exposure to metallic mercury. Int. Arch. Occup. Environ. Health. 59: 551-557.

107. Davis BJ, Price HC, O'Connor RW, Fernando R, Rowland AS, Morgan DL. (2001). Mercury vapor and female reproductive toxicity. Toxicol. Sci. 59: 291-296.

108. Lamperti, A.A. and Niewenhuis, R. (1976). The effects of mercury on the structure and function of the hypothalamo-pituitary axis in the hamster. Cell Tissue Res. 170: 315-324.

109. Saksena, S.K. (1982). Cadmium: its effects on ovulation, egg transport and pregnancy in the rabbit. Contraception. 26: 181-192.

110. Watanabe, T., Shimada, T. and Endo, A. (1979). Mutagenic effects of cadmium on mammalian oocyte chromosomes. Mutat. Res. 67: 349-356.

111. Sánchez DJ, Domingo JL, Llobet JM, Keen CL. (1993). Maternal and developmental toxicity of manganese in the mouse. Toxicol. Lett. 69: 45-52.

112. Murthy, R.C., Junaid, M. and Saxena, D.K. (1996). Ovarian dysfunction in mice following chromium (VI) exposure. Toxicol. Lett. 89(2): 147-154.

113. Elbetieha, A. and Al-Hamood, M.H. (1997). Long-term exposure of male and female mice to trivalent and hexavalent chromium compounds: effect on fertility. Toxicology. 116(1-3): 39-47.

114. NTP (1996a). NTP Technical report on the toxicology and carcinogenesis studies on nickel oxide. (CAS NO. 1313-99-1). National Institute of Health. NTPTRS No. 451.

115. NTP (1996b). NTP technical report on the toxicology and carcinogenesis studies of nickel subsulphide. (CAS No. 12035-72-2) National Institute of Health. NTP-TRS No. 453.

116. NTP (1996c). NTP Technical report on the toxicology and carcinogenesis studies of nickel suphate hexahydrate (CAS No. 10101-97-0) National Institutes of Health. NTP-TRS No. 454.

117. Obone E, Chakrabarti SK, Bai C, Malick MA, Lamontagne L, Subramanian KS. (1999). Toxicity and bioaccumulation of nickel sulfate in Sprague-Dawley rats following 13 weeks of subchronic exposure. J Toxicol Environ Health A. 57(6): 379-401.

118. Schroeder, H.A. and Mitchener, M. (1971). Toxic effects of trace elements on the reproduction of mice and rats. Arch. Environ. Health. 23: 102-106.

119. Holson JF, Stump DG, Ulrich CE, Farr CH. (1999). Absence of prenatal developmental toxicity from inhaled arsenic trioxide in rats. Toxicol. Sci. 51(1): 87-97.

120. Holson JF, Desesso JM, Jacobson CF, Farr CH. (2000b). Appropriate use of animal models in the assessment of risk during prenatal development: an illustration using inorganic arsenic. Teratology. 62(1): 51-71.

121. Holson JF, Stump DG, Clevidence KJ, Knapp JF, Farr CH. (2000a). Evaluation of the prenatal developmental toxicity of orally administered arsenic trioxide in rats. Food Chem. Toxicol. 38(5): 459-466.

122. Nemec MD, Holson JF, Farr CH, Hood RD. (1998). Developmental toxicity assessment of arsenic acid in mice and rabbits. Repod. Toxicol. 12(6): 647-658.

123. Stump DG, Holson JF, Fleeman TL, Nemec MD, Farr CH. (1999). Comparative effects of single intraperitoneal or oral doses of sodium arsenate or arsenic trioxide during in utero development. Teratology. 60(5): 283-291.

124. Gunn, S.A., Gould, T.C. and Anderson, W.A.D. (1968). Selectivity of organ response to cadmium injury and various protective measures. J. Pathol. Bacteriol. 96(1):89-96.

125. Schroeder, H.A. (1967). Cadmium, chromium and cardiovascular disease. Circulation. 35: 570-582.

126. Ferm, V.H. and Carpenter, S. (1968). The relationship of cadmium and zinc in experimental mammalian teratogenesis. Lab. Invest. 18(4): 429-432.

127. Mason, K.E., Young, J.O. and Broww, J.E. (1964). Effectivers of selenium and zinc in protecting against cadmium induced injury of the rat testis. Anat. Rec. 148: 309.

128. Kar, A.B., Das, R.P. and Mukerji, F.N.I. (1960). Prevention of cadmium induced changes in the gonads of rat by zinc and selenium- a study in antagonism between metals in the biological system. Proc. Natl. Instit. Sci. India B 126: Suppl. 40.

129. Gunnarsson D, Svensson M, Selstam G, Nordberg G. (2004). Pronounced induction of testicular PGF (2 alpha) and suppression of testosterone by cadmium-prevention by zinc. Toxicology 200: 49-58.

130. Goyer, R.A. (1997). Toxic and essential metal interactions. Annu. Rev. Nutr. 17: 37-50.

131. Mahaffey, K.R. (1981). Nutritional factors in lead poisoning. Nutr. Rev. 39: 353-362.

132. Oteiza, P.I., Mackenzie, G.G. and Verstraeten, S.V. (2004). Metals in neuro-degeneration: involvement of oxidants and oxidant-sensitive transcription factors. Mol. Aspects Med. 25: 103-115.

133. Groth, D.H., Vignati, L., Lowry, L. *et al.* (1973). In: Trace substances in environmental health-Vi. (D.D. Hemphill, Ed.), pp. 187-189. University of Missouri Press, Columbia.

134. Groth, D.H., Stettler, L. and Mackay, G. (1976). In: Effects and

dose response relationships of toxic metals. (G.F. Nordberg, Ed.). pp. 527-543. Elsevier, Amsterdam.

135. Chen C, Yu H, Zhao J, Li B, Qu L, Liu S, Zhang P, Chai Z. (2006a). The roles of serum selenium and selenoproteins on mercury toxicity in environmental and occupational exposure. Environ. Health. Perspect. 114(2): 297-301.

136. Chen C, Qu L, Zhao J, Liu S, Deng G, Li B, Zhang P, Chai Z. (2006b). Accumulaiion of mercury, selenium and their binding proteins in porcine kidney and liver from mercury-exposed areas with the investigation of their redox responses. Sci. Total Environ. 366: 627-637.

Environmental & Occupational Exposures (2010) *Pages 370–381*
Editors: **Sunil Kumar & R.R. Tiwari**
Published by: **DAYA PUBLISHING HOUSE, NEW DELHI**

Chapter 15

Household Detergents: Their Toxic Potential–Possible Reproductive Effects

*Jaimala Sharma**

Department of Zoology,
University of Rajasthan Jaipur – 302 004

ABSTRACT

Dishwasher detergent, an item of every household and daily use, consists of several chemicals. When washed properly, no harm appears, rather they keep in proper cleaning and sterilization of the utensils. But if used carelessly, potential harm can be caused to the human body, which depends upon route of exposure, type and amount of detergent. Eye and skin irritation are their well-known effects. Their chronic ingestion in small amounts can also cause toxicity in human beings and might affect vital organs including reproductive system of the body.

Gone are the days when utensils were cleaned by using ash of burnt coal or wood. Ash was used for cleaning hands also. In several parts of the world clay was used for bathing and washing of clothes.

* E-mail: sharma_jaimala@yahoo.co.in

Later on soaps, which are esters of fatty acids with alkali emerged as popular cleaning agents. In India it was 7th decade of 20th Century when detergents took over the market of towns. A number of companies marketed various products of detergents for washing of clothes and utensils. In the present time dishwash and other detergents can be seen even in the village households. They are essential part of life in upper and middle class kitchens. Dishwash detergents are available in three forms: (i) Powder (ii) Cake and (iii) Liquid. Liquid detergents are more popular in developed countries where dishwashers are frequent in use. In India cake and powders are more common. Several international, national and local brands of detergents are easily available here.

Detergents are formulations designed to have cleaning properties. Detergents consists of surfactants, builders, boosters, fillers and auxillary compounds. Surfactants mainly include linear alkyl benzene sulfonates (LAS), Alcohol ethoxylates, alkyl phenol exthoxylates and sulfates of alcohol and alcohol ethers. Linear alkyl benzene sulphonates and soaps are used in sizable quantities in India. They constitute 15–30 per cent of the total weight of detergent. Builders constitute 5–30 per cent weight of a detergent. Sodium tripolyphosphate, Trisodium citrate, Sodium nitriloacetate and Zeolite A are major builders used. Fillers that are commonly used are dolomite, China clay, talc and Sodium chloride. They constitute 40–80 per cent of the detergents weight. Auxillaries are colours, perfumes, enzymes, brightners etc. and are present in a very small quantity. Brightners, whiteners and enzymes are called boosters.

Larger amounts of detergents are released in the ecosystem every year. Their consumption is increasing. First of all people in USA started facing problems. Sewage treatment problems begun to arise and foaming problems were experienced on rivers. Benzene was being discharged into the water and was found to be resistant to biodegradation by bacteria due to branched alkyl chain. Then they switched to another surfactants like LAS and alkyl phenol ethoxylates (APE), which are biodegradable and mainly remain in sewage sludge. Soaps, which have C_{12} to C_{18} carbons in chain are readily degraded by the microbes. Similarly fatty acid esters, and alcohol ether sulphates are also biodegradable[1–5].

Despite use of biodegradable detergents, detergents can be a serious environmental problem throughout the world including water pollution by them[6]. They are affecting aquatic ecosystems adversely by causing eutrophication and toxicity to the flora and fauna of the water bodies. Detergents contain Nitrogen and Phosphorus, which is added to the soil and aquatic ecosystems through the drainage of sewage water. It causes overgrowth of some blue green and green algae, which affects the taste and colour of the water. Dead and decomposing algal blooms cause mortality of animals living in the water body[7]. According to WHO publication on their toxicity almost all the kinds of animals are affected. They suffer from acute as well as chronic toxicity. Even those animals, which are not aquatic but drink the polluted water, were found to be affected[8–11].

Detergents when present in small quantity supply of Nitrogen and Phosphorus increases in the soil and crop improves, chronic exposure kills soil microorganisms, and makes it impermeable to water. Porosity of the soil disappears. High dose of detergents hamper seed germination, plant growth and yield of crop plants also decreases. Major source of Phosphorus is Sodium tripoly phosphate (STPP), which is non-toxic to aquatic biota[12].

There are several reports when animals suffered acute toxicity, or death after detergent exposure. Dishwash detergents are common item of household use. The American Association of Poison Control Centre has recorded many exposures to household cleaning substances. According to the record, largest number of occurrences of poisoning in 1993 was due to cleaning products. One million poisonings in Canada each year were due to household cleaner ingestion. Some were fatal. Thousands of children and adults are permanently disfigured or injured through contact with chemicals in the home each year. Cleaners included toilet cleaner, laundry and dishwash detergents, floor cleaners and many more home cleaners. Most of the dish wash detergents contain Chlorine in a dry form that is highly concentrated. Dishwash liquids are labeled "Harmful if swallowed". Each time you wash your dishes, some residue is left on them, which accumulates with each washing. Your food picks up part of the residue, if your meal is hot when you eat it. According to the National Research Council of USA, no toxic information is available for more than 80 per cent of the chemicals in everyday products. They are not tested for acute, chronic, reproductive or mutagenic effects or for their effects on children.

In our laboratory we have conducted toxicity tests for two selected dishwash bars (cakes). A very small amount 0.001 per cent, 0.01 per cent, 0.02 per cent, 0.04 per cent and 0.05 per cent was given to *Swiss albino mice* by gastric intubation daily for 30 days, 60 days and 90 days. Detergent was given in the form of aqueous solution at the rate of 0.02 ml per day. The dose of detergent was selected on the basis of residual amount of detergents left on utensils in one meal of Indians (one full plate, two small bowls and a glass) in the form of per kg body weight and then calculated for mouse accordingly.

The results showed that at all the concentrations used animal weight increased to a great extent (20 per cent–40 per cent) in all the groups; changes in the weight of all the organs were significant. Testes were reduced in size, while adrenal gland increased in size. Long-term treatment affected the brain weight. TSH and T_4 levels in the blood also declined. The effects were more prominent after 90 days treatment. Liver was also affected. LDH, acid and alkaline phosphatase activity and GOT and GPT activity in the serum is found to be affected. Histological damage was also there. Various blood parameters were affected adversely. Haemoglobin content of the blood was reduced[13]. Their effect on selected crop plants like, Pea, Moth, Moong and Gram was also studied. It was observed that at lower concentration *i.e.*, at 0.025 per cent and 0.05 per cent, rate of seed germination and plant growth was good at initial stages. At higher concentrations up to 0.4 per cent germination and plant growth rate both were not good. After yielding the seeds at maturation, if was observed that not only the growth of the plants was affected adversely, the yield per plant was also less and of poor quality in all the four types of crops[14].

Synthetic detergents are toxic to fish in concentration between 0.4 and 400 mg/l. Gill damage is most obvious acute toxic effect. The cause of death may be asphyxiation. Sublethal effects include growth retardation, altered feeding behaviour and inhibition of chemoreceptor organs. Invertebrates and their development are also sensitive to detergents[15]. Nitriloacetic acid (NTA), which is a builder, has caused cancer in the intestinal tract of rats, because of its mutagenic activity[16].

Human skin is sensitive to dish wash detergents. Kein *et al*[17] studied effect of a regular dish wash detergent on human hands. Human hands were exposed to 0.05 per cent solution of a popular dish wash detergent for 15 minutes at 37°C thrice daily. It was observed that within two weeks 13 out of 18 volunteers developed transdermal water loss showing signs of itching, dryness, smarting etc. It shows that very small doses of dish wash detergents can cause skin lesions in substantial proportion of individuals. In some cases they can cause allergy also.

Aqueous cleaners of metal degreasing agents contain linear alkyl benzene sulphonates, alkyl phenol exthoxylates or alcohol ethoxylates, builders (such as hydroxides, phosphates or silicates) surfactants (such as EDTA or NTA) anti corrosive agents (such as ethanolamines) solvents (such as glycol ethers or d-limonene) and other special additives. Generally sold as concentrations, they are typically diluted 3 to 20 times in water, leading to solution containing only a few constituents. The cleaning efficiency depends on physicochemical phenomenon such as wetting, solubilization, emulsification, dispersion, sequestration and saponification[18]. It is enhanced by thermal and mechanical energy. Aqueous cleaners are generally believed to present a low risk to workers health and to the environment. However, some anionic surfactants and strong alkalis are skin and eye irritants, ethanolamines are allergens and several glycol ethers of Ethylene glycol are systemic toxicants that are closely absorbed through the skin. Alkylphenol ethoxylates degrade into persistent and toxic compounds[18].

Surfactants are the chemicals, which are studied commonly for their toxic effects. Even their products after biodegradation are studied for their toxicity and were found harmful. Although all the surfactants are not biodegradable Perani *et al*[19] classified surfactants into three categories:

1. Biocompatible and non-apoptogenic.
2. Surfactants triggering an apoptotic singal without inducing cell necrosis
3 Surfactants triggering an apoptotic signal at low concentrations and destroying the cells by necrosis at higher concentration. The necrosis inducing surfactants also have haemolytic properties.

Oral administration of a liquid dishwash detergent containing anionic surfactant was performed by Scailteeur *et al*[20] on rats. They were unable to observe any microscopic histopathological changes when rats were treated with 2.5 per cent weight wise given for 13 weeks. Peterson[21] also could not detect any adverse systemic effects on haematological parameters. He recorded slight skin irritation at the site of application. Morphology of human blood platelets is also affected by detergents. The platelets showed prelytic, lytic and complete platelet lysis. The cells initially deformed in shape to spiculate disc and finally to a stretched and flat form. Their response to collagen and ADP fibrinogen was also inhibited[22].

Liver is also affected by detergents and their components. Arribus and Castano[23] studied effects of three families of detergents *viz.* Non-ionic–(Triton X-100), Ionic (SDS) and Zwitterionic (CHAPS) on the peptidase activities of the multicatalytic proteinase from rat liver. They observed differential effect of ionic and non-ionic detergents. Triton-X inhibited chymotrypsin and peptidoglutamyl peptide hydrolyzing activities. Nicotinamide deamidase from rabbit liver is inhibited by detergents and thyroxine[24]. Conjunctival cells are affected by various detergents[25]. Benzyalkonium chloride induces corneal epithelial cell dysfunction that can damage the corneal epithelial barrier even at concentration as low as 0.001 per cent and for exposure to over 30 minutes. Corneal epithelium is also affected by detergents[26].

Detergents affect DNA thus are mutagenic also[27]. Fichorava *et al*[28] observed effects of monoxynol-9, benz alkonium chloride, Sodium dodecyle sulphate and Sodium monolourate for their activity against human sperm, HIV and capacity to induce an inflammatory response in human vaginal epithelial cells and rabbit vaginal mucosa. Messinger *et al*[29] found alkyl polyglycosides which are non-ionic surfactants, cause fetotoxicity and teratogenicity.

Several detergents and their products for eg. Nonyl phenol (NP), which is an intermediate from microbial transformation of detergents used throughout the world. Nonyl phenol shows acute toxicity and mimics important hormones resulting in the disruption of several processes by interfering with the signals that control overall physiology of the organism. Organisms like algae, which are on the first level of trophic chain are able to significantly bioaccumulate nonylphenol[30]. These organisms affect the growth of crustaceans and also the hormone levels and metabolic enzymes, which are at the top of the trophic level. Borelli[31] reported that NP is an endocrine disruptor and increases incidence of endocrine dysfunction in several organisms. NP also affects their progeny. It can affect development of immune system and can cause autoimmune diseases. NP affects reproductive system and may be responsible for oligospermia, sperm characteristics, testicular atrophy, increase in weight and proliferation of vaginal epithelium. During critical stages of pregnancy damage to the foetus may be irreversible.

Male fish in detergent contaminated water is reported to express female characteristics, turtles are sex reversed by polychlorinated biphenyls (PCBs), psuedohermaphroditic offsprings are produced by polar bears and seals in contaminated water have an excess of uterine fibroids. In women and wild life also effects of endocrine disruptors can be seen[32]. According to Freyberger and Scholz[33] the detergents, which affect humans and wild life adversely, most likely disturb ligand receptor interactions and/or modification of the receptor protein. Some of the detergents have shown antiandrogenic effects of their components in *in vitro* studies conducted by Freyberger and Scholz[33]. NP is also an uncoupler of oxidative phosphorylation at very low doses suggesting that preferential target of NP are mitochondria[34, 35]. LAS affect activity of respiratory enzymes. When Lactate debydrogenase activity was studied in the gills of a catfish, *Heteropneustus, fossilis*, after 48 hours of LAS exposure, it was strongly increased and aerobic part of metabolism decreased, suggesting influence of LAS[36]. LAS also increase mucous secretion in *Cirrhinia mrigala*[37].

NP competitively inhibits the binding of 17-beta estradiol to estrogen receptor[38]. Serum concentration of T_4 hormone was also found to be decreased in dose dependent manner and serum TSH level was significantly increased. They also observed statistically significant decrease in ovarian weight of female rats treated with Diethylstilbestrol. Diethylstilestrol is found to alter estreous cyclicity in prepubertal female rats. Non-ionic detergents solubilize thyroid peroxidase, which is an intergral membrane protein[39]. 5-nucleotidase which is a membrane enzyme, obtained from pig thyroid cannot be solubilized by TritonX-100, Sodium deoxycholate and Saponin because it is strongly bound to the membrane[40].

Testicular acid and alkaline phosphatase activity in the testes of *Heteropneustus fossilis* in also affected by LAS as per Trivedi *et al*[41–42] (2001). LAS increases acid phosphatase activity, which is suggestive of gross necrosis and dysarchitecture. Decreased activity of alkaline phosphatase indicates reproductive impairment in the fish.

Chronic exposure to detergents affects adrenal glands also. Deevecerski *et al*[43] studied effects of chronic detergent exposure on volumetric and histochemical features of the glomerular zone of adrenal glands in albino rats. They observed that levels of RNA, neutral lipids, triglycerides and phospholipids increased in corticocytes of glomerular zone, while DNA content was decreased. According to them it may be due to onset of the repairing process, as complete neuroendocrine system is affected. Thalamic structures remained activated throghout the exposure as well as the hypophysis. Bovine adrenal chromaffin cells were affected by NP exposure in an experiment conducted by Liu *et al*[44]. NP which also has estrogenic activities is also an inhibitor of endoplasmic reticulum Ca^{2+} ATPase in bovine adrenal chromaffin cells. NP suppressed the Ca^{2+} signalling coupled with Nicotinic acetylcholine receptors and voltage operated Ca^{2+} channels in a dose dependent manner.

References

1. Kravetz L., Salanitro J.P., Dorn P.B. and Guin K.F. (1991) "Influence of hydrophobe–type and extent of branching on environmental response factors of non-ionic surfactants": J.Am. Oil Chem. Soc. 68, 610.
2. Ginkel C.G. Van (1995) "Biodegradability of Cationic Surfactants" in "Biodegradability of Surfactants" Karsa D.R. and Porter M.R. (Eds). Blackie Academic and Professional 183-203.
3. Steber, J., Berger H. (1995) "The biodegradability of anionic surfactants" In "Biodegradability of Surfactants", Karsa D.R. and Porter M.R. (Eds.) Blackie Academic and Professional 134-182.
4. Gode P., Guhl W., Steber J. (1987) "Environmental Compatibility of fatty acid, alphasulfomethyl esters". Fat. Sci Technol, 89: 548–552.
5. Jones F.W. and Westmoreland D.J. (1998) Degradation of nonyl-phenol ethoxylates during the composting of sludges from wool scour effluents. Environ. Sci. Technol. 32, 2623–2627.

6. Roozen I.T.M. (1997) who are really purchasing environmentally friendly detergents? J. Consumer Strd. Home Eco. 21, 237–245.

7. Singh J., Chawla, G. and Viswanathan P.N. (1990) Detergent pollution and aquatic flora. J. Scientific and Industrial Res. 49, 350–353.

8. World Health Organization (1996) Linear alkyl benzene sulfonates and related compounds. International Programme on Chemical Safety, Environmental Health Criteria 169, United Nations Environment Programme, ILO and WHO Publishers, Geneva.

9. Patokar P.L. (1992) Acute, Subacute and chronic toxicity data on anionics. In "Anionic surfactants, Biochemistry, Toxicology, Dermatology". II ed. (C. Gloxhuber and K. Kunstber eds), Surfactant Science Series, Vol. 43: Marecl Dekker Inc., New York, 81-116.

10. Yeh D.H., Penell K.D. and Pavlostathis S.G. (1998). Toxicity and biodegradability screening of non-ionic surfactants using sediment derived methanogenic consortia. Water Science and Technology 38(7), 55–62. 68.

11. Scott M.J. and Jones M.N. (2000) The biodegradation of surfactants in the environment. Biochemika et Biophysica Acta (BBA)–Biomembranes 1508(1-2): 235–251.

12. Lewis M.A. (1990) Chronic Toxicity of surfactants and detergent builders to algae: a review and risk assessmant. Ecotoxicol, Environ Sefty 20, 123–140.

13. Jaimala, Sharma K., Pathak T. and Bhardwaj N. (2008) Toxic effects of dishwash detergents on germination and growth of selected leguminous crop plants (In Press).

14. Jaimala, Sharma K., Pathak T. and Bhardwaj N. (2008), Toxicity of selected dishwash detergents in *Swiss albino mouse*. (In Press).

15. Abel PD (1974) Toxicity of Synthetic detergents to fish and aquatic invertebrates, J. Fish Biol. 6(3): 279–298.

16. Dwyer M., Yeoman S., Lester, J.N. and Petry R. (1990). A review of proposed non-phosphate detergent builders, utilization and environmental assessment. Environmental Technology 11, 263–294.

17. Kein G., Gubauer G., Fitsch P. (2006) The influence of daily diswashing with systhetic detergent on human skin. Brit. J. Dermatol. 127(2): 131-137

18. Lavoue J, Begin D, Geerin M. (2003) Technical Occupational Health and Environmental aspects of metal degreasing with aqueous cleaners, Ann. Occup. Hyg., 47(6): 441–459.

19. Perani A., Gerardin C., Stacey G., Infante MR, Vinardell P., Rodehuser L., Selve C, Maugras M. (2001) Interactions of surfactants with living cells. Induction of apoptosis by detergents containing a beta lactam moiety. Amino acids 21(2): 185–194.

20. Scaitlteur V., Maurer JK, Walker AP, Colvin G. (1986) Subchronic oral toxicity testing in rats with a liquid hand dishwashing detergent containing anionic surfactants. Food Chem. Toxicol. 24(2): 175-181

21. Petersen D.W. (1988) Subchronic percutaneous testing of two liquid hand dishwashing detergents: Food. Chem. Toxicol. 26(9): 803–806.

22. Shiao Y.J., Chen J.C., Wang C.T. (1989) The solubilization and morphological change of platelets in various detergents, Biochim. Biophys. Acta, 980(1): 56–68.

23. Arribas J. and Castano J.g. (1990) Kinetic Studies of the differential effect of detergents on the peptidase activites of multicatalytic proteinase from rat liver J. Biol.Chem. 265(23): 13969-13973.

24. Kirchner J., Watson J.G., Chaykin S. (1965) Nicotinamide deaminase form rabbit liver, 241(4): 953.

25. Piscella P.J. Debbarch C., Harnard P, Geuzot (2004), Conjunctival proinflammatory and proapoptotic effects of latanoprost and preserved and unpreseved timolol: an *ex vivo* and *in vivo* study. Invest. Opthalmol. 45(5): 1360–1368.

26. Parikh CH and Edclhouser HF (2003) Ocular surgical pharmacology: Corneal endotheliol safety and toxicity, Curr. Opin. Opthalmol. 14(4): 178–185.

27. Lleres D. Weibel JM, Heissler D, Zuber C, Duportail G., Mely Y. (2004) Dependence of the cellular internalization and

transfection efficiency on the structure and physico-chemical properties of cationic detergent/DNA/liposomes. J. Gene Med. 6(4): 415–28.

28. Fischorava RN, Bajpai M, Chandra N, Hsiu JG, Spangler M, Ratnam V., Doncel GF (2004) Interleukin IL-1, IL-6, and IL–8 predic mucosal toxicity of vaginal microbicidal contraceptives. Biol. Reprod. 71(3): 761–769.

29. Messinger M., Aulman W., Kleber M, Koehl W (2007) Investigations on the effects of alkyl polyglucosides on development and fertility. Food Chem. Toxicol. 45(8): 1375–82.

30. Correa–Reyes G., Viana M.T., Marquez–Rocha F.J., Kicea A.F., Ponce E., Vazquez–Duhalt R. (2007) Nonylphenol algal bioaccumulation and its effect through the trophic chain, Chemosphere 68(4): 662-670.

31. Borelli I. (2007) Endocrine disruptors, Literature review on toxicology and application field in occupational medicine. G. Ital. Med. Lav. Ergen 29(3 suppl.): 526–528.

32. MC Lachlan J.A., Simpson E., Martin M. (2006) Endocrine disrupters and female reproductive health. Best Pract. Res. Clin. Endocrinol, Metab, 20(1): 63–75.

33. Freyberger A., Scholz G. (2004) Endocrine toxicology–Contribution of *in vivo* methods to the 3R concept. ALTEX, 21 (Suppl.3): 20-27

34. Bragadin M. Perim G. Iero A., Manente S., Rizzoli V., Scutari G. (1999) An *in vitro* study on the toxic effects of nonylphenols (NP) in mitochandria. Chemosphere 38(9): 1997–2001.

35. Bragadin M., Dell' Antone P. (1996) Mitochondrial bioenergetics as affected by cationic detergents. Arch. Environ. Contam. Toxicol. 30(2): 280–284.

36. Zaccone G, Fasula S, Lacascio P, Licata A (1985) Patterns of enzyme activities in the gills of cat fish *Heteropheustus fossilis* (Bloch) exposed to anionoactive detergent N-alkyl-benzene sulphonate (LAS). Histochemistry 82(4): 341–343.

37. Misra V., Lal H., Chawla G., Vishwanathan P.N. (1985). Pathomorphological Changes in gills of fish fingerlings (*Cirrhina mrigala*) by linear benzene sulphonate, Ecotoxiol. Environ. Saf., 1985, 10(3): 302–308.

38. Kim H.S., Shin JH, Moon HJ, Kimts, Kim IV, Seok JH, Pyo MY, Han SX, (2002) Comparative estrogenic effects of p-nonylphenol by 3 day uterotrophic assay and female pubertal onset assay, Reprod. Toxicol, 16(3): 259–268.

39. Neary J T, Davidson B, Armstrong A, Strat H V, Maloof F (1976) Solubilization of thyroid peroxidase by nonionic detergents. J Biol.Chem.25 (18), 2525-9.

40. Piotrowska E., Nied Wiecka J., Jaroszewicy L. (1988-1989). Effect of detergents on the solubilization of 5′ nucleotidase from the thyroid gland, 33–34: 11–21.

41. Trivedi S.P., Kumar M., Misra A., Banerjee I, Soni A (2001) Impact of linear alkyl benzene sulphonate (LAS) on phosphatase activity of testis of teleostan fish, *Heteropneustus fossilis* (Bloch), J. Environ. Biol. 22(4): 263-6.

42. Trivedi S.P., Kumar M., Misra A., Banerjee I, Soni A (2001) Impact of linear alkyl benzene Lewis M.A. (1990) Chronic Toxicity of surfactants and detergent builders to algae: a review and risk assessment. Ecotoxicol, Environ Safty 20, 123–140.

43. Devecerski V., Marjanov M. and Milicevic S. (1992). Reaction of adrenal glomerular zone to detergents, Eur. J. Appl. Physiol. 64: 165–168

44. Liu P.S., Liu G.H., Chao W.H. (2008) Effects of nonylphenol on the calcium signal and catecholamine secretion coupled with nicotine acetylcholine receptors in bovine adrenal chromaffin cells. Toxicol. 244(1): 77–85.

Environmental & Occupational Exposures (2010) *Pages 382–394*
Editors: **Sunil Kumar & R.R. Tiwari**
Published by: **DAYA PUBLISHING HOUSE, NEW DELHI**

Chapter 16

Visual Display Terminal Usage and Adverse Pregnancy Outcomes: An Overview

Rajnarayan R. Tiwari

Scientist C,
Occupational Medicine Division,
National Institute of Occupational Health, Ahmedabad

In an age dominated by technology, computers have become most influential to keep pace with time and progress, as it is a Meta source. Even a child of 8-9 years is looking for net information just for completion of his/her school assignment. The increasing use of personal computer in homes has become an integral part of life. Not only banks and government offices but also private bodies, autonomous institutions and almost every organization are being computerized for smooth and faster flow of data and information. The application of computer technology and the accompanying use of VDTs are revolutionizing the work places and their use will continue to grow in the future. The number of computer users is rising exponentially worldwide and is expected to exceed 1 billion by 2010, up from around 670 million today, fueled primarily by new

* E-mail: rajtiwari2810@yahoo.co.in

adopters in developing nations such as China, Russia and India, according to analysts[1].

The proliferation of video display terminals (VDT), in the modern office setting has generated concern related to potential health hazards associated with their use. These health problems include effects on eyes, musculo-skeletal problems and effects on reproductive system. The effects on reproductive system are important as it not only affects the current generations but also leaves its mark on coming progeny. Visual display terminals were first time implicated with adverse reproductive outcomes in 1980, when a cluster of birth defects was observed among women using VDTs at the Toronto star newspaper. However, this is a debated issue whether such effects occur and to what an extent they result in abnormal reproductive function or outcome. These adverse effects can be summarized according to different sexes. In males the potential reproductive effects can be decreased sperm count and other morphological abnormalities in sperm there by resulting in secondary infertility. The effects in females are generally seen in the form of adverse pregnancy outcomes such as spontaneous abortion. This chapter describes the adverse health effects of visual display terminal usage on reproductive function.

Mechanism of Effect

Three characteristics of VDT use have been proposed as possible explanations for the observed association between VDT use and adverse pregnancy outcomes: physical stress, psychological stress and exposure to electromagnetic fields. Electromagnetic field exposure has been regarded as the most plausible mechanism for possible reproductive effects of VDTs. Two types of electromagnetic fields are produced by the VDT: extremely low frequency (ELF) and very low frequency (VLF) fields.

Pregnancy Outcome

Many epidemiological studies have investigated the claim that work with video display terminals (VDT) is a risk factor during pregnancy. Results have been inconsistent. Firstly in majority of the studies the hypothesis was not supported by the measurement of electromagnetic fields. Secondly, the exposure to magnetic fields from modern VDTs is usually even lower than that from other sources in the office environment, such as printers and photocopying machines[2]. Overall, the studies indicate that VDT operators are not at greater risk than the general population, because very low frequency (VLF) magnetic fields do not appear to be a risk factor and extremely low frequency (ELF) magnetic field exposure is not significantly greater than that experienced in other occupational and residential environments. However, since some studies lend support to the hypothesis that ELF magnetic fields may be a risk factor for pregnancy outcome, studies of subjects exposed to higher than average ELF fields are justified. The studies and their findings with reference to adverse pregnancy outcomes are summarized in Table 16.1.

Miscarriage

A review of ten epidemiological studies[3] examining associations between VDT use and miscarriage concluded that most women in modern offices, work with VDTs does not increase their exposure to electromagnetic fields or increase their risk of miscarriage. However, the miscarriage risk for women who work at high-stress jobs or with older, high-emission VDTs (ELF > 3 mG) is still uncertain. A case-control study of pregnancy outcome found a significantly elevated risk of miscarriage for working women who reported using VDTs for more than 20 hr per week during the first trimester of pregnancy compared to other working women who reported not using VDTs (odds ratio 1.8, 95 per cent CI: 1.2-2.8). Possible explanation for increased risk may have been due to over-reporting of exposure, ergonomic factors; job relates stress or VDT use itself through EMF[4].

Spontaneous Abortion

There are inconsistent findings on the relation between the use of video display terminals (VDTs) and spontaneous abortion. In a case-control study among female telephone operators who used VDTs at work it is reported that the operators who used VDTs had higher abdominal exposure to very-low-frequency (15 kHz) electromagnetic fields (workstations without VDTs did not emit very-low-frequency energy). Abdominal exposure to extremely low frequency fields (45 to 60 Hz) was similar for both operators who used VDTs and those who did not. It also reported no excess risk of spontaneous abortion among women who used VDTs during the first trimester of pregnancy (odds ratio = 0.93; 95 per cent confidence interval, 0.63 to 1.38) and also no dose-response relation was apparent when examined the women's hours of VDT use per week

Table 16.1: Various Studies on VDU Use and Adverse Pregnancy Outcomes

Study	*Outcome*	*Design*	*Cases*	*Controls*	*OR/RR (95%CI)*	*Conclusion*
Kruppa *et al.*[17]	Congenital malformation	Case-control	1475	1475 same age, same delivery date	235 cases, 255 controls, 0.9(0.6-1.2)	No evidence of increased risk among women who reported exposure to VDU or among women whose job titles indicate possible exposure
Ericson and Kallen[16]	Spontaneous abortion,	Case-base	412	1032 similar	1.2(0.6-2.3)	The effect of VDU use was not statistically significant
	Infant died,		22	age and		
	Malformations,		62	from same		
	Very low birth weight		26	registry		
Westerholm and Ericson[18]	Stillbirth,	Cohort	7	4117	1.1(0.8-1.4)	No excesses were found for any of the studied outcomes
	LBW,		–		NR (NS)	
	Prenatal mortality,		13		NR (NS)	
	Malformations		43		1.9(0.9-3.8)	
Bjerkedal and Egenoes[19]	Stillbirth,	Cohort	17	1820	NR (NS)	The study concluded that there was no indication that introduction of VDUs in the center has led to any increase in the rate of adverse pregnancy outcomes
	First week death,		8		NR (NS)	
	Prenatal death,		25		NR (NS)	
	LBW,		46		NR (NS)	
	Very LBW,		10		NR (NS)	
	Preterm,		97		NR (NS)	
	Multiple birth,		16		NR (NS)	
	Malformations		71		NR (NS)	

Contd...

Table 16.1–Contd...

Study	*Outcome*	*Design*	*Cases*	*Controls*	*OR/RR (95%CI)*	*Conclusion*
Goldhaber, Polen and Hiatt[4]	Spontaneous abortion,	Case-control	460	1123	1.8 (1.2-2.8)	Statistically increased risk for spontaneous abortions for VDU exposure. No excess risk for congenital malformations associated with VDU exposure
	Malformations		137	20 per cent of all normal births, same region, same time	1.4 (0.7-2.9)	
McDonald *et al.*[20]	Spontaneous abortion	Cohort	776		1.19 (1.09-1.38)	No increase in risk was found among women exposed to VDUs
	Stillbirth		25		Current/0.97 previous	
	Malformations		158		0.82 current/ 0.71 previous	
	LBW		228		0.94 current/ 112 (89-143) previous1.10	
Nurminen and Kruppa[21]	Threatened abortion,	Cohort	239		0.9	The crude and adjusted rate ratios did not show statistically significant effects for working with VDUs.
	Gestation< 40 weeks,		96		VDU: 30.5%, non: 43.8%	
	LBW		57		VDU: 25.4%, non: 23.6%	
	Placental weight,		NR		Other comp-	
	Hypertension		NR		arisons (NR)	

Contd...

Table 16.1–Contd...

Study	*Outcome*	*Design*	*Cases*	*Controls*	*OR/RR (95%CI)*	*Conclusion*
Bryant and Love[13]	Spontaneous abortion	Case-control	344	647 Same hospital, age, last menstrual period, parity	1.14 (p=0.47) prenatal 0.8 (p=0.2) postnatal	VDU use was similar between the cases and both the prenatal controls and postnatal controls
Windham *et al.*[9]	Spontaneous abortions LBW, IUGR	Case-control	626 64 68	1308 same age, same last menstrual period	1.2 (0.88-1.6) 1.4 (0.75-2.5) 1.6 (0.92-2.9)	Crude Odds ratios for spontaneous abortion and VDU use less than 20 hours per week were 1.2; 95 per cent CI 0.88-1.6, minimum of 20 hours/week were 1.3; 95 per cent CI 0.87-1.5. Risks for low birthweight and intra-uterine growth retardation were not significantly elevated.
Brandt and Nielsen[22]	Congenital malformation	Case-control	421	1365; 9.2% of all pregnancies, same registry	0.96 (0.76-1.2)	Use of VDUs during pregnancy was not associated with a risk of congenital malformations
Nielsen and Brandt[11]	Spontaneous abortion	Case-control	1371	1699; 9.2% of all pregnancies, same registry	0.94 (0.77-1.14)	No statistically significant risk for spontaneous abortion with VDU exposure
Tikkanen and Heinonen[23]	Cardiovascular malformations	Case-control	573	1055 same time, hospital delivery	Cases: 6%, Control: 5%	No statistically significant association between VDU use and cardiovascular malformations

Contd...

Table 16.1–Contd...

Study	*Outcome*	*Design*	*Cases*	*Controls*	*OR/RR (95%CI)*	*Conclusion*
Schnorr *et al.*[5]	Spontaneous abortion	Cohort	136	746	0.93 (0.63-1.38)	No excess risk for women who used VDUs during first trimester of pregnancy and no apparent exposure-response relation for time of VDU use per week.
Brandt and Nielsen[24]	Time to pregnancy	Cohort			1.61 (1.09-2.38)	For a time to pregnancy of greater than 13 months, there was an increased relative risk for the group with at least 21 hours of weekly VDU use
Nielsen and Brandt[25]	LBW, Preterm birth, Small for gestational age, Infant mortality	Cohort	434 443 749 160		0.88 (0.67-1.66) 1.11 (0.87-1.47) 0.99 (0.62-1.94) NR (NS)	No increase in risk was found among women exposed to VDUs
Roman *et al.*[26]	Spontaneous abortion	Case-control	150	297 nulliparous hospital	0.9 (0.6-1.4)	No relation to time spent using VDUs
Lindbohm *et al.*[7]	Spontaneous abortion	Case-control	191	394 medical registers	1.1 (0.7-1.6), 3.4(1.4-8.6)	Comparing workers with exposure to high magnetic field strengths to those with undetectable levels the ratio was 3.4 (95% CI; 1.4-8.6)

Contd...

Table 16.1–Contd...

Study	Outcome	Design	Cases	Controls	OR/RR (95%CI)	Conclusion
Bramwell and Davidson[27]	Spontaneous abortion, fecundability	Cohort	26	–	NR (NS)	No relationship found between VDU use and adverse pregnancy outcomes.
Grajewski *et al.*[28]	Reduced birth weight,	Cohort	24		0.9 (0.5-1.7)	Occupational VDT use does not increase the risk of RBW and
	Preterm birth		30		0.7 (0.4-1.1)	preterm birth.
Luchini L and Parazzini F[29]	Spontaneous abortion, low birth weight, congenital malformation	Systematic review	12 papers		1.0 (0.9-1.0) (pooled OR)	No significant risk emerged for spontaneous abortion, low birth weight and for congenital malformations.

NR: Not reported; NS: Non Significant; LBW: Low Birth Weight; IUGR: Intra-uterine Growth Retardation.

Source: Adapted form ILO Encyclopedia.

(odds ratio for 1 to 25 hours per week = 1.04; 95 percent confidence interval, 0.61 to 1.79; odds ratio for greater than 25 hours per week = 1.00; 95 percent confidence interval, 0.61 to 1.64)[5]. Another study, which measured the EMF exposure, found that on average, the full shift time-weighted average exposures of workers to extremely low frequency (ELF) magnetic fields ranged from 1.0 to 5.6 mG. It also validated spontaneous abortion excess over a 2-year period among 26 women with 32 reproductive events, with rates 1.5-2.5 times the expected[6]. A study among women employed as bank clerks and clerical workers in reported that the odds ratio for spontaneous abortion for working with video display terminals was not increased (odds ratio = 1.1, 95 per cent confidence interval 0.7-1.6). However, the odds ratio for workers who had used a video display terminal with a high level of extremely low frequency magnetic fields (> 0.9 microT) was 3.4 (95 per cent confidence interval 1.4-8.6) compared with workers using a terminal with a low level of these magnetic fields (< 0.4 microT). Adjustment for ergonomic factors and mental workload factors changed the odds ratio for magnetic field exposure only very slightly[7]. A meta-analysis carried out to study the potential association between video display terminal (VDT) use during pregnancy and the outcome provides reassuring evidence on the absence of any major risk of adverse pregnancy outcome as a result of exposure to a VDT[8]. A large case-control study of spontaneous abortions reported a crude odds ratio for SAB and VDT use as 1.2 for use of less than 20 hours per week (95 per cent CI = 0.88, 1.6) as well as for 20 hours or more (CI = 0.87, 1.5), with little change after adjustment for a variety of confounders. The effects of VDT use may vary by the gestational age at SAB, with stronger associations seen in earlier (less than or equal to 12 weeks) compared to later SABs[9]. Similarly, several other studies reported no association between VDT use and spontaneous abortion[10–13].

Birth Defects

Kavet and Tell[14] describe fourteen epidemiological studies seeking to establish a link between VDT use and either spontaneous abortion or birth defects. Of these fourteen studies, one found a significant link between VDT use and spontaneous abortion, and one found a link between VDT use and first trimester spontaneous abortion; the first of these two was later faulted for interviewer bias in a study summarized by Haes and Fitzgerald[15].

Ericson and Kallen[16] identified three cohorts of women categorised as having high, medium or low probability of exposure to VDT electromagnetic fields during 1980-81. There were no statistically significant diffrences in fetal malformation rates or perinatal deaths in these groups of women. In a case control study by Ericson and Kallen using data from their cohort study an association was detected between VDT use and birth defects. However when levels of stress and smoking were taken into account, the association was not statistically significant. Other studies did not detect an association between VDT use and birth defects.

References

1. A billion PC users on the way. Available from: http://news.com.com/A+billion+PC+ users+ on+the+way/ 2100-1003_3-5290988.html. [Last accessed on 2007 Jun 30].
2. Lindbohm ML, Hietanen M. Magnetic fields of video display terminals and pregnancy outcome. J Occup Environ Med. 1995; 37(8): 952-6.
3. Marcus M, McChesney R, Golden A, Landrigan P. Video display terminals and miscarriage. J Am Med Womens Assoc. 2000; 55(2): 84-8.
4. Goldhaber MK, Polen MR, Hiatt RA. The risk of miscarriage and birth defects among women who use visual display terminals during pregnancy. Am J Ind Med. 1988; 13(6): 695-706.
5. Schnorr TM, Grajewski BA, Hornung RW, Thun MJ, Egeland GM, Murray WE, Conover DL, Halperin WE.Video display terminals and the risk of spontaneous abortion. N Engl J Med. 1991; 324(11): 727-33.
6. McDiarmid MA, Breysse P, Lees PS, Curbow B, Kolodner K. Investigation of a spontaneous abortion cluster: lessons learned. Am J Ind Med. 1994; 25(4): 463-75.
7. Lindbohm ML, Hietanen M, Kyyrönen P, Sallmén M, von Nandelstadh P, Taskinen H, Pekkarinen M, Ylikoski M, Hemminki K. Magnetic fields of video display terminals and spontaneous abortion. Am J Epidemiol. 1992; 136(9): 1041-51.
8. Parazzini F, Luchini L, La Vecchia C, Crosignani PG. Video display terminal use during pregnancy and reproductive

outcome–a meta-analysis. J Epidemiol Community Health. 1993; 47(4): 265-8.

9. Windham GC, Fenster L, Swan SH, Neutra RR. Use of video display terminals during pregnancy and the risk of spontaneous abortion, low birthweight, or intrauterine growth retardation. Am J Ind Med. 1990; 18(6): 675-88.
10. Grasso P, Parazzini F, Chatenoud L, Di Cintio E, Benzi G. Exposure to video display terminals and risk of spontaneous abortion. Am J Ind Med. 1997; 32(4): 403-7.
11. Nielsen CV, Brandt LP. Spontaneous abortion among women using video display terminals. Scand J Work Environ Health. 1990; 16(5): 323-8.
12. Ong CN, Thein MM, Berquist U.A review of adverse effects on reproduction amongst female computer terminal workers. Ann Acad Med Singapore. 1990; 19(5): 649-55.
13. Bryant HE, Love EJ. Video display terminal use and spontaneous abortion risk. Int J Epidemiol. 1989; 18(1): 132-8.
14. Kavet R, Tell RA. VDTs: field levels, epidemiology, and laboratory studies. Health Phys. 1991; 61(1): 47-57.
15. Haes DL Jr, Fitzgerald MR. Video display terminal very low frequency measurements: the need for protocols in assessing VDT user "dose". Health Phys. 1995; 68(4): 572-8.
16. Ericson, A and Källén B. An epidemiological study of work with video screens and pregnancy outcome: II. A case-control study. Am J Ind Med 1986; 9:459-475.
17. Kurppa, K, Holmberg PC, Rantala K, Nurminen T, Saxén L, and Hernberg S. Birth defects, course of pregnancy, and work with video display units. A Finnish case-referent study. In Work With Display Units 86: Selected Papers from the International Scientific Conference On Work With Display Units, May 1986, Stockholm, edited by B Knave and PG Widebäck. Amsterdam: North Holland.
18. Westerholm P and Ericson A. Pregnancy outcome and VDU work in a cohort of insurance clerks. In Work With Display Units 86. Selected Papers from the International Scientific Conference On Work With Display Units, May 1986, Stockholm,

edited by B Knave and PG Widebäck. Amsterdam: North Holland.

19. Bjerkedal T and Egenaes J. Video display terminals and birth defects. A study of pregnancy outcomes of employees of the Postal-Giro-Center, Oslo, Norway. In Work With Display Units 86: Selected Papers from the International Scientific Conference On Work With Display Units, May 1986, Stockholm, edited by B Knave and PG Widebäck. Amsterdam: North Holland.

20. McDonald, AD, McDonald JC, Armstrong B, Cherry N, Nolin AD, and Robert D. Work with visual display units in pregnancy. Brit J Ind Med 1988; 45:509-515.

21. Nurminen, T and Kurppa K. Office employment, work with video display terminals, and course of pregnancy. Reference mothers' experience from a Finnish case-referent study of birth defects. Scand J Work Environ Health 1988; 14:293-298.

22. Brandt LPA and Nielsen CV. Congenital malformations among children of women working with video display terminals. Scand J Work Environ Health 1990; 16:329-333.

23. Tikkanen, J and Heinonen OP. Maternal exposure to chemical and physical factors during pregnancy and cardiovascular malformations in the offspring. Teratology 1991; 43:591-600.

24. Brandt, LPA and Nielsen CV. Fecundity and the use of video display terminals. Scand J Work Environ Health 1992; 18:298-301.

25. Nielsen, CV and Brandt LPA. Fetal growth, pre-term birth and infant mortality in relation to work with video display terminals during pregnancy. Scand J Work Environ Health 1992; 18:346-350.

26. Roman, E, Beral V, Pelerin M, and Hermon C. Spontaneous abortion and work with visual display units. Brit J Ind Med 1992; 49:507-512.

27. Bramwell, RS and Davidson MJ. Visual display units and pregnancy outcome: A prospective study. J Psychosom Obstet Gynecol 1994; 14(3): 197-210.

28. Grajewski B, Schnorr TM, Reefhuis J, Roeleveld N, Salvan A, Mueller CA, Conover DL, Murray WE. Work with video display

terminals and the risk of reduced birthweight and pre-term birth. Am J Ind Med. 1997; 32(6): 681-8.

29. Luchini L, Parazzini F. Exposure to low-frequency electromagnetic fields and pregnancy outcome: a review of the literature with particular attention to exposure to video terminals. Ann Ostet Ginecol Med Perinat. 1992; 113(2): 102-13.

Environmental & Occupational Exposures (2010) *Pages 395–405*
Editors: **Sunil Kumar & R.R. Tiwari**
Published by: **DAYA PUBLISHING HOUSE, NEW DELHI**

Chapter 17

Shift and Long Working Hour and Reproduction

*Asim Saha**

Scientist C,
Occupational Medicine Division,
National Institute of Occupational Health, Ahmedabad

ABSTRACT

A number of occupations are being reported to be associated with reproductive dysfunction in both sexes. Some of the occupations may also affect the offspring's if exposed *in utero* through parental exposure. Evidence suggestive of harmful effects of occupational exposure on the reproductive system and related outcomes has gradually accumulated in recent decades, which is further compounded by the persistent environmental endocrine disruptive chemicals. These chemicals have been found to interfere with the function of endocrine system, which is responsible for growth, sexual development and many other essential physiological functions. There are some reports, which indicated the role of shift and long working hours that might affect reproductive health indirectly through the mental/physical or work stress and also factors associated with shift and long working hours such as disruption to normal circadian rhythms etc.

* E-mail: asimsaha2311@yahoo.co.in

Background

Research into occupational exposures and effects on reproductive systems has made important scientific contributions in the past few decades. Early studies mainly focused on possible effects on the foetus rather than the reproductive health of the woman. Later, it was realized that reproductive toxins might also induce hormonal alterations affecting other aspects of reproductive health such as the menstrual cycle, ovulation and fertility. Attention is now shifting from concern for the pregnant woman and the foetus, to the entire spectrum of occupational health hazards among women and the reproductive health of both genders (Figa-Talamanca, 2006)[1]. The work patterns of substantial population of working class people now have variable work schedule *i.e.* evening or night work and rotating shifts etc. Work schedules sometimes showed a tendency to extremely long work shifts. Shift work is defined as work primarily outside of normal daytime working hours. Nowadays the number of shift workers has increased due to technological development as well as demands of certain sectors in odd hours. Shift work is accompanied by a greater incidence of many medical disorders, such as cardiovascular, gastro-intestinal, and neurological disorders. The biological mechanisms that show how shift work acts to induce such disorders in workers are relatively unknown. In this chapter information pertaining to shift work and various diseases especially reproductive heath is discussed.

Shift Work and Injury

Occupational constraints and work schedules were found to relate to an increased risk of work-related injuries (Bourdouxhe *et al.*, 2001)[2]. Working in jobs with overtime schedules was found to be associated with a 61 per cent higher injury hazard rate compared to jobs without overtime. Working at least 12 hours per day was associated with a 37 per cent increased hazard rate and working at least 60 hours per week was associated with a 23 per cent increased hazard rate. Thus, strategies to prevent work injuries should consider changes in scheduling practices, job redesign, and health protection programmes for people working in jobs involving overtime and extended hours (Dembe *et al.*,2005)[3]. Evening and night shift hospital employees were found to be at greater risk of sustaining an occupational injury than day shift workers, with those on the night shift reporting injuries of the greatest severity as measured by disability leave. The injury rate for day shift per 10,000 employees was estimated to be 176 as compared with injury rate estimates of 324 for evening shift and 279 for night shift workers. The average number of days taken off for injury disability was longer for injured night shift workers (46) than for day (38) or evening (39) shift workers (Horwitz *et al.*, 2004) [4]. Saha *et al.* (2007) carried out a study on occupational injury surveillance in a metal smelting industry and highlighted the need of elevated safety status during summer and in evening and night shifts [5].

Shift Work and Pathological Conditions

Shift work exerts major influences on the physiological functions of the human body, which are primarily mediated by the disruption of circadian rhythms since most body functions are circadian rhythmic. There is a large amount of data pointing to an association between shift work and the prevalence of many medical conditions. However, as these disorders are often based on a variety of non-occupational factors, a distinct separation into either occupational (shift-work-related) or non-occupational can be difficult (Mark *et al.*, 2006) [6]. Shift work is associated with various metabolic diseases such as obesity, low concentrations of high-density lipoprotein, elevated lipid levels and disturbed glucose tolerance.

Myocardial Infarction is found to be associated with shift work though the mechanism behind the association is still not clear. Studies have shown that shift work is associated with myocardial infarction in both men and women. Shift work has also been found to be associated with an increased risk of cardiovascular disease (CVD); in particular, night work affects the circadian rhythm. The increased risk of CVD associated with shift work is related to the greater incidence of metabolic syndrome among these workers (Copertaro *et al.*, 2008) [7].

Shift work may also have influence on the prevalence of infections in absence of antioxidative capacity. In comparison to day work, shift work may be associated with differences in health, health behavior, sleep, fatigue and perceived job characteristics, which may also influence the occurrence of infections. Effect of shiftwork on circadian rhythm might affect hormone production and thereby may contribute to many disorders.

Risk Factors in the Workplace Affecting Reproductive Health

Various risk factors are encountered in the work place, which may have adverse effect on reproduction. Generally, occupations involving–manufacture/or application of some of the persistent chemicals that are non-degradable easily as well as bio-accumulative, intensive exposure to heat and radiation, uses of the toxic solvents as well as toxic fumes are reported to be associated with the reproductive dysfunction. Occupational exposure of males to various persistent chemicals have been reported to have male mediated adverse reproductive outcomes in the form of abortion, reduction in fertility etc. with inconclusive or limited evidence (Kumar 2004)[8]. Specific risk factors such as occupational exposure to metals, solvents, pesticides, persistent chemicals, noise and others have negative effect on reproductive health of both male and female. Negative reproductive effects such as increased risk of spontaneous abortions, congenital defects, delay in conception etc have all been observed with the exposure to certain persistent pesticides. Occupational exposure to chemical agents such as organic solvents, aromatic and aliphatic hydrocarbons have negative effects on pregnancy, which can lead to spontaneous abortion, reduced fertility, and birth weight. Various metals such as lead, mercury, and cadmium are shown to have detrimental effect on both male and female reproductive system which includes impaired spermatogenesis, increased risk of spontaneous abortion, stillbirth etc. Prenatal lead exposure increased the risk of pre-term delivery and low birth weight. Environmental persistent chemicals especially endocrine disrupting chemicals may have estrogenic and anti-androgenic effects. Association between noise-induced stress and increased risk in miscarriage, pre-term birth and intrauterine growth retardation were also observed in some studies. Exposure of women to ionizing radiation in the periconceptional period results in foetal death and congenital defects depending upon the dose, duration and developmental stage of the embryo or foetus. Miscarriage, other reproductive outcomes like LBW, pre-maturity and perinatal mortality have been observed in women using Video Display Terminals (VDTs). Women working in the health care sector are also exposed to many potentially harmful chemical agents like disinfectants, anesthetic gases and drugs. Exposures to such toxicants are associated with spontaneous abortion, pre-term birth, embryonic and foetal loss and congenital defects.

Shiftwork and Reproductive Risk

Nonstandard work hours may disturb normal body physiological functions, but their relation to reproductive outcome is poorly understood. Recently published studies suggest an association between rotating shift-work and prolonged waiting time to pregnancy. Most of the studies on spontaneous abortion suggest that some forms of shift work may be associated with increased risk. Moreover, some results have related rotating schedules to intrauterine growth retardation. In the published studies, the type of work schedule examined has varied, and the applied definition of shift work has not necessarily been clear. The main interest areas, however, have been work involving evening and night shifts, rotating or changing schedules, and the irregularity of work patterns. Although the evidence is not ample and remains ambiguous, it is prudent to consider shift work as a potential risk to reproduction (Nurminen, 1998) [9].

A meta-analysis of 29 studies identified shiftwork as a significant risk factor (OR 1.24) for pre-term birth, which further reported that physically demanding work might significantly increase a woman's risk of adverse pregnancy outcome (Mozurkewich *et al.*, 2000) [10]. Costa (1996) [11] and Scott (2000) [12] reviewed the data on shift work and reproduction and summarize evidence-linking shiftwork to adverse pregnancy outcomes (*e.g.* premature births, miscarriages, and low birth weight). Knutsson (2003) mentioned that there is rather strong evidence in support of an association between shift work and pregnancy outcome in terms of miscarriage, low birth weight and preterm birth. Even in the absence of further proof, it would be prudent for women to avoid or be relieved of such work during pregnancy[13]. Uehata and Sasakawa (1982) showed that irregular menstruation and abortions were more common in shift workers[14]. In addition, irregular menstruation have also been linked to shiftwork by Hatch *et al.* (1999) [15].

Labyak *et al.* (2002) further suggested that sleep disturbances may lead to menstrual irregularities, and changes in menstrual function may be a marker of shiftwork intolerance[16]. In Denmark 30 per cent of females in the reproductive age regularly have shift work.

Twenty two epidemiological papers were studied looking at associations between shift work and abortion, stillbirth, preterm birth, and birth weight in which no convincing associations were observed between rotating shift work or fixed nightshift and negative pregnancy outcome. Some epidemiological support was found for a relation between fixed nightshift and late abortions/stillbirth (Schlunssen *et al.*, 2007) [17]. Further, Zhu *et al.* (2004) showed that fixed night work had a high risk of postterm birth; fixed evening work had a high risk of full-term low birth weight; and shift work as a group showed a slight excess of small-for-gestational-age babies[18]. Information on 1475 mothers of infants with selected structural malformations and an equal number of mothers of "normal" babies was analyzed for a possible relationship between shift work and adverse pregnancy outcome or a complicated course of pregnancy by Nurminen in 1989. Threatened abortion and pregnancy-induced hypertension were not associated with rotating shift work alone, but in a noisy work environment moderate risks could not be ruled out. Rotating shift work was associated with a slight excess of babies small for their gestational age independently of noise exposure (Nurminen, 1989) [19]

Another study conducted in women workers of textile mills in China also showed the effect of rotating shiftwork on birth weight. The proportions of pre-term birth (<37 weeks) and low birth weight (<2500 g), respectively, were 20 per cent and 9 per cent for shift workers as compared to 15 per cent and 6 per cent for regular schedule workers (Xu X *et al.*, 1994) [20].

Tuntiseranee *et al.* (1998) has reported that male exposure to long working hours and shiftwork had no association with subfecundity. The OR of subfecundity was highest when both partners worked >70 hours a week irrespective of the cut off point used OR 4.1 in primigravid women; OR 2.0 in all pregnant women. Logistic regressions adjusted for age, education, body mass index, menstrual regularity, obstetric and medical history, coital frequency, and potential exposure to reproductive toxic agents, showed an odds ratio associated with female exposure to long working hours of 2.3 (95 per cent CI) 1.0 to 5.1 in primigravid and 1.6 in all pregnant women[21]. In addition, studies showed that occupational noise at the level of approximately 85 dB Laeq (8 h) or higher and shift work, especially rotating schedules, may have independent negative effects on birth weight and length of gestation and have also been associated with early fetal loss. Moreover, some results have related noise exposure and shift work to menstrual disturbance and infertility. Although the evidence is not ample, it is prudent to consider exposure to high-level noise and shift work as risks to reproduction (Nurminen, 1995)[22].

Fixed evening workers and fixed night workers had a longer time to pregnancy in the study taken place at the Danish National Birth Cohort compared with daytime workers, the adjusted ORs were 0.80 for fixed evening workers, 0.80 for fixed night workers, 0.99 for rotating shift (without night) workers, and 1.05 for rotating shift (with night) workers. The proportions of unplanned pregnancies and contraceptive failures were higher among fixed evening and fixed night workers. But there was no unequivocal evidence of a causal association between shift work and subfecundity (Zhu *et al.*, 2003)[23]. Marino *et al.* (2008) also suggested that any night shift work was found to be associated with a 50 per cent increase in risk of endometriosis, and working more than half of shifts on a job at night was associated with a nearly doubled disease risk. Changing sleep patterns on days off was associated with further increases in disease risk[24].

The studies examining the role of work schedule on the reproductive health of women, often conducted among health care professionals, have not always reached unequivocal conclusions. In an early Swedish study, hospital workers with irregular hours had a slight increase in the risk of spontaneous abortion. No increase in risk, however, was found for night work. Two later case control studies found an increased risk of spontaneous abortion for shift work and night work, and for evening work. Similarly, a study in 3583 Swedish midwives, reported an increased risk in connection with night work and three-shift schedules. A reduction in fecundity was noted for all irregular work hours: the adjusted fecundity ratio for two shifts, three shift and night works were 0.78, 0.77, 0.82, respectively. The same study also found an association of night work and pre-term birth (OR 5-5.6) and to a lesser degree with LBW (Figa-Talamanca, 2006)[1]. Bisanti *et al.* (1996)[25] also showed the association between shiftwork and various unfavorable pregnancy outcomes (*i.e.*, pregnancy loss, spontaneous abortion, low birth weight, etc), which may be due to the interference of shift work with the circadian regulation of human metabolism and, in particular, with the temporal pattern of endocrine function. A low (odds ratio < 2.0) but consistent excess risk of subfecundity has been observed both in a representative sample of the general population of women in reproductive age and in a sample of pregnant women or women who had just given birth. The excess risk was also consistently evident both in the subsample of the first pregnancies and in the subsample of the most recent pregnancies. Only the exposure of women to shift work seemed to affect a couple's fecundity; men working shift work did not modify the fecundity pattern of their own couples.

The known mechanism that induces and promotes cellular damage and results in such disorders is not understood. However, oxidative stress may be one of the causes behind such changes. The antioxidant system is the defense system that neutralizes the free radicals produced in the hazardous oxidative pathway. When the production of free radicals exceeds body antioxidant capacity, oxidative stress occurs (Akbar Sharifian *et al.*, 2005)[26]. Shift work may exert negative influences on the total antioxidant capacity and may therefore be regarded as an oxidative stressor. Thus it may have effect on various cellular functions. Further disruption of circadian rhythms, which in turn altered physiological functions including hormonal activity, might also be likely cause of reproductive impairments among shift workers.

Our knowledge of how occupational exposures affect the reproductive health is not conclusive especially in absence of involvement of reproductive toxins which are not known as there are number of confounding factors associated with the impairment of reproductive health. It appears that for a number of exposures at work, the evidence is sufficient to warrant the maximum protection of the pregnant woman for their exposure to such chemicals. Recent research has advanced the hypothesis that the risk for a negative pregnancy outcome associated with exogenous or endogenous factors may be modified by the presence of other maternal risk factors, including genetic variation in metabolic detoxification activities. This might explain why work-related negative reproductive effects are observed in some women but not in others. Another reason for the uncertainty of the epidemiologic evidence is related to methodological problems (Figa-Talamanca, 2006)[1]. The data on shift work and reproductive health is still not conclusive but positive data suggest the precautions to be taken during pregnancy against such work pattern. Knutsson (2003) also recommended that women should avoid shiftwork during pregnancy[10].

References

1. Irene Figa-Talamanca. Occupational risk factors and reproductive health of women. *Occup med*, 2006; 56: 521-531.
2. Bourdouxhe M, Toulouse G. Health and safety among film technicians working extended shifts. *J Hum Ergol* (Tokyo), 2001; 30(1-2): 113-8.
3. Dembe AE, Erickson JB, Delbos RG, Banks SM. The impact of overtime and long work hours on occupational injuries and illnesses: new evidence from the United States. *Occup Environ Med*, 2005; 62(9): 585.
4. Horwitz IB, McCall BP. The impact of shiftwork on the risk and severity of injuries for hospital employees: an analysis using Oregon workers' compensation data. *Occup Med*, 2004; 54(8): 556-63.
5. Saha Asim, Kumar Sunil, Vasudevan DM. Occupational injury surveillance: A study in a metal smelting industry. Indian J Occup and Environ Med 2007; 11: 103-107
6. Anke van Mark, Michael Spallek, Richard Kessel, and Elke Brinkmann. Shiftwork and pathological conditions. *Occup Med Toxicol*, 2006; 1: 25.
7. Copertaro A, Bracci M, Barbaresi M, Santarelli L. Assessment of cardiovascular risk in shift healthcare workers. *Eur J Cardiovasc Prev Rehabil*, 2008; 15(2): 224-9.
8. Kumar, S. Occupational Exposure and reproductive dysfunction. *Journal of Occup Health* 2004; *46*: 1-19.
9. Nurminen T. Shiftwork and reproductive health. *Scand J Work Environ Health*, 1998; 24(suppl 3): 28-34.
10. Mozurkewich EL, Luke B, Avni M, and Wolf F M. Working conditions and adverse pregnancy outcome: a meta-analysis. *Obstetrics and Gynecol*, 2000; 95: 623-635.
11. Costa, G. The impact of shift and night work on health. *Applied Ergonomics*, 1996; 27: 9-16.

12. Scott, A. J. Shift work and health. *Primary Care,* 2000; *27:* 1057-1070.

13. Knutsson A. Health disorders of shift workers. *Occup Medicine,* 2003; 53*:* 103-108.

14. Uehata T, Sasakawa N. The fatigue and maternity disturbances of night workwomen. *J Hum Ergol,* 1982; 11(Suppl.): 465–474.

15. Hatch, M C, Figa Talamanca I, and Salerno S. Work stress and menstrual patternsamong American and Italian nurses. *Scandinavian J Work, Environ and Health, 1999; 25*: 144-150.

16. Labyak, S., Lava, S., Turek, F., and Zee, P. Effects of shiftwork on sleep and menstrual function in nurses. *Health Care for Women International,* 2002; 23: 703-714.

17. Schlunssen V, Viskum S, Omland O, Bonde JP. Does shiftwork cause spontaneous abortion, pre-term birth or low birth weight?. *Ugeskr Laeger* 2007; 169(10): 893-900.

18. Jin Liang Zhu, Niels H Hjollund, Jorn Olsen. Shiftwork, duration of pregnancy, and birth weight: The National Birth Cohort in Denmark. *American Journal of Obstetrics and Gynecology,* 2004; 191(1): 285-291.

19. Nurminen T. Female noise exposure, shift work, and reproduction. *J Occup Environ Med,* 1995; 37(8): 945-50.

20. Xu X, Ding M, Li B, Christiani DC. Association of rotating shiftwork with preterm births and low birth weight among never smoking women textile workers in China. *Occup Environ Med,* 1994; 51(7): 470-4.

21. Tuntiseranee P, Olsen J, Geate A, Kor-Anantakul O. Are long working hours and shift work risk factors for fertility? A study among couples from southern Thailand. *Occupational and environmental medicine,* 1998; 55(2): 99-105.

22. Nurminen T. Shift work, fetal development and course of pregnancy. *Scand J Work Environ Health,* 1989; 15(6): 395-403.

23. Zhu JL, Hjollund NH, boggild H, Olsen J. Shift work and subfecundity: a causal link or an artefact?. *Occup Environ Med,* 2003; 60(9): E12.

24. Marino JL, Holt VL, Chen C, Davis S. Shift work, hCLOCK T3111C Polymorphism, and Endometriosis Risk. *Epidemiology*, 2008, ahead of print.

25. Bisanti L, Olsen J, Basso O, Thonneau P, Karmaus W. Shift work and subfecundity: a European multicenter study. European Study group on Infertility and Subfecundity. *J Occup Environ Med*, 1996; 38(4): 352-8.

26. Akbar Sharifian, Saeed farahani, Parvin Pasalar, Marjan Gharavi, and Omid Aminian. Shift work as an oxidative stressor. *Circadian Rhythms*, 2005; 3: 15.

Index